*Practice and theory of
enzyme immunoassays*

LABORATORY TECHNIQUES IN BIOCHEMISTRY AND MOLECULAR BIOLOGY

Volume 15

Edited by

R.H. BURDON - *Department of Bioscience and Biotechnology, University of Strathclyde, Glasgow*
P.H. van KNIPPENBERG - *Department of Biochemistry, University of Leiden, Leiden*

ELSEVIER
AMSTERDAM · LONDON · NEW YORK · TOKYO

PRACTICE AND THEORY OF ENZYME IMMUNOASSAYS

P. Tijssen

Centre de recherche en médecine comparée
Institut Armand-Frappier
Université de Québec
531, boulevard des Prairies
Ville de Laval, Québec, Canada H7V 1B7

ELSEVIER
AMSTERDAM · LONDON · NEW YORK · TOKYO

ELSEVIER SCIENCE PUBLISHERS B.V.
Sara Burgerhartstraat 25
P.O. Box 211, 1000 AE Amsterdam, The Netherlands

Library of Congress Cataloging in Publication Data

Tijssen, P.
 Practice and theory of enzyme immunoassays.
 (Laboratory techniques in biochemistry and
molecular biology ; v. 15)
 Includes bibliographical references and index.
 1. Immunoenzyme technique. I. Title. II. Series.
QP519.L2 vol. 15 574.19′2′028 s [616.07′56] 84-28634
[QP519.9.I44]

ISBN 0-444-80633-4 (pocket edition)
ISBN 0-444-80634-2 (library edition)
ISBN 0-7204-4200-1 (series)

1st edition	1985	5th impression	1988
2nd impression	1986	6th impression	1990
3rd impression	1987	7th impression	1992
4th impression	1987	8th impression	1993

This book is printed on acid-free paper.

Printed in The Netherlands

Preface

Enzyme immunoassays have become solidly entrenched in many fields. Unfortunately, they are often performed in a haphazard way. This is not altogether surprising since this powerful assay technology transcends several discipline boundaries and is extensively applied as a tool in fields other than enzymology and immunology. The fast flow of new ideas and assay designs and the rapid progress in the application of this technique may be reasons why comprehensive reviews on this subject are still missing.

It is attempted in this book to provide both the basic understanding of these techniques and a practical guideline for the choice and experimental details of enzyme immunoassays. Another goal of this review has been to be sufficiently provocative to leave the very diverse group of veteran or would-be assayists (clinicians, applied and basic scientists) with a healthy distrust of the, frequently misleading, accepted wisdom abounding in EIA-logy. I hope that this effort will be useful since researchers in the life sciences are frequently concerned with the detection or discrimination of minute amounts of resembling compounds, not seldom at the limit of detectability.

Intricate interactions among different assay parameters (sensitivity, detectability, specificity, etc.) and differences in their concepts have been emphasized and uniformly used throughout the text to avoid the confusion reigning in the literature. This attempt to prevent confusion necessitated the introduction of a few new terms, which I hope, will be inoffensive.

Comments or suggestions from readers are invited.

Dedication

To the memory of my mother and my father-in-law who both passed away while this book was in press.

To Trics, Andrew, Janice, and our relatives in Elden, Utrecht, Raalte, Elst, Deventer, Alphen a/d Rijn, and Leiden.

Acknowledgements

I am particularly grateful to my wife, Trics, for her extensive editorial help and many valuable suggestions, and to Dr. L. Gyenes, who, in addition to his encouragements, gave freely of his time and talents to critique and upgrade early drafts up till the final manuscript. I must thank both my family and Mrs. G. Gyenes for their patience during those many evenings, weekends, and holidays which were consumed with the preparation and correction of this review.

Among my other, previous colleagues at the Université de Montréal, I am thankful to Drs. P. Crine and S. Garzon for reviewing various chapters. I wish also to thank Drs. Andrew and Jennifer Scott for the use of their computer and Dr. P. Viens and his co-workers, in particular Andrée l'Ecuyer, for their keyrole in the word-processing of the manuscript.

Finally, I wish to express my gratitude to Dr. R. Ruppanner, chairman of the 'Centre de recherche en médecine comparée' at the Institut Armand-Frappier. I am greatly indebted to Prof. E. Kurstak, Director of the Comparative Virology Research Group of the Faculty of Medicine of the Université de Montréal, for his criticism and encouragement in the preparation of this volume. I have been most fortunate to have been associated with Professor Kurstak and his Research Group from the beginning of the development of enzyme immunoassays, first as a Ph.D. student and then for some time as a member of this Group. I have thereby benefited from grants to Professor Kurstak's projects from the Medical Research Council of Canada, from the National Sciences and Engineering Research Council of Canada, and from the National Cancer Institute of Canada. I thank the Editors of this series and the editorial staff of Elsevier Science Publishers (Biomedical Division) for their patience and constructive suggestions.

Contents

List of abbreviations

AA	Activity amplification
Ab	Antibody
AB	Antibody (anti-Ig)
ABC	Avidin–biotin complex
ABM	Aminobenzyloxymethyl
ABTS	2,2′-Azino-di(3-ethylbenzthiazolinesulfonic acid)
AEC	3-Amino-9-ethylcarbazole
Ag	Antigen
AM	Activity modulation
AMETIA	Antibody-masking enzyme tag immunoassay
AMP	Adenosine 5′-monophosphate
AMSA	S-Acetylmercaptosuccinic anhydride
APAAP	Alkaline phosphatase anti-alkaline phosphatase (enzyme–antibody) complex
APase	Alkaline phosphatase
5-AS	5-Aminosalicylic acid
ATP	Adenosine 5′-triphosphate
BAEE	$N\alpha$-Benzoyl-L-arginine ethyl ester
BBHZ	(+)-Biotin bromoacetyl hydrazide
B-cap-NHS	(+)-Biotin γ-aminocaproic acid N-hydroxy-succinimide ester
BDB	Bis-diazotized benzidine
BGase	β-Galactosidase
BHZ	(+)-Biotin hydrazide
BNHS	(+)-Biotin-N-hydroxysuccinimide ester
BNP	(+)-Biotin p-nitrophenyl ester
BRAB	Bridged avidin–biotin (method)
BSA	Bovine serum albumin

BSNHS   Bis-succinic acid *N*-hydroxysuccinimide ester
BUdR   5-Bromo-2′-deoxyuridine
C   Concentration
CA   Caprylic acid
CBB   Coomassie Brilliant Blue
CDI   Carbodiimide
CHM-NHS   *N*-(4-Carboxycyclohexylmethyl)-maleimide
             N-hydroxysuccinimide ester
Con A   Concanavalin A
CM   Carboxymethyl
CN   4-Chloro-1-naphthol
CV   Coefficient of variation
DAB   3,3′-Diaminobenzidine
DBM   Diazobenzyloxymethyl
DCC   *N,N*′-Dicyclohexylcarbodiimide
DEA   Diethanolamine
DEAE   Diethylaminoethyl
DI   Detectability index
DIG   Diffusion-in-gel
DMAB   3-Dimethylaminobenzoic acid
DMEM   Dulbecco's modification of Eagle's minimum
             essential medium
DMF   *N,N*-Dimethylformamide
DMSO   Dimethyl sulfoxide
DNA   Deoxyribonucleic acid
DNase   Deoxyribonuclease
DNBS   2,4-Dinitrobenzene sulfonate
DNFB   2,4-Dinitro-1-fluorobenzene
DPT   Diazophenylthioether
ECF   Ethyl chloroformate
ED   Effective dose
EDC   1-Ethyl-3-(3-dimethylaminopropyl)carbodi-
             imide
EDTA   Ethylenediaminetetraacetic acid
EGTA   Ethyleneglycol-bis-(β-aminoethyl ether)-
             N,N,N′,*N*′-tetraacetic acid

EIA	Enzyme immunoassay
ELISA	Enzyme-linked immunosorbent assay
EMIT	Enzyme-multiplied immunoassay technique
EMMIA	Enzyme modulator mediated immunoassay
FA	Formaldehyde
FAD	Flavin adenine dinucleotide
FBS	Fetal bovine serum
FMN	Flavin mononucleotide
FNPS	Bis(4-fluoro-3-nitrophenyl)-sulfone
GA	Glutaraldehyde
GAase	Glucoamylase (= amyloglucosidase)
GAPITC	Glut-azo-hydroxyphenylisothiocyanate
GOase	Glucose oxidase
GPDase	Glucose-6-phosphate dehydrogenase
GU	6-7-β-Galactosyl-coumarin-3-carboximido)-hexylamine (= galactosyl umbelliferyl)
HAT (HT) medium	Medium containing hypoxanthine, aminopterin, and thymidine (HT: without aminopterin)
HEPES	N-2-Hydroxyethylpiperazine-N'-ethanesulfonic acid
HGPRT	Hypoxanthine-guanine phosphoribosyl transferase
HPPA	2-Hydroxy-3-phenylpropionic acid
HVA	Homovanillic acid
IEF	Isoelectric focusing
Ig (IgA, IgG, etc.)	Immunoglobulin (with α, γ, etc., heavy chain)
i.p.	Intraperitoneal
ITP	Isotachophoresis
IU	International units (in immunology)
LAB	(Covalently enzyme-)linked avidin bridge
LPS	Lipopolysaccharides
MBS	m-Maleimidobenzoyl-N-hydroxysuccinimide ester
MBSA	Methylated bovine serum albumine
MBTH	3-Methyl-2-benzothiazolinone hydrazone

MC	Methyl cellulose
MDase	Malate dehydrogenase
2-ME	2-Mercaptoethanol
MHC	Major histocompatibility complex
MMBI	Methyl-4-mercaptobutyrimidate
MONA	Multiple of normal activity
m-PMS	*m*-Phenazine methosulfate
MPOase	Microperoxidase
4-MU	4-Methylumbelliferone
4-MU-P	4-Methylumbelliferyl phosphate
MW	Molecular weight
NAD$^+$	Nicotinamide adenine dinucleotide
NADH	Nicotinamide adenine dinucleotide (reduced)
NADP$^+$	Nicotinamide adenine dinucleotide phosphate
NADPH	Nicotinamide adenine dinucleotide phosphate (reduced)
NAG	*N*-Acetylglucosamine
NAM	*N*-Acetylmuramic acid
NBM	Nitrobenzyloxymethyl
NBPC	1-(3-Nitrobenzyloxymethyl)pyridinium chloride
NHS	*N*-Hydroxysuccinimide
NHS-FBA	*N*-Hydroxysuccinimide ester of *p*-formylbenzoic acid
NMR	Nuclear magnetic resonance
NPP	Nitrophenyl phosphate
NSF	Non-specific factors
ODA	*o*-Dianisidine
o-NP	*o*-Nitrophenol
o-NPG	*o*-Nitrophenyl-β-D-galactopyranoside
o-NPP	*o*-Nitrophenyl phosphate
OPD	*o*-Phenylenediamine
OPDM	*N,N'-o*-Phenylenedimaleimide
OT	*o*-Toluidine
PAGE	Polyacrylamide gel electrophoresis

PAP	Peroxidase-anti-peroxidase (enzyme–antibody) complex
PAPS	Polyaminopolystyrene
PBQ	p-Benzoquinone
PBS	Phosphate-buffered saline
PEG	Polyethylene glycol
pI	Isoelectric point
PIPES	Piperazine-N,N'-bis(ethanesulfonic acid)
PLP	Periodate-lysine-paraformaldehyde (fixative)
POase	Peroxidase
PVC	Poly(vinyl chloride)
QAE	Diethyl-(2-hydroxypropyl)-aminoethyl
RAPITC	Ars-azo-hydroxyphenylisothiocyanate
RBC	Red blood cells
RF	Rheumatoid factors
RIA	Radioimmunoassay
RNA	Ribonucleic acid
RNase	Ribonuclease
RZ	Reinheitszahl ('purity number')
s.c.	Subcutaneous
SC	Secretory component
SD	Standard deviation
SD_m	Standard deviation of mean
SDS	Sodium dodecyl sulfate
SpA	Protein A
SPDP	3-(2-Pyridyldithio)propionic acid N-hydroxy-succinimide ester
TBS	Tris-buffered saline
TCA	Trichloroacetic acid
TCM	Thymocyte-conditioned medium
TDIC	Tolylene-2,4-diisocyanate
T_H	T-helper cells
TK	Thymidine kinase
TMB	3,3',5,5'-Tetramethylbenzidine
TN	Turnover number

t-NBT	t-Nitroblue tetrazolium chloride
Tris	Tris(hydroxymethyl)aminomethane
T_S	T-suppressor cells
U	International units (in enzymology)
UV	Ultraviolet

CHAPTER 1

Introduction

Enzyme immunoassays (EIA) are based on two important biological phenomena: (i) the extraordinary discriminatory power of antibodies, based on the ability of the immune system of vertebrates to produce a virtually unlimited variety of proteins (antibodies), each with an affinity for a specific foreign compound (antigen or hapten); and, (ii) the extremely high catalytic power and specificity of enzymes, which may quite often be detectable with great ease. EIA consist thus of a two-pronged strategy: the reaction between the immuno-reactants (antibody with the corresponding antigen) and the detection of that reaction using enzymes, labeled to the reactants, as indicators.

A plethora of other labels has been employed, such as radioactive tracers (radioimmunoassays, RIA), chemiluminescent and fluorescent labels, metal atoms and sols, stable free radicals (measured by elec-tron spin resonance), latexes and bacteriophages. Among these, RIA are extremely useful both for diagnostic purposes and basic research. They have, however, a number of important disadvantages: (i) expen-sive equipment is needed to measure radioactivity; (ii) the reagents have a short shelf-life; (iii) they represent potential health hazards, and often require licensing; and, (iv) necessitate special disposal of radioactive wastes. EIA have similar specificities and potentially even higher detectabilities, and offer, in addition, important advantages over RIA (Table 1.1), but may also carry some minor disadvantages (Chapter 18).

TABLE 1.1
Advantages of enzyme immunoassays

- Very high sensitivity, detectability, and specificity are possible.

- Equipment required is relatively cheap.

- Assays may be very rapid and simple.

- Reproducibility is high and evaluation is objective.

- Feasible under field conditions.

- No radiation hazards.

- Reagents are relatively cheap and generally of long shelf-life.

- Versatility of assays may be significantly increased by the great variety and specific properties of enzymes.

- Full advantage of the properties of monoclonal antibodies may be achieved with EIA.

1.1. History of enzyme immunoassays

EIA were developed in the mid-sixties for the identification and localization of antigens in histological preparations, analogous to immunofluorescence methods, and for the identification of precipitation lines obtained by immunodiffusion and immunoelectrophoresis (Nakane and Pierce, 1966, 1967; Avrameas and Uriel, 1966). These enzyme immunohistochemistry (EIH) methods were recognized as very useful in other fields (Tijssen and Kurstak, 1974; Kurstak et al., 1975, 1977; Sternberger, 1979; Farr and Nakane, 1981; Polak and Van Noorden, 1983).

   The observation that antigens or antibodies can be immobilized on solid phases made it possible to apply similar methods for the quantitative detection of immunoreactants in test tubes (Engvall and Perlmann, 1971; Van Weemen and Schuurs, 1971), not only enlarging enormously the number of haptens, antigens or antibodies that could be assayed, but also providing a much higher concentration of immobilized antigen than generally obtained with relatively cumbersome cell cultures.

Rubenstein et al. (1972), subsequently, developed a homogeneous system in which the enzyme is labeled, generally with a hapten, without seriously affecting its activity. This method is applicable if the antibody reacting with the hapten either reduces or increases enzyme activity. The presence of free hapten in the added sample lowers the fraction of antibody able to react with enzyme–hapten conjugate and thus lowers the effect of the antibody on the enzyme.

The development of methods to produce monoclonal antibodies (Köhler and Milstein, 1975; Section 5.4) not only enhanced the possibility of a more stringent standardization of EIA with higher specificity and sensitivity, but also contributed to new assay designs.

In addition to the detection of antigens and antibodies, EIA will, undoubtedly, play an increasingly important role in molecular biology. For example, the 'bio-blot' method (Leary et al., 1983) for the detection of DNA–DNA or DNA–RNA duplexes on nitrocellulose membranes offers important advantages over conventional procedures in which radioactive probes are used and autoradiographic detection. In this method, biotinylated DNA probes are prepared by nick translation (Rigby et al., 1977) in the presence of biotinylated analogs and hybridized with the DNA or RNA on filters. Biotin is then detected by avidin-labeled enzyme (Section 3.1).

1.2. Purpose and organization of this volume

The bases of EIA are found in immunology and enzymology. However, the advantages of EIA extended these assays to many areas which do not usually involve enzymology or immunology. For these reasons, and to give the necessary theoretical basis, the background of EIA is described in somewhat more detail than for other methods dealt with in the preceding volumes of this series.

Reagents for EIA and EIH are generally obtained from commercial suppliers at prices which reflect their costs for overhead, marketing, etc. Most of these products, however, can be prepared in the laboratory at a 5–10 times lower cost. For example, the widely used horseradish peroxidase (POase) may be prepared from a crude extract in less than an hour by a very simple method (Section 10.2.1.2), saving hundreds of dollars and yielding enzyme with a higher activity, and which is better suited for EIA, than the commercially offered pure enzyme.

Enzyme conjugates should be prepared in the laboratory (Chapter 11 and Chapter 12), since: (i) commercial preparations are restricted with respect to antigens, antibodies or enzymes; (ii) it is much cheaper; (iii) quality may be better controlled; and, (iv) conjugates can be prepared which are commercially not available.

EIA often makes use of solid phases. The relative merits and disadvantages of such techniques, as well as ways to optimize them will be discussed. An important aspect, which has not yet been investigated in detail for EIA, is the influence immobilization of enzymes has on enzyme kinetics. The solid-phase may cause strong local differences in the microenvironment of the enzyme, the implications of which can only be inferred from studies on immobilized enzymes in solid-phase biochemistry (Chapter 9). Major or minor flaws in EIA design, which may discredit an otherwise perfectly valid EIA, will be discussed.

Homogeneous assays, which are not submitted to separation steps, pose different requirements for optimal results, such as the absence of endogeneous enzyme or inhibitors in the sample, substrate depletion, and cross-reactivity.

The criteria of standardization as well as the methods of calculation and presentation of results of EIA deserve obviously close attention. However, automation is discussed more briefly since this could be useful only to a relatively small but well-informed group of readers.

This volume has three central chapters dealing with the quantitative assay of biological compounds (Chapter 14), the detection and identification of molecules separated by electrophoresis (Chapter 16), and the localization of particular molecules in cells (Chapter 17), and ramifications are made for particular procedures or theoretical considerations. A general overview (Chapter 2) and a discussion of non-immunologic recognition systems used in EIA (Chapter 3) are presented. Various aspects related to antigens and haptens (Chapter 4), physicochemical properties of antibodies, their biosynthesis, and purification (Chapters 5–7), the reaction between antibody and antigen, particularly with reference to features important in EIA (Chapter 8) and the basics of enzymology (Chapters 9–10) are also included.

1.3. The use of terms in enzyme immunoassays

Accuracy, precision, and sensitivity are very loosely used terms, generating considerable confusion. Obviously, results of EIA cannot be meaningfully interpreted nor can theoretical considerations be made if such important basic concepts are not clearly distinguished. Unfortunately, this confusion persists even in advanced theoretical treatments or in data processing.

Sensitivity is defined by the dose–response curve: it corresponds to the change in response (dR) per unit amount of reactant (dC) and equals dR/dC (not necessarily constant). It is used in this sense throughout this monograph. It should be stressed that publications carrying the word 'ultrasensitive' in their title nearly always describe a method which requires only small amounts or low concentrations of material for detection. This property is defined and used here as detection limit or detectability (= ability to detect). Fig. 1.1 shows the essential difference between these two concepts. If meaningful results are obtained only between two similar response limits (e.g., in the usual sigmoidal dose–response curves), a high sensitivity will decrease the span of concentrations which can be determined reliably. Unfortunately, the controversy over these terms is particularly strong among radioimmunologists.

A great deal of confusion also surrounds the terms accuracy and precision (Fig. 1.1). Accuracy is the conformity of a result to an accepted standard value (reference accuracy) or to a true value. Precision reflects either the calculated result with standard deviation (Section 15.1) or the number of digits or decimals in which a result is expressed and may be of very low accuracy; e.g., in tests with two-fold serial dilutions, the results may be stated as, e.g., 16384. This titre, due to the frequent subjectivity of such tests, may easily be higher or lower by a factor of 2 and the precise number may be totally inaccurate.

In order to achieve satisfactory accuracy, it is essential to avoid errors. However, distinction should be made between experimental errors and mistakes. Mistakes are the type of errors ('blunders') which necessitate the repetition of the test, whereas experimental errors are inherent to the test and may result from random error, from bias or from both. Random errors may be due to slight fluctuations in measuring enzyme activity, variations in temperature, ionic composition of the sample, etc., and can be minimized by the use of standards. Bias is a systematic error (storage effects, improper

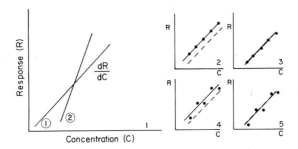

Fig. 1.1. The different concepts of sensitivity ($= dR/dC$) and detectability (detection limit) are represented in frame 1. System (1) has a higher detectability (ability to detect small amounts) than system (2), whereas the latter is more sensitive (more responsive to slight changes in the concentration). The different concepts of precision (i.e., with its relative scatter; Section 15.1) and accuracy (i.e., conformity with theoretical results) are illustrated in frames 2–5 in which the broken lines show the theoretical relation and the dots with the solid lines represent the experimental results. Frame 2 shows high precision (small standard deviation) but low accuracy, 3 high precision and high accuracy, 4 has low precision and low accuracy, whereas 5 shows results having low precision but high accuracy.

calibration of pipets, etc.) which can be minimized by regular evaluation of the reagents. Important types of bias in EIA are binding of non-specific immunoreactants, enzymes, inhibitors, ions which influence enzyme activity, etc., present in the sample.

Specificity, another frequently misused term in EIA, should refer to the degree of discrimination of the assay between negative and positive samples (i.e., relative affinities of two systems).

The synonymous use of the terms immunogen and antigen is not justified. An immunogen is a substance which is able to induce an immune response in an animal, whereas an antigen is a substance which is able to react with the antibody, and need not to be identical with immunogen. The term allergen is used here for antigens reacting with IgE antibodies.

Many names and acronyms are in use to identify the various assays. This is avoided here, mainly to eliminate the ambiguities when similar acronyms are used for different tests, e.g. CELISA for cellular enzyme-linked immunosorbent assay (Morris et al., 1982), for chemiluminescent enzyme-linked immunosorbent assay (Pronovost et al., 1981), and for complement enzyme-linked immunosorbent assay (Tandon et al., 1979).

Mainly two types of abbreviations are used: for often-used organic chemicals an acronym (GA for glutaraldehyde, etc.), and for enzymes contractions of their names ending with 'ase' despite the fact that for some enzymes other abbreviations are more widely used (e.g., POase instead of HRPO for peroxidase).

Outline of the strategies for enzyme immunoassays

2.1. Classification of enzyme immunoassays

The development of various EIA procedures has led to confusing terminology and classifications, which are often misleading concerning their fundamental features and tend to obscure their relative merits. Not surprisingly, many comparative studies produced inconclusive results. The frequent comparison of the relative merits of radioactive and enzyme labels, as evaluated in RIA by saturation analysis and in ELISA by immunometric analysis, is basically faulty since the underlying principles of these assays are different (Ekins, 1980). Here, EIA will be classified according to their essential differences to expose the inherent limitations and potentials of each assay: EIA are based either on Activity Amplification (AA) or Activity Modulation (AM).

EIA have not received the intense theoretical and statistical evaluation to which RIA have been subjected. The following considerations will, hopefully, eliminate some of the confusion currently besetting EIA.

2.2. Sensitivity and detectability of activity amplification and activity modulation assays

Both in homogeneous and heterogeneous AA assays, a large excess of immunoreactant is used to obtain a maximum signal for the compound to be tested. The law of mass action (i.e., the rate of complex formation is proportional to the concentration of the reactants) implies that, even at very low concentrations of the molecules, a high fraction will react if the immunoreactant is added in excess. The theoretical limit of the number of molecules detectable by AA methods is thus 1. In practice, this has not been achieved (down to about 10^4 molecules), though Rotman (1961) measured enzyme activity of single molecules of β-galactosidase.

AM methods, in contrast, depend on the modulation of the enzyme signal by competition of the test molecule for the same immunoreactant. Contrary to AA methods, the sensitivity of AM assays increases with lower immunoreactant concentrations since at low concentrations a variation in the amount of competing molecules has a larger impact on the interaction with the labeled species. According to the law of mass action, the low antigen and antibody concentrations reduce considerably the rate of complex formation. Moreover, at very low concentrations the accuracy tends to be poor.

It is obvious that a constant amount of antibody requires less antigen to become 50% saturated if the affinity is higher. The affinity constant K, which has dimensions of the reciprocal of concentration (i.e., M^{-1}; Section 8.3), is, therefore, of utmost importance in AM assays. It is practical to express antigen and antibody concentrations in $1/K$ (i.e., M) units. The detection limit attainable in AM-type assays also depends on the relative experimental error, E_e, so that the minimal amount of reactants that can be detected is given by E_e/K. For example, the detectability of an antigen–antibody system with a K of 10^{10} M^{-1} and a relative error of 5% is $0.05/10^{10}$ M^{-1} = 5×10^{-12} M (about 10^8 molecules/ml). Among others, E_e depends on the ease with which the enzyme is detected and on the fractional modulation in enzyme activity maximally possible. The detectability of AA-type EIA is, therefore, potentially far superior to that of AM methods. Enzymes may be quite sensitive to environmental factors (temperature, ionic strength, inhibitors, activators, or proteases present in biological fluids) which may further decrease the sensitivity of EIA. Generally, the accuracy and the detectability of AM assays is less than obtainable with radioactive labels in RIA. On the other hand, AA methods have potentially much higher detectabilities than saturation analysis by RIA, often by several orders of magnitude.

2.3. Specificity of activity amplification and activity modulation assays

The specificity of these EIA is determined by the uniqueness of the interaction between antibody and antigen, as well as to environmental factors. Non-specificity of the immune reaction can be traced to two phenomena, shared reactivity and cross-reactivity, discussed in Section 8.6. Specificity of a polyclonal antiserum is generally higher than that of its component antibodies, due to the specificity bonus (Section 8.6).

In AA procedures, antigens which share reactivity towards the same antibody will be complexed in a ratio proportional to their concentrations (appear equipotent) since the antibodies are present in large excess. Environmental influences have relatively little effect.

In AM procedures, however, the relative potency (i.e., the molar concentrations yielding an identical bound/free ratio) of cross-reactants or competitors is important since antibodies are not present in excess. The apparent affinity constants determine to a large degree the maximum specificity attainable. Cross-reactants usually bind less avidly than the specific antigen. Consequently, AM-type procedures are often more specific than AA assays.

2.4. General characteristics of enzyme immunoassay designs

The practical implications of the considerations discussed above are compiled in Table 2.1. Most EIA are either of the AA- or the

TABLE 2.1
Practical implications for activity amplification (AA) and activity modulation (AM) assays

---

– AA assays have inherently a potential detectability several orders of magnitude higher than AM asssays.

– AM assays have an intrinsically higher specificity than AA assays.

– Monoclonal antibodies have a high positive impact on specificity of AA assays.

– The use of two different antisera in 'sandwich' methods may increase specificity in AA assays.

– AA assays are faster than AM assays at their limiting detectabilities due to the excess of antibodies in AA assays and to the law of mass action.

– The detectability of AM assays is not better than that of saturation analysis RIA, in contrast to AA assays.

AM-type; these terms are not strictly synonymous to non-competitive and competitive assays, respectively. The variety of solid-phase EIA (Chapter 14) may appear confusing, both with respect to their arrangement and the requirements desired (i.e., testing for antigen or antibody, with high specificity or high detectability). However, an analysis of the various solid-phase EIA reveals that, irrespective of design, three stages can be distinguished: (i) attachment of the capture immunoreactant to the solid phase; (ii) incubation with the test sample so that the target molecules are always found in or compete for the second layer; and, (iii) an amplification step in AA assays, which may contain many layers of immunoreactants (Fig. 2.1). This amplification step is possible both in non-competitive and in indirect competitive assays. Except for rare occasions (Section 17.2.2.5), only one layer of antigen is used, either as capture molecule (R_1), or in the sample (R_2), or in the amplification step (R_3) in the case of the Ig-class capture methods (Section 2.5.1). The detectability and specificity of these designs follow the rules discussed in Sections 2.2 and 2.3. For example, in non-competitive virus assays

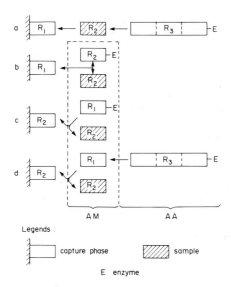

Fig. 2.1. Design of solid-phase EIA. One of the immunoreactants (R_1 or R_2, generally antibody or antigen) is immobilized on the solid phase and serves to capture the complementary reactant from the sample ('immunoextraction'). In EIA, the substance to be assayed is thus added in the second layer. Amplification of the signal of reaction between R_1 and R_2 is achieved with R_3 which may consist of several layers.

(i.e., R_1 = antibody, and R_2 = viral antigen), the direct use of labeled immunoreactant in R_3 produces much higher specificity than the use of the indirect method (i.e., antibody and labeled anti-IgG antibody) for R_3. This expectation is corroborated by numerous publications in virology, in which the indirect method detected related virus strains whereas the direct method detected only the specific strain (Barbara and Clark, 1982). A compromise should, therefore, be made with respect to specificity and detectability.

2.5. Designs of enzyme immunoassays

2.5.1. Non-competitive, solid-phase enzyme immunoassays

These AA-type methods, which are among the most popular EIA, may be subdivided according to the immunoreactant immobilized on the solid phase. Immobilization of antigen on solid phase is popular for detecting IgG or IgA antibodies (Fig. 2.2a). This method has high detectability due to the fact that several labeled anti-Ig molecules react with each primary antibody molecule and that the anti-Ig is obtained from hyperimmune serum. It is possible to increase detectability using a bridge method in which non-immunologic (avidin-biotin, protein A) or immunologic recognition systems further increase the enzyme/test molecule ratio in the complex (Section 14.5.1.2). These designs are sometimes named a-ELISA (a = amplified; Butler et al., 1980). In the immunologic bridging systems, enzyme molecules are complexed with anti-enzyme antibodies raised in the same species as the antibody of the last layer in the immobilized antigen–antibody complex. These two complexes are then linked with an anti-Ig from another species (Fig. 2.2b). It is theoretically possible to introduce a whole series of antibodies (e.g., double bridge, Section 17.3.2.2) to improve detectability with each subsequent layer. Methods using non-immunologic bridges are essentially similar.

It is also possible to immobilize the sample antigen followed by detection with labeled antibodies. This method yields higher specificity but suffers from high background staining and high dependence on dilution factors: optimum results are obtained only within a restricted range of dilutions due to competition by non-specific proteins or to the insufficiency of the antigen to cover all available sites on the solid phase.

A general approach for the detection of antigens is to create a so-called antibody sandwich (immobilized antibody, antigen, antibodies; Fig. 2.2c). If the indirect method is used to detect the captured antigen, the second antibody should be from a different species, to prevent the reaction of the labeled anti-Ig with the first, immobi-

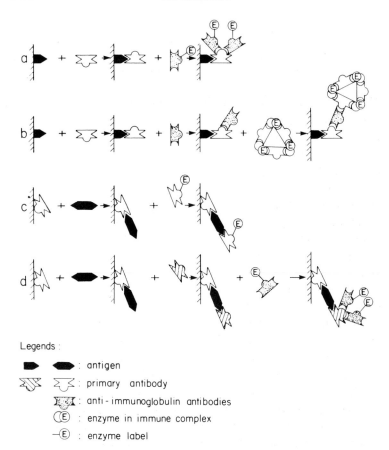

Legends:

▶ ◀▶ : antigen

⤳ ⤳ : primary antibody

▨ : anti-immunoglobulin antibodies

Ⓔ : enzyme in immune complex

─Ⓔ : enzyme label

Fig. 2.2. Non-competitive, solid-phase EIA. During the first stage, antigen (a and b) or antibody (c and d) is immobilized on the solid phase. These captured molecules extract the corresponding immunoreactants from the sample in the second step. Different detection methods can be used in the third stage, such as direct detection with labeled antibody (a and c) or by bridge (b) or more elaborate indirect (d) procedures.

lized antibody (Fig. 2.2d). This problem can often be circumvented by immobilizing Fab fragments, since anti-Ig are mostly directed to Fc fragments. In principle, it is possible to reduce the number of incubation steps by using monoclonal antibodies against different epitopes on the antigen. Such monoclonal antibodies would not compete for the same site and thus antigen and labeled antibody may be incubated simultaneously for the reaction in Fig. 2.2c. In practice, this theoretical shortcut may encounter difficulties (Section 14.5.3).

A recently developed variant of this method is the class-capture technique useful in the diagnosis of infectious diseases. This method is based on the observation that after the first infection primarily IgM antibodies (Section 5.1.1) are produced which are gradually replaced by IgG antibodies in chronic or recurrent infections. Various laborious methods have been developed to separate IgG from IgM and to establish the relative proportion of antibodies in the two classes. In the very simple but powerful class-capture method, the presence of IgM can be detected by immobilizing an anti-IgM antibody which will capture the IgM from the serum. If the IgM contains antibodies, they will, in turn, be able to capture the antigen, which can be revealed by the methods shown in Figs. 2.2c or 2.2d. The titres of IgM and IgG antibodies can be established in parallel experiments.

2.5.2. Non-competitive, homogeneous enzyme immunoassays

These AA-type EIA are performed without a solid phase and they do not require the separation of free and bound label. The distinction between bound and free conjugate is achieved by labeling two monoclonal antibodies directed against different epitopes of the antigen with two enzymes selected so that one produces the substrate for the other (e.g., glucose oxidase, (GOase) and peroxidase (POase); Fig. 2.3). Significant enzyme activity in such systems is detected only when the two labeled antibody preparations react with the antigen, bringing their labels close. This technique (Ngo and Lenhoff, 1981) is still in its infancy but may offer new useful assay systems. A selection of indicator molecules with their corresponding substrate, intermediate product and final product is given in Table 2.2.

TABLE 2.2

Proximal linkage systems for enzyme immunoassays (adapted from Sevier et al., 1981)[a]

System	Indicators (I_1/I_2)	Substrates	Products (P_1/P_2)
Proximal enzymes	hexokinase/GPDase	ATP/glucose NAD$^+$	glucose-6-phosphate/ gluconolactone-6-phosphate + NADH
Proximal enzymes	GOase/POase	glucose/H-donor	peroxide/oxidized H-donor
Bioluminescence	NAD oxidoreductase/ luciferase	NADH/FMN	FMNH$_2$/hv
Allosteric activation	phosphofructokinase/ phosphoenol pyruvate carboxylase	fructose-6-phosphate/NADH/ (MDase)	phosphoenol pyruvate/NAD$^+$
Allosteric inhibition	aspartate aminotransferase/phosphoenol pyruvate carboxylase	oxalacetate/glutamate/NADH	phosphoenol pyruvate/NAD$^+$ and oxalacetate
Enzyme/ substrate	POase/luminol	peroxide	hv

[a] I_1 and I_2 are the indicators labeled to the two antibodies: P_1 is the intermediate product and P_2 the final product. Abbreviations: GPDase, glucose-6-phosphate dehydrogenase; GOase, glucose oxidase; POase, peroxidase; H-donor, hydrogen donor; hv, emission of light.

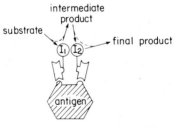

Fig. 2.3. Proximal linkage system for EIA. An antigen with two different epitopes is recognized by the corresponding antibodies (symbol as in Fig. 2.2), which are coupled with two selected enzymes (Table 2.2) of which the second (I_2) increases the production of measurable, final product due to the close vicinity of I_1 producing the substrate for I_2. The formation of product is low if these labels are not brought together, i.e., in the absence of antigen.

2.5.3. Competitive, homogeneous enzyme immunoassays

Several general systems, all of the AM type, are known in this group. The first was developed by Rubenstein et al. (1972) for the detection of a hapten, using an enzyme–hapten conjugate as antigen. This method is widely known under the trade name EMIT (Syva Co.). The activity of the conjugated enzyme is modulated by the reaction of anti-hapten antibody with the haptenated enzyme, either by steric hindrance or by a change in the configuration of the enzyme. Competing free hapten will decrease this modulation (Fig. 2.4a).

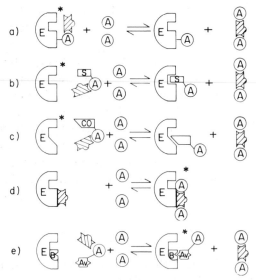

Fig. 2.4. Competitive, homogeneous EIA. The symbol E represents enzyme, A antigen or hapten, S and CO substrate and enzyme cofactor, and Av and B avidin and biotin. Enzymes indicated with * have 'modulated' (increased or decreased) activities. In (a) hapten is conjugated to the enzyme and reaction with the antibody (shaded structure) modulates the enzyme activity. This interaction is, however, prevented if antigen is present in the sample. Similar principles apply if substrate (b) or cofactor (c) are conjugated with the antigen. In (d) antibody is directly linked to the enzyme, and the reaction of this antibody, particularly with high-molecular weight antigens, will block the active site of the enzyme. In (e) antibody, directed to haptens labeled to avidin, prevents avidin from inhibiting the biotin-containing enzyme, unless antibody is neutralized by the same hapten present in the sample.

Depending on the system, both activation or inhibition may occur. It will be seen later (Section 10.2.2) that the same antiserum may contain a fraction of antibodies which activates the enzyme and a fraction which inhibits the enzyme.

Instead of the enzyme, the substrate may be conjugated to the antigen (Burd et al., 1977). The antibody reacting with the antigen–substrate conjugate then prevents the substrate being used by the enzyme. The addition of free antigen (for standard curve or as test sample) prevents some antibody from reacting with substrate-bound antigen (Fig. 2.4b). A third possibility may be the conjugation of the antigen to an enzyme cofactor (Carrico et al., 1976). Enzyme activity is blocked by the antibody unless free antigen is competing for the antibody (Fig. 2.4c). It is also possible to conjugate the enzyme to the antibody, a method conceptually similar to EMIT. The substrate is prevented from serving the enzyme when the antibody reacts with its antigen (Wei and Reibe, 1977; Fig. 2.4d). Another variant (Bacquet and Twumasi, 1984) is based on avidin's capacity to bind biotin-containing enzymes (resulting in inhibition) even if a hapten is conjugated to the avidin. Antibodies to this hapten inhibit sterically this enzyme inactivation, unless hapten present in the sample competes for the limited number of antibody sites (Fig. 2.4e).

2.5.4. Competitive, solid-phase enzyme immunoassays

The first EIA described (Van Weemen and Schuurs, 1971; Engvall and Perlmann, 1971) belong to this group. In this assay the antibody is immobilized on the solid phase and the antigen is labeled with the enzyme. In the test, binding of the antigen–enzyme conjugate by the immobilized antibody is inhibited by the addition of free antigen (to obtain a standard curve or present in the test sample). Since a restricted number of antibodies are available, the enzyme activity is lowered (Fig. 2.5a). The product concentration is, therefore, inversely proportional to the concentration of the free antigen (standard or test) added. This assay is of the AM type.

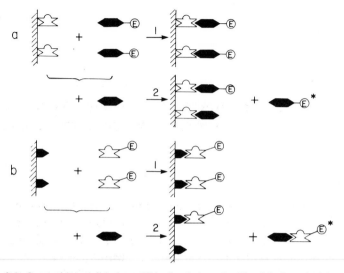

Fig. 2.5. Competitive, solid-phase EIA. Symbols as in Fig. 2.2. In principle, two approaches are possible: (a), antibody is immobilized on the solid phase which binds enzyme-labeled antigen (1) or, if present, antigen contained in the sample (2); and, (b), antigen is immobilized and may react with enzyme-labeled antibody (not in excess!). Free antigen in the sample will compete for this antigen and lower the amount of enzyme bound. The * indicates that in system (a) labeled antigen is eliminated by washing, whereas in system (b) labeled Ag is removed in the form of immune complexes.

Alternatively, the antigen may be immobilized and the antibody is labeled with the enzyme. The test or standard antigen, added together with the labeled antibody, competes for the restricted amount of antibody and thus lowers the final activity (Fig. 2.5b). This is also an AM procedure. It is possible to increase the detectability of this assay by making an indirect test of the procedure depicted in Fig. 2.5b. The free antigen is added with diluted antiserum instead of labeled antibodies. The free antigen competes with the immobilized antigen and thus prevents a certain fraction of the antibodies from being immobilized. The immobilized antibodies are, in a subsequent step, detected by labeled anti-Ig antibodies, or with one of the bridge-methods. This assay (Fig. 2.1d) is, therefore, a mixed or sequential AM- and AA-type procedure.

Non-immunologic molecular recognition systems used in immunoassays

A high capacity of molecular recognition is at the basis of the structure and operation of all living systems. Many of these substances can be exploited for assays in connection with, or similar to, EIA. Currently, a few (avidin/biotin, protein A, lectins) are used to great advantage, and will contribute considerably to increase the applicability of EIA.

3.1. The avidin/biotin system

The avidin/biotin system is rapidly becoming an important tool for EIA since: (i) avidin has an exceptionally high affinity for (+)-biotin (10^{15} M^{-1}); (ii) (+)-biotin is very easily coupled to antibodies and to many enzymes often without any loss of activity; and, (iii) avidin is very stable and has several binding sites so that it may be used as a bridging molecule between two biotinylated molecules. The use of the avidin/biotin system produces superior detectabilities and low background levels.

Biotin is one of about a dozen water-soluble factors of the vitamin B complex and is a coenzyme for enzymes involved in carboxylation reactions. The carboxyl group of the valeric acid side chain of (+)-biotin is covalently linked through an amide bond to the ε-amino group of a lysyl residue of those enzymes. The antibacterial function of avidin by binding biotin and inhibiting all biotin-enzymes is plausible. Avidin is isolated from egg white which contains several antibacterial proteins (lysozyme, conalbumin). Due to some sequence homology, it has been suggested that avidin and lysozyme may have common ancestors (Green, 1975). A protein very similar to avidin, streptavidin, from *Streptomyces avidinii*, is still little used, but has an important edge over avidin with respect to background staining. Avidin is stable over a wide range of pH and temperature values, and the avidin–biotin complex has an even higher stability to heat and proteolytic enzymes. Affinity chromatography to purify either biotin or avidin, using immobilized avidin or biotin, has not been successful due to the very high affinity. However, analogs with considerably lower affinities can be used successfully in affinity isolation procedures (see below). Though avidin is a very basic glycoprotein with an isoelectric point (pI) of 10.5 (Fraenkel-Conrat et al., 1952), it can be crystallized from strong salt solutions only in the pH range of 5 to 7.

Native avidin has a mass of 15600 daltons for each of the 4 subunits (Green, 1975). The optical density of a 1 mg/ml avidin solution is 1.54 cm^{-1} at 282 nm (Green and Toms, 1970). It is sensitive to strong light (György et al., 1942) and oxidation (Fraenkel-Conrat, 1952). Glass commonly adsorbs basic solutes strongly, and avidin is no exception (Costello et al., 1979). Silanization solves the problem only partially; slightly less adsorption is observed on polyethylene.

One unit of avidin combines, by definition, with 1 μg of (+)-biotin, and since it can be calculated that 1 mg of avidin binds a maximum of 14 μg of (+)-biotin, 14 U/mg would be the highest attainable specific activity of avidin. Each subunit is able to bind biotin in the pH 2–13 range (Green, 1963, 1975). A random binding (no allosteric interaction) has been observed (Green, 1975) with an association rate constant of 7×10^7 M^{-1} sec^{-1} and a very small dissociation rate constant of 5×10^{-8} sec^{-1} (an extremely long half life of the complex of about 160 days). The binding sites are deep in the avidin: the carboxyl group of the valeric acid of bound biotin lies 0.8–0.9 nm beneath the van der Waals surface of the molecule. There is reason to believe that current applications of avidin/biotin in EIA, which fail to take the depth of the binding site into account, lead to suboptimal results (Section 3.2.4). Almost every atom in the biotin molecule appears to contribute to the interaction with avidin and many analogs or small fragments of (+)-biotin (urea, glycol, tetra-hydrofuran, caproic acid) may be bound or compete in the interaction (Green, 1975). This engulfment of biotin may, at least partially, be responsible for the high affinity. The 4 binding sites are not evenly distributed but two sites are close together so that each pair of sites binds only one biotinylated protein (Green, 1975). Since there are 2 pairs of binding sites, the avidin molecule is capable of acting as a bridging agent between two biotinylated proteins, but not, as commonly stated, as an amplifying factor.

3.2. Preparation of avidin and biotinylated immunoassay reactants

3.2.1. Purification of avidin

In the classical method (Melamed and Green, 1963; Green and Toms, 1970) avidin is adsorbed to carboxymethylcellulose at high pH, fol-lowed by elution with a stepwise gradient of $(NH_4)_2CO_3$, rechroma-tography on CM-cellulose, and crystallization. This time-consuming method is efficient for large quantities. Starting with 5 l frozen egg white, which can be obtained commercially, about 50 mg avidin is obtained.

A very simple method (Heney and Orr, 1981) using affinity chro-matography on 2-iminobiotin agarose or 2-iminobiotin-6-aminohex-yl-Sepharose 4B (for both, 2-iminobiotin is incorporated via a spacer) yields pure avidin in a single step with over 90% recovery. This technique is based on the strong binding of avidin by the cyclic guanidino analog of biotin, 2-iminobiotin, in its free base form (above pH 9.0), but not in its salt form. Though this method can be used directly for the isolation of avidin from homogenized egg white (almost 1 mg avidin/egg), it is preferable to use a crude extract if large quantities are to be purified.

Egg whites, obtained from large fresh eggs by the careful breaking of the shell and separation from the yolk, are homogenized and diluted with a half volume of distilled water. The solution at 4°C is brought slowly to 2.8 M $(NH_4)_2SO_4$ (enzyme grade) and stirred for 2 h. The precipitate is removed by centrifugation for 20 min at $8000 \times g$. Ammonium sulfate is added to saturation (about 4 M; take volume increase into account) and the mixture is stirred at 4°C overnight. Avidin precipitates during this step and is collected by centrifugation for 30 min at $8000 \times g$. The pellet is resuspended in distilled water (40 ml) and dialyzed extensively against distilled water.

2-Iminobiotin-Sepharose or -agarose (5–10 ml; commercially available) is equilibrated with a solution containing 50 mM Na_2CO_3, pH 11, and 1 M NaCl. The pH of the diluted homogenized egg white or of the crude extract is raised to 11 with NaOH and NaCl is added to 1 M. The extract corresponding to 10–15 egg whites is applied on the equilibrated column which is then washed with the equilibrating buffer (10 ml/h) until the absorbance at 282 nm is zero. Avidin is eluted by converting 2-iminobiotin to the salt form with a 50 mM ammonium acetate buffer, pH 4.0, containing 500 mM NaCl. The yield (usually 8–12 mg) is determined from the absorbance of avidin at 282 nm (Section 3.1). The column can be used many times.

3.2.2. Purification of streptavidin

Streptomyces avidinii can be obtained from the American Type Culture Collection (ATCC 27419) and grown in a medium according to Stapley et al. (1963) on 2% agar plates at 30°C. Spores from four plates are used to inoculate 4 l of medium, which is then incubated for 3 days at 30°C. The medium is clarified by centrifugation (10 min, $10000 \times g$) and concentrated in an Amicon concentrator (PM 10 membrane) to 400 ml. To this solution at 0°C, $(NH_4)_2SO_4$

is added to 70% saturation and the precipitate is dissolved in 20 ml water and dialyzed twice (6 h) against 1 l water. The sample is centrifuged for 20 min at $35000 \times g$, the supernatant recovered, and the pH adjusted to 11 (with NH_4OH). An equal volume of 50 mM $(NH_4)_2CO_3$, pH 11.0 and containing 500 mM NaCl, is added. Streptavidin is purified from this solution on 2-iminobiotin AH-Sepharose 4B as described for avidin (yield: 10–14 mg per 4 l culture, Hofmann et al., 1980).

3.2.3. Spectrophotometric assay of avidin or biotin

A simple spectrophotometric assay for avidin and biotin is based on the binding of the dye, 4'-hydroxy-azobenzene-2-carboxylate, to avidin giving a new absorbtion band at 500 nm (molar extinction coefficient, $34500 \ M^{-1} cm^{-1}$) and a change of color from yellow to red (Green, 1965). Biotin readily displaces the dye, which has a K of 5.8×10^{-6} M, from avidin. To measure the displacement of the dye by biotin, 1.3 mg avidin in 2 ml of 20 mM sodium phosphate buffer, pH 7.0 is mixed with 0.1 mM dye solution to saturate all binding sites. The decrease of extinction at 500 nm due to added biotin is measured. A change of optical density of 0.1 (1 cm optical pathway) is produced by either 50 μg avidin or 0.65 μg biotin. Many biological solutions, including tissue culture media, may contain biotin and thus interfere.

Another procedure, which is based on the fluorescence quenching of tryptophan when biotin binds to avidin, has a detectability of as little as 20 ng biotin (Lin and Kirsch,1977).

3.2.4. Preparation of biotinylated proteins

Biotin moieties may be conjugated to proteins by rendering the carboxyl group of biotin reactive towards the free amino groups of proteins (Fig. 3.1). Though avidin may be conjugated directly to one of the immunoreactants, full advantage of this system is only obtained by using avidin as bridge-molecule between biotinylat-

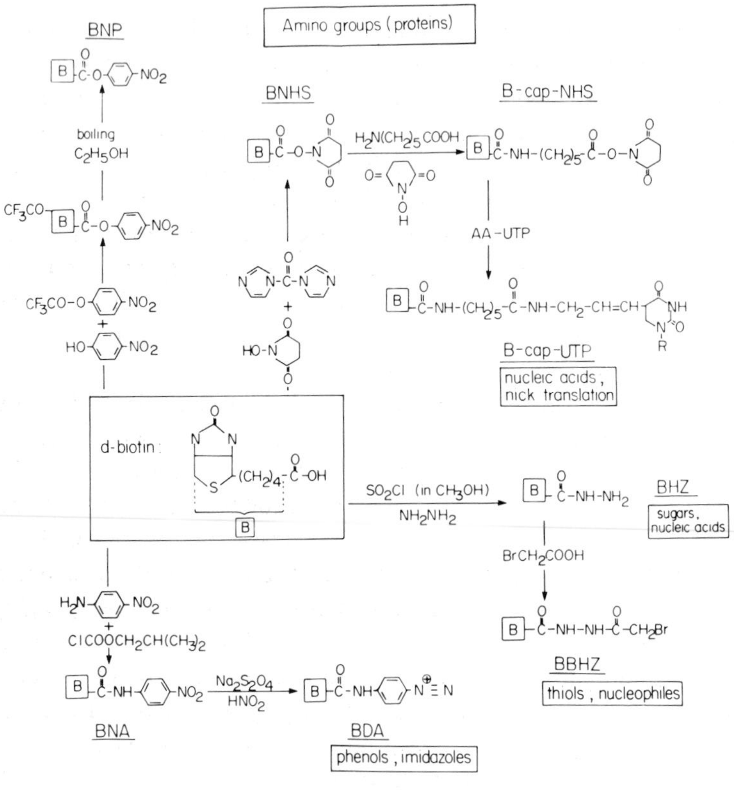

Fig. 3.1. Pathways to render (+)-biotin reactive to different groups on macromolecules. Most common is the synthesis of biotinyl-*p*-nitrophenyl (BNP) ester, details of which are given in Section 3.2.4.1, and biotinyl-*N*-hydroxysuccinimide (BNHS; Section 3.2.4.2), easily conjugated to amino groups, e.g., in proteins. Caproylamido-BNHS ester (B-cap-NHS; Section 3.2.4.3) is expected to give considerably better results for EIH and EIA than the commonly used BNP or BNHS and can be conjugated to 5-(3-amino)allyldeoxyuridine triphosphate (Langer et al., 1981). B-cap-UTP is introduced in DNA by nick translation. Alternative pathways to prepare biotin derivatives active with groups other than amino groups are given in Table 3.2. The derivative, biotinyl-diazoanilide (BDA), prepared from biotinyl-nitroanilide (BNA), reacts with phenols or imidazoles, whereas biotinyl-bromoacetyl hydrazide (BBHZ) prepared from biotinyl hydrazide (BHZ) reacts with sulfhydryls or other nucleophiles. The latter reagent can also be made reactive to sugars and nucleic acids.

ed enzyme and biotinylated immunoreactants. Avidin, however, can be directly conjugated to enzymes which are inactivated by biotinylation (e.g. alkaline phosphatase – APase). Two different esters of biotin with high reactivity towards the amino groups are commonly used to biotinylate proteins: biotinyl-*p*-nitrophenyl (BNP) ester and biotinyl-*N*-hydroxysuccinimide (BNHS) ester. BNHS is much more water-soluble, and, therefore, easier to handle, but should be stored desiccated to prevent hydrolysis. Both esters were originally prepared with dicyclohexylcarbodiimide (DCC). However, dicyclohexylurea, which is difficult to remove, may accumulate as a by-product, and alternative methods are preferable.

The depth of the binding sites of avidin may impede its reaction with biotin if large ligands are directly bound to the carboxyl group of biotin. Green et al. (1971) prepared dimeric biotin probes by inserting spacers (extenders) of different lenghts. The length of this spacer-chain had to exceed 12 C-C bonds before this probe could link two avidin molecules, though they failed to consider the weakening of the interaction due to the repulsion arising from juxtaposing highly positively charged avidin molecules. Nevertheless, improvement of the avidin/biotin interaction by the introduction of an ε-amino caproic acid (spacer between the carboxyl group of biotin and the reactive NHS group; Costello et al., 1979) was recently confirmed by Hofmann et al. (1982) and Leary et al. (1983).

3.2.4.1. Synthesis of biotinyl-p-nitrophenyl ester (BNP)   To 2.44 g of finely powdered (+)-biotin suspended in 60 ml pyridine, 1.4 g *p*-nitrophenol and 10 g *p*-nitrophenyl trifluoroacetate (Aldrich) are added. After stirring for 1 h at 50°C, the clear solution is cooled to room temperature and the solvent removed in vacuo. The residue is dried over P_2O_5 overnight. The semi-solid mass is triturated with 20 ml ether, filtered and washed with 10 ml ether, 20 ml water, and 20 ml ether. The dried product is suspended in 30 ml 95% ethanol and heated to boiling until all material is dissolved. Cooling yields crystals, which are washed with ice-cold 95% ethanol. The yield is about 75%, the melting point is 160–163°C (Bodanszky and Fagan, 1977).

3.2.4.2. Synthesis of biotinyl-N-hydroxysuccinimide ester (BNHS)
For the synthesis of BNHS, N,N-dimethylformamide (DMF; ACS grade) is dried over molecular sieves (Fisher Co, type 3A beads). N-hydroxysuccinimide (NHS) and $(+)$-biotin are dried separately over P_2O_5 in vacuo.

Biotin (1 g) is dissolved in 20 ml DMF by gentle heating at 80°C in a dry flask and 665 mg N,N'-carbonyldiimidazole (Aldrich) are added. Heating is stopped when the evolution of CO_2 ceases. The mixture is stirred for 2 h at 25°C and 475 mg NHS (in 10 ml DMF) are added. Stirring overnight in a sealed flask dissolves the precipitated intermediate and produces the NHS ester. Solvent is removed in vacuo and the product is recrystallized from refluxing isopropanol. The yield of BNHS (colorless) is about 75%; the melting point is 210°C (Jasiewicz et al., 1976). BNHS should be stored desiccated.

3.2.4.3. Synthesis of caproylamido-BNHS ester (B-cap-NHS)
B-cap-NHS is prepared by dissolving BNHS (as prepared above) in 3 ml dry DMF and mixing with 131 mg γ-amino caproic acid in 4 ml of 100 mM $NaHCO_3$ solution. The mixture is stirred for 4 h at room temperature and most of the solvent is eliminated under reduced pressure in a rotary evaporator. The oily white residue is suspended in 10 ml citric acid (10% w/v), collected on Whatman no 1 filter paper and washed 5 times with cold water. The precipitate is dried at 45°C under reduced pressure over P_2O_5 for 3 days. The intermediate (300 mg) is dissolved in 20 ml dry DMF at 95°C (in a round-bottom flask) and 160 mg carbonyldiimidazole in 5 ml DMF are added at once with stirring. The temperature is maintained at 95°C for 30 min. The flask is then cooled to room temperature and 100 mg NHS are added 2 h later. The flask is sealed and stirred overnight. The DMF is removed under reduced pressure in a rotary evaporator. The pale-yellow oil is added to 15 ml isopropanol. Several hours later, an off-white precipitate forms; the supernatant is discarded and the precipitate is dissolved in 25 ml dry isopropanol by gentle heating. The volume is then reduced to about

10 ml and the flask is cooled. The very fine white crystals which develop, are dried at reduced pressure overnight over P_2O_5 at 60°C. The yield is about 240 mg or 60%; the melting point is about 150°C (Costello et al., 1979).

3.2.4.4. Biotinylation of immunoreactants   At low protein concentrations (1 mg/ml) most of the added ester hydrolyzes instead of coupling to the protein. Therefore, a standard concentration of about 10 mg/ml in 100 mM carbonate buffer, pH 8.5, should be used. BNP, BNHS or B-cap-NHS is dissolved (immediately prior to use) in dry DMF of DMSO (for NHS) so that the required amount is contained in less than 0.1 volume of the protein solution (Table 3.1). The two solutions are mixed, incubated for 4 h or overnight with gentle stirring. The protein is then desalted on Sephadex G-25 or by extensive dialysis until free of biotin. Alternative methods (Fig. 3.1; Table 3.2) in which biotin is activated towards groups other than amino groups should find wide application in EIA. For

TABLE 3.1

Percentage of amino groups substituted after reaction with biotin *N*-hydroxysuccinimide (BNHS)[a]. From Guesdon et al. (1979)

Molar ratio BNHS/amino group	Sheep IgG	GOase	POase	APase	BGase
1 : 10	26[b]	4		3	
1 : 2		35		34	
1 : 1	42	50			
2 : 1		71		90	55
4 : 1	95				
10 : 1	100		72	100	84

[a]GOase: glucose oxidase (20–30 free amino groups; 150 kDa); POase: peroxidase (2–4 amino groups; 44 kDa); APase: alkaline phosphatase (50–70 amino groups; 100 kDa); BGase: β-galactosidase (100 amino groups; 465 kDa). The sheep IgG (80 amino groups; 150 kDa) was anti-rabbit IgG antibody. Suggested amounts of activated biotin (at 100 M in dry DMF) to be added to 1 ml 100 mM $NaHCO_3$, containing 10 mg protein are 57 µl for IgG, 20 µl for GOase, 5 µl for POase, 22 µl for BGase. It is not recommended for APase (rapid inactivation).

TABLE 3.2

Preparation of biotin derivatives active with groups other than amino groups (reactions shown in Fig. 3.1)

A. *Biotinyl-diazoanilide (BDA)* (Bayer and Wilchek, 1980).

Biotinyl-nitroanilide (BNA) is prepared (steps 1–6) by the mixed anhydride method (Section 12.3.1); its transformation to BDA (steps 7–10) should be performed immediately before use.

1. Dissolve 1 mmol (244 mg) biotin in 3 ml dry (Section 3.2.4.2) DMF and add 0.14 ml triethylamine.
2. Cool solution to 10° C and add 0.16 ml isobutyl chloroformate.
3. After 5 min add 150 mg *p*-nitroaniline.
4. Incubate overnight at room temperature.
5. Precipitate BNA with ethyl acetate.
6. Collect BNA and recrystallize from isopropanol.
7. Dissolve BNA in 2 ml DMF and add water until suspension becomes slightly turbid.
8. Add excess of crystalline $Na_2S_2O_4$ (about 0.2 g) and acidify after 10 min with 1 N HCl to pH 2.0.
9. Treat with $NaNO_2$ at 0° C (Table 12.4, step 2,3).
10. Bring the pH of the solution to 8.0 and use BDA immediately for conjugation (see Table 12.4, steps 5 and 6) (the appearance of a deep yellow or reddish color is a sign of reaction).

B. *Biotin hydrazide (BHZ)* (Heitzmann and Richards, 1974; Bayer and Wilchek, 1980).

1. Add slowly 1 ml thionyl chloride to 10 ml chilled methanol (in ice–saline bath).
2. Add 1 g of biotin and incubate overnight at room temperature.
3. Evaporate to dryness, dissolve in 10 ml methanol, evaporate again to dryness, and redissolve in 5 ml methanol.
4. Add 1 ml hydrazine hydrate and incubate overnight at room temperature, and collect precipitate (BHZ) by filtration.
5. Concentrate filtrate (another precipitate of BHZ will appear) and wash combined precipitates with ether.
6. Recrystallize from DMF.

C. *Biotinyl-bromoacetyl hydrazide (BBHZ)* (Givol et al., 1971; Bayer and Wilchek, 1980).

1. Dissolve 260 mg BHZ (prepared according to method above) in 10 ml 500 mM $NaHCO_3$ and chill to 0° C.
2. Add 520 mg bromoacetic anhydride in 4 ml dioxane at 0° C.
3. Collect precipitate after 15 min by filtration.
4. Dissolve in isopropanol and precipitate again with ether.

---

example, biotin hydrazide (BHZ) or biotinyl-bromoacetyl hydrazide (BBHZ) is very reactive with aldehyde groups which can be generated with ease (Section 11.2.2) in sugars or glycoproteins.

3.3. Protein A (SpA)

SpA, isolated from the cell wall of *Staphylococcus aureus* (usually Cowan 1 strain), has an affinity for Fc fragments of many Ig (Forsgren and Sjöquist, 1966; Kronvall et al., 1974). Among the Ig from 65 mammalian species, 37 precipitated SpA, whereas the other 28 inhibited precipitation with other sera. Of the sera from 72 birds investigated, only 2 primitive species inhibited the precipitation. This reactivity towards Ig (like anti-Ig antibodies) makes SpA a very powerful tool for the isolation or selective removal of IgG (or its subclasses) or of immune complexes, and as tracers in EIA or EIH. Estimates of the molecular weight of SpA vary between 42000 and 56000 (Björk et al., 1972). The isoelectric point (pI) is 5.1 (Lindmark et al., 1977) and the extinction coefficient is 1.65 at a concentration of 10 mg/ml, at 275 nm and 1 cm optical pathway (Sjöquist et al., 1972). The high frictional ratio and intrinsic viscosity (Björk et al., 1972) are indicative of an extended rather than a globular shape. This elongated protein contains 4 highly homologous domains, each capable of binding Ig (Sjödall, 1977). Though, usually only 2 sites react with soluble IgG, other ratios have been reported (Gruhn and McDuffie, 1979; Langone, 1982). The presence of at least 2 active sites on the SpA molecule and its multispecificity make it tailor-made for the use as a linker between two unrelated Ig. SpA contains little or no sugar or phosphate and is stable over a wide range of pH (2–10).

The reactivity of SpA towards Ig depends on species, on the class and subclass of the Ig and on ionic conditions (Section 7.1.8.1). SpA binds Ig predominantly with the Fc portion of IgG molecules. It should be noted, however, that normally occurring antibodies to staphylococcal proteins are very common (Espersen and Schitz,

1981) and even highly purified SpA isolated from bacteria grown in horse serum media may induce antibodies which react specifically with equine IgG (Lind, 1974).

The association constant K of SpA for rabbit IgG is around 10^8 M^{-1} (Langone, 1982) and equilibrium is generally reached fast. Dissociation is usually negligible but may increase strongly at an excess of IgG (O'Keefe and Bennett, 1980). Temperature influences are minor between 4 and 50°C. The K of SpA with IgG varies considerably both with the species and the pH, but binding of the antigen at the Fab sites enhances the affinity between the Fc portion of the IgG and SpA, a phenomenon shown to depend on the antigen-induced aggregation (Sandor and Langone, 1981). This is very fortunate for solid-phase EIA and EIH since weakly binding IgG, such as from goat and sheep, complex with SpA several 100-fold more in the assay when absorbed to the antigen than in the free form (Langone, 1982). Complexing is not affected by EDTA or low concentrations of detergents (Tween, Triton X-100, or Brij 97) used in EIA.

The binding site for SpA is at the C_H2-C_H3 interface for human and guinea pig IgG (Langone, 1982) and may be similar in other species. Consequently, IgG–SpA interaction does not inhibit the antigen–antibody reaction. Moreover, a single enzyme conjugate may be used for a wide range of Ig, with an affinity which is frequently superior to that of anti-Ig antibodies. Enzyme-labeled SpA produces generally a lower background than enzyme-labeled anti-Ig. For obvious reasons SpA is not recommended for tissues with abundant Ig in their interstitia or having numerous IgG-containing plasma cells.

3.3.1. Purification of protein A

SpA can be isolated from *Staphylococcus aureus* strain Cowan 1 in high yields (Sjöquist et al., 1972). A common yield is about 150–170 mg SpA per 100 g wet bacteria. Bacteria are grown by the method described in Table 3.3, steps 1, 2. A stirred fermentor

TABLE 3.3

Preparation and fixation of protein A-bearing staphylococci for use as immunosorbents (Kessler, 1981)[a]

---

1. Grow *Staphylococcus aureus* bacteria (pathogenic!) strain Cowan 1 (ATCC 12598. NT.CTC 8530), in CCY broth in stirred fermentor (Arvidson et al., 1971) or in fortified Penassay broth in shake flasks (Kessler, 1976). The latter method is simpler but yields only about 2/3 of that usually obtained in stirred fermentor (limiting factor being aeration). Bacteria are grown on agar slant cultures and non-contaminated cultures are transferred to blood agar Petri dishes (24 h at 37° C) before seeding (inoculum 1% of total volume). Growth at 37° C is monitored by absorbance (scattering) at 525 nm.

2. Avoid stationary growth phase which would significantly reduce the amount of protein A.

3. Harvest cells by low speed centrifugation (avoid tight packing) i.e. at about $7000 \times g$ for 5 min and 6×250 ml Sorvall GSA or Beckman YA-14 rotor.

4. Wash pellets twice with 40 mM phosphate buffer, pH 7.2, containing 150 mM NaCl and 0.05% NaN_3 (PBS-N).

5. Fix bacteria by adding 1.5% formaldehyde (original concentration 37%) to 10% (w/v) bacterial suspension in PBS-N and stirring for 90 min.

6. Collect the fixed bacteria by centrifugation. Resuspend cells immediately to 10% (w/v), transfer to a big Erlenmeyer flask (depth of liquid phase should not exceed 2 cm), immerse flask in a 80° C water bath and shake rapidly.

7. After 5 min all bacteria should be dead. Grainy clumps, which may be formed if the cells are not rapidly resuspended after centrifugation in step 6, should have disappeared. Wash twice with PBS-N and store the fixed cells at $-70°$ C.

---

[a] Ying (1981) used a slightly different method by heat-killing the bacteria (7 min at 80° C) at the end of fermentation (step 4) and not after fixation (step 5).

---

with a working volume of 10 l will produce about 200–250 g wet bacteria which can be immediately processed after two washings with 0.9% NaCl or stored as a paste at $-30°$C.

About 100 g of wet bacteria are suspended in 1 l 50 mM Tris–HCl buffer, pH 7.5, containing 145 mM NaCl and placed in a shaking water bath at 37°C. After equilibration, about 5 mg lysostaphin (Sigma) and 1 mg DNase are added. The rate of digestion is monitored by the absorbance (scattering) at 525 nm of aliquots diluted with 0.9% NaCl, which should become constant after about 2 h. The suspension is then cooled to 4°C and clarified by low-speed centrifugation, the pellet is washed once with water and centrifuged again. The pH of the combined supernatants is lowered to 3.5 with 5 M HCl and centrifuged again to remove the precipitate formed. The pH is subsequently raised to 7.0 with 5 M NaOH and the SpA is precipiated by slowly adding 550 g of $(NH_4)_2SO_4$ per l (80% saturation). After 1 h of stirring the precipitate is collected by centrifugation, resuspended in 100 ml distilled water and dialyzed extensively against water at 4°C.

The dialyzed crude extract is centrifuged to remove the usual slight precipitate and ammonium bicarbonate is added to a final concentration of 100 mM. This sample is applied to an equilibrated DEAE-Sephadex A-50 column (150 ml; see Section 7.1.3.3) at a rate of about 60 ml/h. The column is washed with 2 volumes of 100 mM ammonium bicarbonate and SpA eluted with ammonium bicarbonate, pH 8.0, using a linear gradient between 100 to 400 mM (150 ml of each solution). Fractions are monitored at 275 nm and their SpA activity measured by a sandwich EIA (SpA forms a bridge between solid-phase IgG and enzyme-conjugated IgG) (Section 14.2.2). The fractions containing SpA are often contaminated with high-molecular weight components, which , after concentration of the samples, can be removed on a Sephadex G-150 column (1.5×50 cm; 50 mM Tris–HCl buffer, pH 8.0, containing 1 M NaCl).

Instead of purified SpA, fixed SpA-bearing bacteria (Table 3.3) can also be used as immunosorbent (Sections 7.1.8.1 and 13.5.2). Binding by 1 ml of a 10% suspension is about 1.2–1.6 mg IgG (of the proper species). Fixation of bacteria with trichloroacetic acid instead of formalin may offer some advantages (Section 13.5.2).

3.4. Lectins: specific carbohydrate-recognizing glycoproteins

The glycoproteins responsible for hemagglutinating activity of seed extracts have been termed agglutinins, phytohemagglutinins, and more recently, lectins, since their origin is not restricted to plants (reviews: Gold and Balding, 1975; Goldstein and Hayes, 1978). Lectins are generally extracted from finely ground seed meal, precipitated with $(NH_4)_2SO_4$ and purified by affinity chromatography which exploits the specific sugar-recognizing capacity (Lis et al., 1974).

The nomenclature of lectins is not systematic, some derive their name from the genus name of the plant of origin (Concanavalin A, or Con A, from *Canavalia ensiformis*; ricin from *Ricinus communis*), others are designated by the latin name of their origin (*Helix pomatia* agglutinin), whereas still others are simply called pea lectin or soybean lectin. In Table 3.4 lectins are listed according to the sugar groups they recognize (Goldstein and Hayes, 1978). Some lectins are very toxic.

The detailed discussion of the various lectins is not within the scope of this volume; at least two volumes have been published on Con A (Cohen, 1974; Bittiger and Schnebli, 1976). However, the preparation and characterization of Con A, which is important for EIA due to its reactivity to POase, is given as an example.

Con A is purified by the simple method of Agrawal and Goldstein (1967) and obtained in high quantities (2–2.5 g from 100 g of jackbean meal). Jack-bean meal (General Biochemicals) is suspended in 150 mM NaCl (200 g meal in 1 l) and stirred overnight at 4°C. The suspension is then strained through cheese-cloth and the residue re-extracted. The combined extracts are centrifuged at $15000 \times g$ (30 min) and the pellet is discarded. It is important to keep the pH at 7–8 during the subsequent steps. The supernatant is first brought slowly to 30% saturation with $(NH_4)_2SO_4$ (Section 7.1.2). The supernatant is recovered after centrifugation and saturation with $(NH_4)_2SO_4$ is raised to 80%. The pellet obtained after centrifugation is dialyzed against 1 M NaCl. Insoluble material is removed by

TABLE 3.4
Major lectins and their specificity

D-mannose- and D-glucose-binding lectins
1. *Canavalia ensiformis* (Jack bean: concanavalin A)
2. *Lens culinaris* syn. *esculenta* (lentil)
3. *Pisum sativum* (pea)
4. *Vicia faba* (fava bean)

2-Acetamide-2-deoxy-D-glucose-binding lectins
1. *Bandeiraea simplicifolia* (type II, see also D-galactose-binding lectins)
2. *Cytious sessilifolius*
3. *Triticum vulgaris* (wheat germ)
4. *Solanum tuberosum* (potato)
5. *Ulex europaeus* II (gorse; see also L-fucose-binding lectins)

2-Acetamide-2-deoxy-D-galactose-binding lectins
1. *Bauhinia purpuria* (binds also other sugars)
2. *Dolichos biflorus* (horse gram)
3. *Glycine max* (soybean)
4. *Helix pomatia* (snail)
5. *Phaseolus lunatus* syn. *limensis* (lima bean)
6. *Sophora japonica* (pagoda tree)

D-galactose-binding lectins
1. *Abrus precatorius* (jeguirity bean)
2. *Arachis hypogaea* (peanut)
3. *Bandeiraea simplicifolia* I
4. *Maclura pomifera* (Osage orange)
5. *Ricinus communis* (Castor bean, two types)

L-Fucose-binding lectins
1. *Anguilla anguilla* (eel)
2. *Lotus tetragonolobus* (asparagus pea)
3. *Ulex europaeus* (furze, gorse)

centrifugation and discarded. The observation that Con A interacts with Sephadex provides a convenient basis for its purification by affinity chromatography. The crude preparation of Con A is applied on a large column of Sephadex G-50 in 1 M NaCl (4 × 50 cm) at a rate of about 30 ml/h. The column is then washed for 2 days with 1.5–2 l of 1 M NaCl. Con A is desorbed from the column with 100 mM glucose in 1 M NaCl and is monitored at 280 nm. Extensive dialysis (18–20 times) against large volumes of 1 M NaCl is required.

Con A consists of 26000 dalton subunits which readily form tetramers (Edmundson et al., 1971). Each subunit contains one Mn^{2+} and one Ca^{2+} which are needed for its activity and has one carbohydrate-binding site (Becker et al., 1971b). Excess of metals, however, abolishes activity (Agrawal and Goldstein, 1967).

The use of lectins in EIA largely depends on the avidity bonus (Section 8.5), since their intrinsic affinities are often significantly lower than those of antibodies and insufficient for EIA.

CHAPTER 4

The nature of immunogens, antigens, and haptens

Two fundamental requirements must be met by a molecule to be immunogenic: (i) it should be foreign to activate the defense mechanism; and, (ii) it must be of a certain complexity to react with the different components of the immune system necessary to induce the immune response. Immunogenicity, i.e. the ability to stimulate the production of specific antibodies, is not an inherent property, such as the molecular weight, but is dependent on the experimental conditions. Studies with partially hydrolyzed antigens have demonstrated that only restricted portions of the macromolecules are involved in antigen–antibody interaction. These regions, named epitopes (or antigenic determinants), are rather small (5–7 amino acids) in order to fit in the antigen-binding sites (paratopes) on the antibody. Macromolecules may contain many epitopes per molecule; proteins usually contain one epitope per 40–80 amino acids. Thus, antigens carry a number of epitopes, which are usually different so that each is able to react with a different antibody. Immunogens carry, in addition to these epitopes, carrier determinants which play a role in the immune response.

Epitopes do not act as templates for the formation of antibodies. Instead, antibodies are synthesized against all antigenic conformations the immune system could possibly encounter, before the actual contact with the immunogen. The precursor of each antibody-forming lymphocyte (derived from B cells) makes Ig of only one specificity which is inserted in the cell membrane as a surface receptor to commit this cell for the synthesis of Ig with this specificity if the need arises. The signal for this need is conveyed by the binding of the immunogen to this surface-bound receptor (clonal selection). For the large majority of immunogens this precursor cell proliferates into specific antibody-secreting cells and a clone of memory cells (responsible for the faster and stronger secondary response) only if the immunogen is also recognized via its carrier determinant by a T cell. For example, glucagon (a pancreatic hormone of 29 amino acids) can be digested by trypsin to yield the epitope portion (N-terminal) and the carrier portion (C-terminal) which react with B and T cells, respectively. Both determinants must be foreign to the host (important consideration for the linkage of haptens to carriers). In addition, the immunogen should be taken up and processed by macrophages (Section 5.1.2). This processing is essential for the immune response and might be the reason for the poor immunogenicity of polymers of D-amino acids (Sela and Fuchs, 1973). Small molecules are, hence, not immunogenic except when conjugated to a larger protein molecule.

Epitopes can be either sequential or conformational. Elements structurally projecting from the core of the molecule are often immunodominant in the epitope. Charged groups make large contributions to the affinity between the two reactants, but often lead to lower specificity. Immunogenicity is better when both negative and positive charges are present on the same molecule (Gill et al., 1967). Immunodominance in an epitope may be due to: (i) differences in conformation, i.e. in the protruding groups (Sela, 1969); (ii) differences in accessibility, i.e., a gradient of binding energies to the most exposed subunit; and, (iii) alternatives in optical configuration; in general no cross-reactivity is obtained between enantiomorphic epitopes.

The phylogenetical relationship of the immunogen to the host is important. A close relationship means that, at best, only a few determinants of the immunogen are different, leading to a weaker response which, however, is more specific. As a general rule, the species to be immunized is chosen depending on whether a strong response or a weaker but more specific response is required. For example, chickens are a convenient source of antibodies against mammalian immunogens (serum proteins), but they produce antibodies against determinants common to several or many species. Widely distributed proteins, e.g. cytochrome c, generally are poor immunogens.

Protein structures have a large number of different amino acid residues, whereas nucleic acids have a smaller number of different bases. Therefore, a larger diversity can be obtained in epitopes of protein than of nucleic acids. Some residues, such as aromatic amino acids, are much more immunogenic than others (Sela and Arnon, 1960). In general, proteins, conjugated haptens and polysaccharides are strongly immunogenic, whereas lipids, steroids, and nucleic acids are weakly immunogenic. Carbohydrates generally interact poorly with T cells (Section 5.1.1).

Haptens which do not induce immune responses but can react with their antibodies are rendered immunogenic by conjugation to a carrier. Though very often haptens are small molecules, immunogenicity and not size is the criterion. In fact, large non-immunogenic molecules may act as haptens and rendered immunogenic after conjugation to a suitable carrier. Virtually any compound may serve as an antigenic determinant if coupled to a suitable carrier. Too many hapten molecules per carrier may, however, lead to tolerance.

After their administration, immunogens are degraded by the usual catabolic pathways. Globular proteins seem to be recognized before extensive degradation: the antibodies raised against them react with these proteins in the native state (conformational determinants). Other epitopes are recognized after degradation by macrophages. Some haptens may become reactive with other proteins and induce an immune response, such as in penicillin allergy (change from penicillin to penicilloyl–protein conjugates).

Production of antibodies

An understanding of the basic principles of the biology of the immune response and its regulation is a prerequisite for the successful experimental production of antibodies. This enables the investigator to induce a vigorous antibody production, instead of obtaining highly unpredictable results and undesired effects, such as tolerance (immune unresponsiveness).

Some highly recommended reviews are Eisen (1980), Roitt (1980), Benacerraf and Unanue (1981), Golub (1981), and Klein (1982).

5.1. Biology and regulation of the immune reponse

5.1.1. Primary and secondary immune response

Humoral immune responses can be divided into two types: primary and secondary responses, which reflect the cellular dynamics of the immune system and the immune state of the host. A primary response is caused by the first exposure to a given immunogen and results in the appearance of predominantly IgM antibodies after a relatively long lag period, followed by a peak and a decline of antibody formation. After a lapse of time, another exposure to the immunogen produces a quite different, secondary response which is characterized by a shorter lag period, a stronger response with predominantly IgG antibodies and, after a peak has been reached, a slower decrease.

Moreover, antibodies of the secondary response usually have a higher affinity which may increase even more with time (maturation, see Section 8.5). The immune system stores information of the first contact with the immunogen ('priming') in so-called memory cells.

Some immunogens cause no secondary responses (only IgM) and the immune response to these immunogens is not helped by T cells, as to other immunogens. These T-independent immunogens have the capacity to stimulate directly B lymphocytes, probably because they often have repeating structures, such as in the case of polysaccharides from bacterial origin. In non-responder animals T-dependent immunogens may also give rise to primary but not to secondary responses.

The IgM–IgG transition in response to T-dependent immunogens involves Ig-class switching while conserving the same antigen binding specificity and affinity. This is based on a change in the molecular process of antibody production, in which the gene coding for the paratope is recombined with another gene coding for the rest of the peptide chain of another Ig class. Affinity maturation, however, involves the selection of high-affinity clones since each clone of lymphocytes produces antibody of only one particular specificity and affinity. The slow increase in affinity of the antiserum (e.g., 10000 times) may be due to several mechanisms: (i) selection of lymphocytes producing higher-affinity antibody since they compete more efficiently for a low dose of immunogen; and, (ii) effective competition of high-affinity antibodies with lymphocytes containing receptors with low affinity for the same immunogen.

5.1.2. Cellular aspects of the immune system

The lymphoid tissues include primary (or central) lymphoid organs (bone marrow, thymus and bursa of Fabricius in birds), and secondary (or peripheral) lymphoid organs (lymph nodes, spleen, tonsils, appendix, Peyer's patches).

Lymphocytes, erythrocytes, macrophages, granulocytes and platelets are all derived from a pluripotent hemopoietic stem cell. This stem cell proliferates into other stem cells which further differentiate into progenitor and, subsequently, precursor cells in different micro-environments. Lymphocytes differentiate into B and T lymphocyte sets according to the primary organ in which they mature. The inductive organ for B cells in mammals is probably the bone marrow itself. The two populations of lymphocytes can then interact in the primary lymphoid organs. Removal of the primary lymphoid organs at birth showed that B cells are involved in antibody production whereas T cells are required for both the cell-mediated and humoral immunity. In addition to these cells, accessory cells (macrophages) are required for antibody formation.

Lymphocytes are small spherical cells, many of which circulate continuously in body fluids (blood, lymph). T and memory (T and B) cells circulate more efficiently than B cells, which tend to reside in the spleen. T cells are either cytotoxic or regulatory. Regulatory cells are divided into a few (Mitchison, 1981) or many subsets (Gershon et al., 1981). The different subsets of lymphocytes can be distinguished by surface markers, e.g., antigens of the Ly or Qa series (McKenzie and Potter, 1979). Among the cells involved in an immune response, both the T and B cells recognize specifically a given immunogen, in contrast to the macrophage.

Mononuclear phagocytes ('monocytes') also recirculate continuously until a local inflammation activates and transforms them into regularly shaped macrophages when they become resident (Van Furth, 1980). Though macrophages were first thought to be mere scavengers, they have several roles in the humoral response, such as the antigen presentation to T lymphocytes and T–B cell cooperation (Unanue, 1981).

Apart from these three groups of cells, the peripheral lymphoid organs and the blood and lymphatic circulation play an important role in the immune response. Lymph nodes and spleen intercept foreign substances by their resident macrophages. The localized immunogen can enter in contact with the most appropriate lymphocyte from a continuously recirculating pool. Secondary lymphoid organs have distinct T- and B-cell areas which is surprising since their interaction is required. The enlarged plasma cells, derived from the stimulated B cells, produce antibodies which are then excreted and transported through the body. Antibody-producing cells can, therefore, be obtained from the spleen (the most usual source of cells for producing hybridomas; Section 5.4), whereas antibody can be obtained from the body fluids.

5.1.3. Genetic control of the immune response by the major histocompatibility complex (MHC)

The availability of inbred mice with different haplotypes (combination of a given allele at different loci) permitted the recognition of genetic loci involved in the control of immune responses (I region). This analysis demonstrated that MHC genes control many functions of the immune response. The MHC seems essentially similar for all vertebrates, though differences in their organization exist (Jackson et al., 1983). The MHC in the mouse is known as H-2, that of man is called HLA and is a composite of several multiallelic genes with a polymorphism not seen with any other genetic locus (Klein, 1979). The actual number of alleles is unknown but may be in the hundreds, so that combination of the different loci results in an extraordinary polymorphism. Another striking feature of the MHC is that their products provoke unusually strong responses in other individuals of the same species with an alloreactivity of the order of 10^4 times stronger than with other immunogens.

The MHC contains several major regions which in turn consist of several subregions. The products of these loci fall into three classes (Klein, 1979): class I products are strong surface alloantigens expressed on essentially all cells, class II products (restricted to B cells, macrophages and some sets of T cells; Bach et al., 1976) are responsible for the control of immune responses and regulate cell interactions, whereas class III genes code for components of the complement pathway (Shreffler, 1976) and control their levels in the serum.

The ability to produce antibodies against a given antigen is determined by the haplotype of the I region of H-2 or the D region of HLA. A given haplotype will produce immune responses to a series of antigens but not to others. In the mouse the I-region has at least 5 subregions, i.e. immune response genes Ir-1A, Ir-1B, the immune suppression gene I-J expressed on T suppressor (T_S) cells (Benacerraf and Germain, 1978) and the I–E and I–C loci. Many of the products of these genes (cell surface antigens) have been analyzed and have been named Ia-(I-associated) antigens (Gonwa et al., 1983). These antigens act particularly at the level of cellular interactions (Klein, 1982).

Each individual inherits one MHC haplotype from each parent and transmits one to its progeny, which are expressed codominantly.

5.1.4. Immunoregulation

Feedback mechanisms are important in the regulation of the quantity of antibody produced.

Clonal selection of the appropriate B cell occurs through the reaction of the cell-surface antibody with the corresponding epitope on the immunogen. However, for most immunogens the involvement of T cells is essential (Section 5.1.1). These T-dependent immunogens have at least two types of determinants (Raff, 1970), one for the B cells (the haptenic determinant or epitope) and one for the T cells (the carrier determinant). If an animal is primed with a hapten conjugated to a carrier, e.g., ovalbumin, a second injection of the same immunogen at a later date results in the usual secondary response. However, if this time the hapten is coupled to another carrier (e.g., serum albumin), there is no secondary response to the hapten since the T cells will not recognize the carrier. Transfer of serum albumin-primed T cells from another animal with the same MHC constitution would induce a secondary response in this experimental system, i.e. the carrier effect is transferable. Since the primary–secondary response switch concurs with an IgM–IgG switch, T cells seem to be important for the control of this phenomenon. The requirement for at least two sites of recognition poses restrictions on the minimum size of an immunogen, explains the failure of haptens to elicit immune responses by themselves, and shows that in the production of antisera it is necessary to use the same carrier throughout.

A dichotomy exists in the functions of T cells: some cells (T_H) promote the production of antibody, whereas others $(T_S$ cells) suppress it (Gershon et al., 1981).

Macrophages not only present the immunogen to the T cells but their MHC products also interact with receptors for these molecules on the T cells. Thus, T cells must have the same MHC expression (one of the two parental haplotypes in heterozygotes) as the macrophage (Kappler and Marrack, 1976). This interaction results in the activation of T_H cells, which interact with and activate the B cell. The latter, under the effect of the immunogen, proliferates and matures into antibody-secreting plasma cells and memory cells. Immunogen not bound to macrophage might stimulate T_S cells leading to the suppression of the immune response.

The Ir genes (Section 5.1.3) which control the response of B cells to T-dependent immunogens seem to determine the recognition of carrier determinants. This might explain why the response of one animal is much stronger to a given immunogen than to another. These genes, therefore, seem to determine whether an immunogen induces the activation of mainly T_H or T_S cells. Another mechanism of control has been advanced by Jerne (1974). Antibodies generated in response to an immunogen may reach high concentrations (e.g. 1 mg/ml) and their idiotype (Section 6.2) behave as foreign to the host, causing in turn the production of anti-antibodies, anti-anti-antibodies, etc., and so cause the development of an interlocking network which then becomes part of the overall regulatory mechanism. Though this anti-idiotype network mechanism is generally accepted, it is difficult to assess the extent of its operation. Among the set of anti-idiotype antibodies, some will mimic the immunogen in that their structure is an internal image of the epitope. Recently, Kennedy et al. (1984) showed that anti-idiotype antibodies could be used to raise antibodies against hepatitis virus. A similar approach was taken by Koprowski et al. (1984) in cancer therapy.

T-independent immunogens (reviewed by Feldmann, 1974) usually have multiple copies of the same determinant and are, therefore, capable to react with several receptors on the same B cell ('capping'), which activates the cell. At high concentrations, T-independent immunogens may become polyclonal activators of B cells and act as mitogens of B cells. T-dependency may vary with the host: haptenated polyacrylamide beads are T-independent in the mouse (Feldmann et al., 1974) and T-dependent in man (Galanaud, 1979).

Soluble factors, such as lymphokines and monokines, produced by T cells and monocytes, respectively, influence B-cell activation. Thymocytes also produce soluble factors which stimulate and support growth of B cells in vitro (Andersson et al., 1977). This forms the basis for the in vitro immunization and production of monoclonal antibodies (Reading, 1982). Soluble factors can be specific or non-specific for the antigen (Volkman and Fauci, 1981). The antigen-specific factor may represent secreted T-cell receptors. Some monokines may also replace lymphokines in the immunization procedure in vitro (Jonak and Kennett, 1982).

5.1.5. Tolerance

Tolerance to self-antigens is learned by the immune system, not inherited as self-nonself discrimination (Bretscher and Cohn, 1970). Auto-antibodies against a large number of self-antigens may occur in sera of normal individuals. Their levels can be raised by stimulation with polyclonal B-cell mitogens.

Tolerance and immune response are opposite attributes of the immune system in as much as after an initial exposure to a given molecule the second contact will result in an increased or decreased response. This phenomenon is under the control of the cells involved in the regulatory circuits. Molecules with epitopes inducing an enhanced immune response are called immunogens, whereas molecules with epitopes inducing a tolerant state are called tolerogens. Tolerance is also specific to particular epitopes and can, therefore, be defined as the acquired inability of an individual to generate an immune response against a specific molecule (tolerogen). As a rule, tolerance induction by an epitope is inversely related to its immunogenicity.

The mechanisms most often proposed for tolerance are: (i) clonal deletion (elimination of the tolerogen-specific clone); and, (ii) excessive activation of T_S cells.

Tolerance against a given epitope is not a desired trait if immune sera have to be produced. A number of conditions which promote tolerance should, therefore, be avoided. An important factor is the quantity of immunogen used for immunization. T-independent immunogens may act as tolerogens if injected at high doses (e.g., 100 times the usual dose; Parks et al., 1979). T-dependent immunogens can induce the so-called low-zone and high-zone tolerance, i.e. the epitope is immunogenic only between these two concentrations (Gershon and Kondo, 1971). These two responses to the same epitope reflect the observation that T cells are made tolerant at much lower concentration levels than B cells. Since many self-antigens (mostly T-dependent) are present at low doses, self-tolerance may be equivalent to low-zone tolerance (lack of T_H activity). The route of administration and the physical form of the antigen are also important. Soluble and small immunogens may become tolerogenic when applied intravenously. A given protein may be tolerogenic for an animal, although its aggregated (polymeric) form may be immunogenic. Consequently, it is difficult to induce tolerance to particulate antigens, such as viruses, bacteria and parasites.

Immunological unresponsiveness can also be induced in newborn or fetal animals who have not yet developed immunological competence. This was first shown with dizygotic cattle twins (Owen, 1945). Permanent tolerance to foreign cells (skin grafts) can be induced by injection of allogeneic cells into embryos (Billingham et al., 1953). Tolerance can, therefore, be used advantageously to obtain more specific antisera. For example, in the production of antibodies against cell-associated tumor antigens by immunization with cancer cells, antibodies will be raised not only against the tumor antigens but also against normal cell constituents. However, injection of very young animals with normal cells could render them tolerant to these antigens and subsequent immunization with tumor cells would induce the production of antibodies only against the tumor antigens (Billingham et al., 1953; Gold and Freedman, 1965).

Tolerance can be abrogated spontaneously if the tolerogen disappears or by different experimental manoeuvres which stimulate T_H cells. A cross-reacting immunogen may also break the tolerance if it has carrier determinants not shared with the tolerogen: tolerance against a hapten can be abrogated by the use of another carrier which will generate other T_H cells. The same principle may apply for antigens presented in different forms (denatured or native). In vitro immunization, e.g. to proteins which are in most animals recognized as 'self-antigens', may also circumvent the problem of tolerance.

5.2. Production of polyclonal antisera

5.2.1. Preparation of immunogens

Immunization is largely empirical and may be influenced by many factors (Table 5.1). The consistency in the quality of the antisera

TABLE 5.1
Factors determining the antibody response (and Sections of discussion)

Immunogen
   Nature of immunogen (4); purity of immunogen and relative immunogenicity (5.2.1); relation to host (4; 5.1.1; 5.1.2); physical form (4; 5.1.5; 5.2.2); adjuvants (5.2.2; 5.2.3); manner and amount of administration (5.2.4); side effects (5.1.2).

Immune system
   First or subsequent contact with immunogen (5.1.1; 5.4.4); affinity of receptors on both T and B cells and relative quantities of T_H and T_S cells (5.1.2; 5.1.4); possibility of tolerance (5.1.5); response maturation (5.2.1).

Animal
   Age, species, health condition (5.1.2); genetic composition (5.1.3); immunogenic experience with related substances (5.1.4).

forms the essential basis of all immunoassays and can be best controlled by an in-house production. Often, the desired antisera may not be offered commercially.

It is impossible to discuss in some detail the preparation of immunogens in this limited space. Moreover, most investigators are familiar with the purification of the immunogens of their interest. Some general, excellent treatises were edited by Williams and Chase (1967) and Sela (1973–1982). Some characteristics of immunogenic preparations should, nevertheless, be stressed here.

The degree of purity of an immunogen is not necessarily related to the specificity of the antibody produced, since traces of very immunogenic impurities may overwhelm the response to the principal antigen. An example important in EIA is the presence of a potent immunogenic non-peroxidase glycoprotein in commercial ('pure') horseradish POase (Moroz et al., 1974). On the other hand, the ease with which antibodies are produced against highly immunogenic impurities can be used for their removal. Purity of antigen is less important for the production of monoclonal antibodies (Section 5.4) since each clone of lymphocytes produces one particular clonotype of antibodies. The expression 'biochemical purity' may also be misleading: proteins separated by PAGE and stained with Coomassie blue may seem to contain unique bands, but subsequent staining with the 100-fold more sensitive silver stain may reveal many additional bands. It is possible to inject protein bands cut directly from polyacrylamide gels even if they contain sodium dodecyl sulphate (SDS; Strauss et al., 1975; Blomberg et al., 1977). A simple method is to place the SDS-gel in a 4 M sodium acetate solution (at 25°C about 10 min) and visualize it under fluorescent light under an angle of about 30° and with a dark background (sensitivity similar to that of Coomassie blue staining). Protein bands stained with Coomassie blue or amido black can also be used directly (Boulard and Lecroisey, 1982). After the bands are cut out, they are equilibrated in distilled water for about 20 min, homogenized in saline and injected subcutaneously into a rabbit (about 100 µg) or mouse (a few micrograms). SDS–PAGE does not resolve proteins of the same molecular weight (e.g. see Gilbert, 1978). If this problem is encountered, two-dimensional electrophoresis should be used (O'Farrel, 1975). A disadvantage of using immunogen fragments generated by proteolysis and separated by SDS–PAGE (Section 16.1.2; Tijssen and Kurstak, 1983) for immunization is the lack of antibodies against conformational epitopes and possible loss of carrier determinants.

Immunoprecipitates in agarose gels obtained by one of the many methods available (see Clausen, 1980, vol. 1, pt. III in this series) are also excellent immunogens to raise specific antibodies. These immunoprecipitates can be cut out from the gel and, after washing in neutral saline, used directly for immunization (Bradwell et al., 1976). This method may alleviate the problems of difficult purification procedures in that antibodies generated against impurities in the first immunization will not coprecipitate with the specific antibodies under certain conditions. This method, however, requires two succeeding immunizations to generate specific antisera.

The purification of larger particles, such as viruses, poses generally fewer problems, though the complexity of these particles may in turn require their dissociation and fractionation to decrease the number of epitopes.

5.2.2. Adjuvants

A common method to enhance the humoral response to weak immunogens is the admixture of the immunogens with so-called adjuvants. These adjuvants are immunopotentiators which activate one or more sectors of the immune system resulting in an enhanced immune response. A rigid classification of adjuvants or a unifying concept of the mechanism of their action is, therefore, impossible (Dresser, 1977).

Adjuvants, such as aluminum salts or mineral oils, alter the physical state of water-soluble immunogens by forming depots and lower the rates of elimination. This results in a prolonged persistence of the immunogen in tissues and a continuous stimulation of the immune system, which can be mimicked by daily injections of very small amounts of immunogen (Herbert, 1966).

Some adjuvants (endotoxin and poly(A.U)) increase synthesis of proteins. Other adjuvants stimulate different cellular compartments of the immune system: (i) mycobacteria, retinol, and poly(A.U) expand T-cell populations; (ii) endotoxin and *Bordetella pertussis* stimulate B cells; and, (iii) many adjuvants of bacterial origin mobilize macrophages. Complete Freund's adjuvant causes local formation of granulomas which are rich in macrophages and immunocompetent cells.

The increased cooperation between T cell, B cell, and macrophage also depends on the immunogen and the host. For molecules with low immunogenicity, adjuvants favor the induction of immune response at the expense of tolerance. Extensive reviews on adjuvant action have been presented by Jolles and Paraf (1973), WHO report No. 595 (1973) and Borek (1977).

5.2.3. Preparation of adjuvants and admixture with immunogens

Generally, all soluble immunogens or protein–hapten conjugates are mixed with, emulsified in or adsorbed onto adjuvants. The most widespread adjuvants are: (i) Freund's adjuvants; (ii) aluminum salts and bentonite; (iii) methylated bovine serum albumin; and, (iv) heat-inactivated *Bordetella pertussis*.

5.2.3.1. Freund's adjuvant (FA)   FA is a mineral oil with a stabilizer (emulsifier included) to yield stable water-in-oil emulsions with the immunogen and is commercially available (Difco) as 'incomplete FA'. The complete FA (Difco) contains, in addition, a dispersion of dried, heat-killed *Mycobacterium tuberculosis* in the oil phase (0.5 mg/ml). FA is best stored at $-20°C$.

The immunogen dissolved in saline or distilled water (sterile) should not exceed a maximum concentration of about 75 mg/ml to obtain stable emulsions; whole serum should be diluted at least 50 times. The failure to make a proper emulsion leads to disappointing results of immunizations. A simple way to prepare stable emulsions (Herbert, 1973) is to place the two solutions (same volumes) in two immunologically clean glass vials and to inject vigorously(!) with a 2 ml glass syringe (plastic syringes are often lubricated with Tween 80) with a fine-bore needle (0.5 mm), small fractions of the antigen solution into the FA while the opening of the needle is held below the surface of the oil. Between each addition, the bottle is shaken and no aqueous phase should appear at the bottom of the vial (otherwise this aqueous phase is reinjected into the oil). After all immunogen is injected, the emulsion is further mixed using a syringe with larger needle, since higher dispersion also increases viscosity.

Another simple method, suitable for small volumes, is the double-hubbed needle method (Berlin and McKinney, 1958), though on rare occasions it may fail to generate stable emulsions. Two Luer-lock syringes are fitted to a double-hubbed (bore 1 mm) needle so that fluid expulsed from one syringe will enter the other. One syringe is filled (less than half) with immunogen solution, the other with FA. The first stroke pushes the immunogen into the FA and the mixture is pushed back and forth until the proper viscosity is reached. Other commercial equipment (Mulsichurn, Virtis homogenizer) may also be suitable. Before use, the emulsions are tested by allowing a drop of the emulsion to fall into cold water. Though the initial drop may spread over the surface, subsequent drops should remain as discrete white drops on or below the surface. This indicates that the water phase is well established within the oil drop. If a cloud of tiny particles is formed, the emulsion is oil-in-water from which no or little adjuvant action can be expected.

5.2.3.2. Aluminum salts   The slightly toxic aluminum salts can be divided into two groups, the insoluble (oxide, hydroxide, and phosphate) and the soluble (sulfate, alum) salts. The soluble salts precipitate proteins or cause them to form aggregates which subsequently release immunogen slowly to activate continuously the immune system. Insoluble aluminum salts provide a large sorptive area (limits diffusion) and mobilize phagocytic cells by providing particulate attraction.

The most convenient form is the aluminum hydroxide adjuvant. A 10% aqueous solution of potassium alum, $AlK(SO_4)_2 \cdot 12H_2O$ (Mallinckrodt's 'photopurified' granular product) is sterilized by filtration. To 10 ml of this solution 22.8 ml of 250 mM NaOH is added while stirred vigorously. The suspension is centrifuged at low speed to avoid hard packing and the supernatant is discarded. The pellet is washed twice and resuspended in physiological saline to 10 ml. Immunogens are adsorbed by mixing equal volumes. Efficiency of adsorption should be checked.

5.2.3.3. Methylated bovine serum albumin (MBSA)   MBSA is an excellent adjuvant by its ability to complex with negatively charged substances (proteins, polynucleotides) due to its high positive charge (Sueoka and Cheng, 1962). MBSA is prepared by dissolving 1 g BSA in 100 ml absolute methanol and adding 0.84 ml concentrated HCl. This solution is left for at least 3 days in the dark at room temperature. MBSA precipitates gradually, is collected by centrifugation, washed twice with methanol, dissolved in water, neutralized and lyophilyzed. MBSA can be stored as a sterile neutral solution.

Immunogen is complexed by the addition of an equal amount (w/w) of MBSA and the precipitate is resuspended to a concentration of 0.25 mg/ml before it is emulsified with Freund's adjuvant.

5.2.3.4. Bordetella pertussis for use with alum-precipitated proteins   *B. pertussis* is heat-inactivated and mixed with alum-precipitated protein (10^9 cells with 0.1 mg immunogen). Alum-precipitated protein is prepared by the drop-wise addition of 2.5 ml 10% $AlK(SO_4)_2 \cdot 12H_2O$ (Section 5.2.3.2.) to 1.5 ml 1 M $NaHCO_3$ and 2.5 ml (1 mg/ml) protein solution. The flocculent precipitate is centrifuged at low speed and washed with saline.

5.2.4. Immunization procedures

Two fundamental rules should be followed: (i) a blood sample should be taken before immunization to detect pre-existing antibodies; and, (ii) antisera should not be pooled.

The shorter the immunization, the more specific the antibodies tend to be, but the antisera are also less potent. The skin should always be sterilized with alcohol before injections.

Immunization programs tend to be overdone, particularly with adjuvants. The maximum response with water-in-oil emulsions occurs after several weeks, and booster injections should be given subcutaneously at intervals of 1 month when primary response starts declining. Affinity of antibodies generally increases with time and with greater intervals between boosts. Trial bleedings should be made. Boosters are most efficient with inocula lacking adjuvants and should be given about 2 weeks after the last injection rather than the 1–2 months of the adjuvant-based inocula.

The choice of animal is mostly one of convenience rather than necessity. A notable exception is the production of anti-insulin antibodies for which guinea pigs should be used. Generally, rabbits, goats and sheep are used for polyclonal antisera and mice and rats for monoclonal antisera. As a rule of thumb, about 15 µg of immunogen or 5×10^6 cells per kg of body weight suffices.

Intravenous (i.v.) inoculation is used preferentially for soluble or particulate immunogens. For alum-precipitated immunogens it is used in combination with a subcutaneous (s.c.) injection. Though the response is rapid, it is not sustained. Usually a small amount is given on 3 succeeding days, a double dose 4 days later and a threefold dose after another 4 days.

Intramuscular inoculations are suited for antigens in complete FA, generally in the thigh muscles of the hind legs of mammals or the breast of fowl.

Subcutaneous inoculations are convenient but the response is slower than by the intramuscular route. It is recommended for boosters since it decreases the chances of an anaphylactic shock. The needle (bevel up) is inserted into the fold of the skin, lifted between thumb and forefinger, until the tip of the needle feels free. After the injection the needle track should be pinched to prevent loss of inoculated material. Little can be gained by inoculations at many sites.

The intradermal route is excellent if small volumes (1 ml or less) of scarce antigen are used. Complete FA will cause granulomas within a few days. Foot-pad inoculations should be avoided. No air bubbles should remain in the hypodermic needle of the immunogen-filled syringe. The point of the needle (bevel up) is forced through the shaven skin folded between forefinger and thumb, while the point should remain just visible below the surface. The inoculum should feel like a hard swelling.

Intraperitoneal (i.p.) inoculations are common with mice. The mouse, starved overnight (only water), is anesthesized before injection and kept in the palm of the hand with the tail between the fingers. The needle should be inserted into the abdomen to the side of the umbilicus with a stabbing movement, to a depth of no more than 5 mm.

A detailed review of inoculation techniques has been presented by Herbert (1973).

5.2.5. Bleeding procedures

Bleeding is not always necessary to obtain antibodies. The hen provides conveniently packaged antibodies in large quantities (10–15 mg/ml) in the egg yolk and the difference in skill required between bleeding rabbits and collecting eggs needs hardly be emphasized (Jensenius et al., 1981). One egg may provide the equivalent of more than 15 ml serum. The IgY (Section 6.1.6.1.) content of the yolk is actually higher than that of the hen's serum (Rose et al., 1974). Bar-Joseph and Malkinson (1980) inoculated the hen intravenously (100 μg of virus) and observed peak levels in yolk one week later, which persisted for 1 to 2 weeks. Immunization with adjuvants (Jensenius et al., 1981) sustains high antibody levels over prolonged periods.

Animals should be fasted for 12 h prior to bleeding but should be provided with water. The rabbit can be restrained in a special box or by wrapping the animal rapidly in a large blanket with its head sticking out but preventing escape. To bleed the rabbits from the marginal ear vein, the posterior side and the edge of one of the ears is shaven, dried and smeared with a thin layer of petroleum jelly to prevent premature clotting. A diagonal cut is made across the vein (not severed) and a bottle is immediately placed under the ear. The base of the ear can be squeezed to prevent venous return. Immediately after the cut, the blood flow may be little, but should begin after a few minutes. Clots which may form may be rubbed off with a cloth. If the flow is, nevertheless, irregular, xylol may be applied distal to the incision (admixture to the blood causes hemolysis!). Up to 50 ml may be collected at 1 month intervals. Cardiac puncture is simple, but should not be attempted by unexperienced personnel. Gordon (1981) recently described a simple method for repeated bleeding of rabbits from the central ear artery. The dorsal surface of the ear is moistened with 70% alcohol, shaven, the terminal 1 cm of the ear wetted with xylol (upper and lower surface) and the ear briskly massaged over the central artery. An 18-gauge hypodermic needle with the hub removed, is inserted 5–10 mm into the central ear artery and blood collected in a centrifuge tube. The first time about 40 ml is collected and in subsequent bleedings (1–2/week) up to 100 ml.

Rats may be bled conveniently from the tail vein (Shek and Howe, 1982). Other simple methods suitable to obtain small quantities of serum from mice are from the tail-tip and from the retro-orbital plexus (Herbert, 1973). For large animals the jugular vein is convenient. The blood samples are allowed to coagulate for about 2 h at room temperature and then incubated overnight at 4°C. The serum is decanted, clarified by low-speed centrifugation and stored in conveniently sized aliquots at −20 or −70°C.

5.3. The relative merits of polyclonal and monoclonal antibodies in enzyme immunoassays

A clone of B cells produces antibody of only one specificity i.e.

the clonotype. An immunized animal produces generally a random number of clonotypes and its antiserum becomes polyclonal. It has been estimated that $10–40 \times 10^6$ distinct clonotypes can theoretically be generated by a BALB/c mouse which contains about 2×10^8 B cells (Klinman and Press, 1975). About 1 out of every 10000 clonotypes seems to recognize a given epitope with varying degrees of affinity. Thus, several thousand clonotypes could be produced by an animal against a given epitope (Klinman and Press, 1975; Köhler, 1976). In practice, however, only a random few (up to about 10) B-cell clones are activated and only few distinct antibodies are generated out of this large repertoire of randomly formed specificities (Briles and Davie, 1980). It is, therefore, practically impossible to make reproducible reagents against any epitope. The complex immunoregulatory mechanisms further increase the variations in the idiosyncratic responses. Even antisera from the same animal taken at different times differ in their properties. In contrast, monoclonal antibodies are produced by a single clone of B cells and, consequently, have the same specificity and affinity. Monoclonal antibodies can be produced in virtually unlimited quantities and pure immunogen is not required for the immunization due to cloning and selection during the production.

The strategy of the immune system to produce polyclonal antibodies yields two important bonus effects, i.e. the 'affinity bonus' (or avidity) and the 'specificity bonus', both of which are eliminated by cloning (Sections 8.4 to 8.6). The specificity of monoclonal antibodies may sometimes prove to be not as high as expected. Some may cross-react, and this cross-reactivity cannot, in contrast to polyclonal antisera, be removed with immunosorbents (Brodsky et al., 1979). A monoclonal antibody is unable to distinguish different antigens if they bear the same epitope. For example, Bundesen et al. (1980) encountered this problem with a peptide sequence common to several hormones. Kurstak et al. (1983) emphasized problems with monoclonal reagents in virus diagnosis.

Monoclonal antibody production is time consuming, particularly for weak immunogens which require many fusion experiments to obtain a producing hybrid. Excellent immunogens usually yield 5–20 producing hybrids per fusion. The number of species to produce monoclonal antibodies is limited. Fusion of myeloma cells with cells of other species leads to rapid segregation of chromosomes (Yarmush et al., 1980). Each monoclonal antibody may have very specific properties, quite different from the average of polyclonal Ig of the same subclass. Monoclonal antibodies may also have biological functions different from the corresponding polyclonal antisera and may be much more sensitive to inactivation by freezing and thawing, changes in pH or other physical properties (Mosmann et al., 1980), important for their purification.

A general comparison of monoclonal antibodies and polyclonal antisera is given in Table 5.2. The lower avidity bonus (Section 8.5) of monoclonal antibodies and the small fraction of high-affinity

TABLE 5.2
Comparison of some properties of monoclonal and polyclonal antibodies

	Monoclonal	Polyclonal
Purity of immunogen	not of prime importance	important
Time and expense	initially high	little
Useful antibody content	0.5–5 mg/ml (ascites) 5–40 µg/ml (medium)	< 1 mg/ml–few mg/ml
Irrelevant Ig	0.5–1 mg/ml (ascites)	about 10 mg/ml
Physicochemical properties	individual	spectrum which changes
Cross-reactivity to copurify-ing immunogens	–	+
Cross-reactivity removable?	no	mostly
Number of epitopes recog-nized	1	many
Affinity	homogeneous	heterogeneous

antibodies (dominant in polyclonal sera) among the antibodies generated are probably the reasons for their frequent lower detectability in EIA when compared with polyclonal antisera, despite the lower concentration of antibody in the latter (Zweig et al., 1979; Kendal, 1980) and makes the selection of high-affinity monoclonal antibodies mandatory. Pooling of different monoclonal antibodies to gain avidity has given conflicting results (Ehrlich et al., 1982; Yolken, 1982), reflecting most probably the relative spacing of the epitopes. On the other hand, monoclonal antibodies make new designs of EIA possible, e.g. in simultaneous two-site immunometric assays (Section 2.5.1) and the proximal linkage immunometric assays (Section 2.5.2). The most important advantage monoclonal antibodies offer for EIA is the possibility to standardize the assay methods, specificities, detectabilities and sensitivities.

5.4. Production of monoclonal antibodies

5.4.1. Strategy for the production of monoclonal antibodies

Lymphocytes, activated in vivo or in vitro to produce antibodies, do not have the ability to grow in vitro. Essentially this problem may be overcome by two different methods: (i) transformation of B cells in vitro, e.g. by oncogenic viruses; or, (ii) fusion of antibody-producing cells with myeloma cells to confer immortality to the B cells.

Direct transformation of human B lymphocytes with Epstein Barr virus seems to hold great promise since a high percentage of the cells may be transformed. This method met also with some success for rabbit cells, using SV_{40} virus, but less with murine cells (Zurawski et al., 1978; Steinitz et al., 1980; Reading, 1982).

Most current protocols use the approach of fusion with mutant myeloma cells according to a strategy in which the mutant cells are rescued from death by hybridization with lymphocytes in a medium otherwise lethal for this mutant (Littlefield, 1964; Ephrussi and Weiss, 1969) in which only the hybrids survive. Usually only a few hybrids produce the desired antibodies.

The two most popular myeloma cell lines used for this purpose are those lacking hypoxanthine–guanine phosphoribosyl transferase (HGPRT) or thymidine kinase (TK). Other kinds of mutants can be used as well, such as those resistant to ouabain (in combination with HGPRT⁻; Baker et al., 1974). Myeloma cells treated with biochemical inhibitors can also be rescued by fusion with untreated lymphocytes (Wright, 1978).

Myeloma cells lacking HGPRT are selected by growing them in the presence of 6-thioguanine or 8-azaguanine. Cells having HGPRT incorporate these base analogs into their DNA and die since these analogs interfere with transcription. Cells lacking HGPRT do not incorporate these lethal drugs since their nucleic acids are formed by the de novo pathway. In a similar way TK⁻ cells may be selected by bromodeoxyuridine (BUdR). The selection of HGPRT⁻ cells is easier than that of TK⁻ cells since HGPRT is coded for by a gene on the single active X-chromosome of mammalian cells, whereas the loss of TK activity would require two simultaneous mutations in the TK genes (autosomal) on both chromosomes (Goding, 1980). Both mutants are unable to produce nucleic acid precursors by the salvage pathway and would die in a medium containing folic acid antagonists (aminopterin, amethopterin, or methylamethopterin), which block the de novo pathway (Fig. 5.1).

Lymphocytes, which do not have the capacity to grow in vitro, contain enzymes for both the de novo and salvage pathway. In the presence of aminopterin, the lymphocyte can produce nucleic acid precursors by the salvage pathway. By fusion, the myeloma cell confers upon the lymphocyte an unknown element for its in vitro growth, whereas the lymphocyte provides the salvage pathway enzymes, conferring to the hybrid cell the capacity to grow in the presence of aminopterin. To stimulate this salvage pathway, the medium is supplemented with exogenous hypoxanthine and thymidine (*H*ypoxanthine, *A*minopterin, and *T*hymidine; 'HAT' medium).

For the production of stable hybridomas, ontogenetically related cells should be used (Köhler, 1981) from the same species (Yarmush et al., 1980) and at a similar stage of differentiation (Ringertz and Savage, 1976).

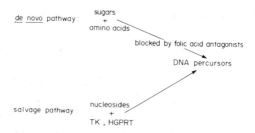

Fig. 5.1. Two pathways in normal cells to synthesize DNA precursors. The mutant myeloma cell line, which has the capacity to grow indefinitely in vitro and can confer this property on antibody-producing lymphocytes through cell fusion, lacks the salvage pathway (no thymidine kinase (TK) or hypoxanthine-guanine phosphoribosyl transferase (HGPRT)). This cell line would, therefore, not grow in the presence of folic acid antagonists. Fused cells, however, may grow since the antibody-producing cells contribute the salvage pathway.

Regardless of the fusion method used, only a small fraction of the hybridoma cells actually produce the desired antibody. Without proper precaution such cells are soon overgrown by the faster dividing non-producers.

For the production of monoclonal antibodies, immunization may be achieved either in vivo (most common) or in vitro. Immunization in culture and subsequent production of monoclonal antibodies may carry several important advantages (reviewed by Reading, 1982): (i) the period required for immunization is very short (only 5 days); (ii) self-antigens can be used as immunogens; (iii) immunogen concentration is easily controlled; (iv) the production of antibodies can be sampled regularly; and, (v) it is possible to study the fundamental mechanisms of the humoral response. A disadvantage of in vitro immunization is that usually only a primary response is obtained (IgM production) since the secondary response is dependent on the restimulation of memory B cells (North and Askonas, 1976).

Practical aspects of tissue culture techniques have been reviewed by Adams (1980).

5.4.2. Methodology for the production of hybridomas

5.4.2.1. Choice of animals and myeloma cell lines

Many inbred mouse strains are suitable. However, the myeloma cells are mainly of BALB/c origin, and BALB/c mice have a reasonably large spleen so that the obvious choice for immunization is the BALB/c mouse. The hybridoma cells producing the desired antibodies can later be injected i.p. into BALB/c mice where they grow into a tumor and produce larger quantities of the desired antibody than would be obtained by in vitro cultures. For some immunogens, other mouse strains (e.g., C57BL or SJL) may be necessary to obtain an immune response due to differences in the Ir genes (Section 5.1.3). The hybridomas poduced will then have characteristics of both parental strains and in vivo maintenance of the ascites tumors requires the use of F_1 hybrids (e.g., SJL × BALB/c F_1 mice).

Rats are also suitable for the production of monoclonal antibodies on a 10-times larger scale (Galfrè et al., 1979). The Y3 myeloma (κ-producing) of Lou rats can be used and ascites tumors can be obtained two weeks after an i.p. injection of 0.5 ml pristane by the i.p. injection of $5 × 10^7$ hybridoma cells. A minor disadvantage is the unreactiveness of rat IgG2a with protein A (Rousseaux et al., 1981). The use of rabbit spleen cells with mouse myelomas has not yet been successful.

Female animals are easier to handle and mice should be 8–10 weeks old.

Several satisfactory plasmacytoma cell lines are available (Table 5.3). All the early lines produced myeloma proteins, so that hybridomas secreted three types of Ig: the original myeloma proteins, the specific antibodies, and hybrid molecules. The X63 plasmacytoma, which produces a fully sequenced IgG1, was used in the original technique of Köhler and Milstein (1975). These X63 cells may undergo spontaneous fusion with each other and can be grown at very low cell densities making it relatively easy to clone hybrids. Several variant lines have been selected from this line (NS-1, Sp2, F0) some of which do not synthesize or secrete heavy or light chains. Sp2

TABLE 5.3
Some myeloma cell lines used for monoclonal antibody production

Cell line	Common designation	Resistance to drug	Ig chains produced	References
P3X63-Ag8	X63	8-Ag	γ_1, κ	Köhler and Milstein, 1975
P3NS-1/1Ag4-1	NS-1	8-Ag	$-$[a]	Köhler and Milstein, 1976
Sp2/0-Ag14	Sp2	8-Ag	$-$	Shulman et al, 1978
S194/5XXO.BU1	S194	BUdR	$-$	Trowbridge, 1978
P3X63-AG8.653	653	8-Ag	$-$	Kearney et al., 1979
F0	F0	8-Ag	$-$	Fazekas de St. Groth and Scheidegger, 1980
210.RCY3.Ag1.2.3	Y3	8-Ag	κ	Galfrè et al., 1979
GM15006TG–A12	A12	6-Tg	γ_2, κ	Croce et al., 1980

FO, which is a Sp2 + Sp2 hybrid, may require frequent recloning; Y3 is a rat myeloma, A12 a human myeloma, the others are from mouse. Drug resistance: 8-Ag and 6-Tg: 8-azaguanine and 6-thioguanine (cells lack hypoxanthine phosphoribosyl transferase); BUdR: 5-bromo-2-deoxyuridine (cells lack thymidine kinase).
[a] Sp2 may occasionally re-express light chain.

is less effective than X63 for cloning at lower densities (Fazekas de St. Groth and Scheidegger, 1980), has a longer generation time and yields less stable hybrids. The F0 line overcomes many of these problems but, being itself a hybrid, requires frequent recloning. The 653 line is an excellent choice, it has a high fusion frequency ($2–5/10^4$ myeloma cells) and its hybrids are stable.

The hybridoma success rate can be increased by the inclusion of feeder cells (Fazekas de St. Groth and Scheidegger, 1980; Miner et al., 1981), e.g., mineral oil-induced peritoneal exudate cells, which enhance the survival of hybrid cells early after fusion, perhaps through the action of monokines produced by macrophages (Reading, 1982).

Fusion efficiency is highest when the viability of the myeloma line is high (at least 90%) and cells are in exponential growth. For this purpose, $1-2 \times 10^4$ cells are seeded per ml tissue culture medium and cultured in an atmosphere of 5% CO_2. The viability and growth is established by counting the cells daily with a hemocytometer. The cells are subcultured every few days to obtain vigorously growing cultures when the maximum density is reached (about 10^6 cells/ml). Caution is necessary with antibiotics which may obscure contamination with mycoplasmas (McGarrity and Coriell, 1971). The latter should be avoided (Section 5.4.5) since it may pose serious hazards to the cell lines (Stanbridge and Schneider, 1976) and even reverse their sensitivity to HAT selection (Shin and van Diggelen, 1977). Care must also be taken to avoid cross-contamination between cultures (very common).

Revertants of myeloma cells may occasionally occur. It is good practice to culture the cells 2 or 3 times a year in the presence of the drug to which the cell line is resistant (e.g. 2×10^{-5} M 8-azaguanine).

Myeloma cells do not need trypsinization for subculturing since they grow either in suspension or are only lightly adherent. They can be released by a gentle flushing with a pipet.

5.4.2.2. Preparation of media   A $100 \times$ stock solution of hypoxanthine and thymidine and a $100 \times$ stock solution of aminopterin can be purchased or prepared in the laboratory: (i) dissolve 136.1 mg hypoxanthine in 100 ml distilled water by heating to 45°C for about 1 h; 37.8 mg of thymidine is then added, the solution is cooled to room temperature, sterilized by filtration and frozen in small aliquots at $-20°C$; and (ii) aminopterin, 1.76 mg, is suspended in 90 ml distilled water and dissolved by adding drop-wise 1 N NaOH (about 0.5 ml); this $100 \times$ stock solution is then neutralized with 1 N HCl, adjusted to 100 ml, sterilized by filtration and frozen at $-20°C$ in 5 ml aliquots.

Aminopterin is very toxic and must be protected from light. Deterioration of this drug leads to growth of the non-hybridized myeloma cells. Hypoxanthine precipitated during storage may be redissolved by heating in a boiling water bath.

The saline solution contains 8 g NaCl, 0.4 g KCl, 1.77 g $Na_2HPO_4 \cdot 2H_2O$, 0.69 g $NaH_2PO_4 \cdot H_2O$, 2 g glucose and 10 mg phenol red in 1000 ml distilled water. The pH of this solution is stable at room temperature.

Among the tissue culture media used, Dulbecco's Modified Eagle's Medium (DMEM) and Iscove's Medium yield by far the best results (Davis et al., 1982). For in vitro immunization, DMEM supplemented with glucose (4.5 g/l) is used (Reading, 1982). Several other supplements have been found to be beneficial. Beside the addition of glutamine (which is rather unstable), 2-mercaptoethanol (2-ME) enhances antibody production (Click et al., 1972). 2-ME-treated fetal bovine sera are mitogenic for T cells (Opitz et al., 1977) and produce polyclonal B-cell activation (Goodman and Weigle, 1977). Other additives are sodium pyruvate (just before use), $NaHCO_3$, and sometimes, non-essential amino acids and HEPES (see below). Bacterial lipopolysaccharide (LPS), a potent B-cell mitogen, increases the success rate (Davis et al., 1982). The medium additives are prepared as concentrated ($100 \times$) solutions: 100 mM sodium pyruvate, 5 mM 2-ME, 10 mM non-essential amino acids, 100 mM L-glutamine, and (if used) penicillin-streptomycin (10000 units and 10 mg/ml) and LPS (from Difco) at 5 mg/ml, sterilized by filtration and stored in aliquots at $-20°C$. Just before use, these sterile solutions are added to the medium to a concentration of 1%. HEPES at 0.18 mM is sometimes used to improve pH control.

The medium is supplemented with serum, though Iscove and Melchers (1978) defined a synthetic medium. Significant differences may exist among various batches of fetal bovine serum (FBS), perhaps with only 1 in 5 or 10 batches being satisfactory. Addition of 2% horse serum may improve poor FBS (Schreier and Nordin, 1977). Addition of 20% FBS to media significantly increases hybridomas compared to the lower concentrations used (Davis et al., 1982). Only 2% rabbit serum was used in the studies of Reading (1982).

5.4.2.3. Preparation of polyethylene glycol (PEG) for fusion
Virtually all fusions are achieved with PEG. Different PEG preparations from different companies have been compared by Fazekas
de St. Groth and Scheidegger (1980). The lower molecular weight
(MW) preparations have the drawback of toxicity and the higher
MW preparations of high viscosity. A very satisfactory compromise
proved to be the PEG 4000 for gas chromatography (Merck, No.
9727). Kodak 1450 PEG may be superior.

PEG is melted and sterilized by autoclaving, cooled to 50°C (still
liquid) and combined with an equal volume of PBS, pH 7.0. Since 1 g
PEG gives very close to 1 ml, this produces a 50% (w/v) solution.
The PEG solution can be stored frozen.

The optimum concentration of PEG (30–50%) for fusion is very
close to the toxic concentration (at or above 50%). Toxicity of the
different batches of PEG may vary considerably. It can be advantageous to include 5% dimethylsulfoxide (DMSO) in the PEG preparation (Norwood et al., 1976; Fazekas de St. Groth and Scheidegger,
1980).

5.4.2.4. Preparation of spleen and feeder cells   The mouse killed
by cervical dislocation is rinsed with 70% alcohol and its spleen
removed aseptically. Cells are squeezed from the capsule with a
spatula trough a sterile 50-mesh stainless steel screen into 10 ml
saline or in a plastic Petri dish containing 10 ml saline. After clumps
of cells are dispersed by pipetting up and down, the suspension
is transferred to a 15 ml centrifuge tube and allowed to settle for
10 min at room temperature. About 10 ml supernatant is removed
without disturbing the settled cells. The suspension is mixed and
an aliquot of 50 µl is transferred to 1 ml trypan blue solution
to establish the number and viability of cells (should be more than
95%). The cell suspension is diluted and centrifuged for 10 min
at about 200 g. The pellet is taken up in saline to a concentration
of 10^7 cells/ml. On the average, a mouse spleen yields 10^8 cells.

The necessity for feeder cells for the first few days after fusion
is undisputed, but not the nature of these cells. Köhler (1978) used

normal spleen cells, whereas Fazekas de St. Groth and Scheidegger (1980) used macrophages. Davis et al. (1982) did not detect a beneficial effect of these widely used cells, but, in contrast, found that either LPS or thymocytes yielded 10 times more colonies, and their combination about 30 times more. With a properly functioning feeder layer, the cell input can be reduced about 50 times, more diluted cell suspensions can be used and positive cultures are obtained from single hybrids. In combination with microtrays, this eliminates much of the cloning labor.

Peritoneal macrophages are prepared from normal BALB/c mice by the method of Fazekas de St. Groth and Scheidegger (1980). The abdominal skin is removed after rinsing with 70% alcohol and the peritoneal cavity is flushed with 4 ml 340 mM sucrose by entering a 18-gauge 4 cm needle directly above the symphysis and resting the tip over the right lobe of the liver. The fluid is withdrawn after gentle massage of the abdomen. The yield is about $1-3 \times 10^6$ macrophages which should be washed in standard medium and used within 30 min. About 50% of the cells are lymphocytes. The macrophages (from 5 mice) are prepared the day before fusion, suspended in HAT medium at a concentration of 8×10^4 cells/ml, incubated in a humid chamber (90% saturation) containing 5% CO_2 and distributed in 0.05 ml aliquots over the 96 flat-bottom wells of the tissue culture microtray, each containing 0.15 ml HAT medium.

Thymocytes are obtained from the thymus of BALB/c mice. Contamination by cutting of the oesophagus or the trachea should be avoided. The glands are rinsed with non-supplemented medium and a cell suspension is prepared by forcing the cells into 10 ml supplemented medium (see below). Cell clumps are dispersed by pipetting and the suspension is diluted to 8×10^6 cells/ml.

5.4.2.5. Mixed leukocyte (or thymocyte) culture-conditioned medium
Thymocytes produce lymphokines which stimulate and support growth of B cells (Andersson et al., 1977). These factors may be non-specific (NSF) or specific for the immunogen (Kilburn and Levy, 1980). These NSF represent a heterogeneous group of molecules

(Farrar et al., 1977) and may replace T cells (Schimpl and Wecker, 1972). Stimulation with alloantigens is an excellent method to obtain NSF (Amerding and Katz, 1974) due to the high immunogenicity of MHC antigens (Section 5.1.3).

Reading (1982) adapted this to obtain concentrates of NSF for in vitro immunization. For this purpose, thymocytes are prepared (Section 5.4.2.4) from both BALB/c and C57BL/6 mice and equal numbers are mixed to a final concentration of 5×10^6 cells/ml and cultured in plastic culture flasks in DMEM supplemented with 4.5 g dextrose/l, MEM non-essential amino acids, sodium pyruvate, 2-ME, HAT, HEPES, and 2% rabbit serum. After 48 h, the cells and other debris are pelleted and the supernatant (thymocyte-conditioned medium, TCM) is filtered (200 nm) and stored at $-70°C$ in aliquots of 10 ml.

5.4.2.6. Semi-solid or viscous media for cloning   Though both agar (Sharon et al., 1979) and methyl cellulose (MC; Iscove and Schreier, 1979) can be used, MC gives considerably better results (Davis et al., 1982). These media differ in their properties, agar becomes semi-solid, whereas MC remains liquid and immobilizes cells by its high viscosity. MC cannot be pipetted and should be added with a syringe without a needle. It has a number of advantages: it is chemically inert, has no mitogenic activity, it is relatively easy to retrieve cells from this medium, and small colonies can be easily located since all cells are on the bottom of the plate.

The MC stock solution is prepared according to Iscove and Schreier (1979). MC (Methocel MC A4M, premium grade, 4000 cP, Dow Chemicals) is added to distilled water just boiling over a Bunsen burner (20 g/450 ml), and the previously weighed 2 l Erlenmeyer flask is removed from the flame, covered with aluminum foil and shaken vigorously until all the MC is dispersed. The suspension is heated again just to boiling and cooled to about 45°C. Prolonged boiling or autoclaving should be avoided since it hydrolyses, but this momentary boiling suffices for sterility. After the addition of 500 ml double-strength medium and water to 1 l and thorough mixing, the final 2% stock solution is obtained, which is immersed in ice for 2 h to hydrate the MC. This viscous solution is stored at $-20°C$ in aliquots of 50 ml, thawed before use and kept for two days at 4°C to further hydrate the MC (some transparent fibers will remain; not serious).

5.4.2.7. Production of ascites tumors

About 10^6 cells from a stable hybridoma clone are injected i.p. into a histocompatible (or nude) mouse which was treated 1–2 weeks earlier with 0.5 ml pristane (2,6,10,14-tetramethylpentadecane) i.p. The tumor becomes evident after 2–3 weeks. When the peritoneal cavity is distended, ascites fluid is collected by the method used for the retrieval of macrophages, replacing the 4 ml 340 mM sucrose with 3×6 ml of serum-free medium. The cells are removed from the pooled fluid and the antibodies purified (Section 7.3). A yield of 50 mg/mouse is common. If tumors fail to appear, light irradiation (350 rad) may help.

5.4.2.8. Storage of hybridoma cells by freezing

Cells in an exponential growth phase are collected (4 ml) and pelleted at low speed. The cells are taken up in 2 ml complete medium, 40% FBS and 10% DMSO added, distributed over 4 cryotubes, and gradually frozen by placing them overnight in a styrofoam container at $-70°C$, or in the vapor phase of a container with liquid nitrogen. The cells are then transferred to liquid nitrogen where they may be stable for years. The key to the highest recovery of cells is quick thawing (under hot tap). The cells are then pelleted, washed with serum-free medium, and cultured directly with complete medium. Recovery is usually higher than 50%.

5.4.3. Production of monoclonal antibodies after in vivo immunization

The methods leading to the isolation of fused cells are fairly standard. Two different methods are used for cloning: (i) limiting dilution; or, (ii) cloning on semi-solid or in viscous media. Once the desired clones are obtained, antibodies may be produced in vitro or in vivo. The in vivo production is based on the formation of ascites tumors which produce large quantities of antibodies.

5.4.3.1. Preparation of hybridomas from spleen cells of immunized animal and myeloma cells   Immunization protocols differ from laboratory to laboratory, but hyperimmunization is not a good approach (Oi et al., 1978). Immunization is not only important to expand the desired clones of B cells, but also to induce their differentiation into cells which are much more efficient in fusion (Andersson and Melchers, 1978). A single injection is sometimes preferred while others use conventional immunization protocols (Sections 5.2.3 and 5.2.4). A boost is given intravenously (i.v.) usually after 4–6 weeks (50 µg in saline) repeated i.v. on the 3 succeeding days with 150 µg in saline. Stähli et al. (1983) obtained a high frequency of hybridomas by increasing the dose in the week prior to fusion (200–400 µg, on days 7, 4, 3, 2, 1 i.p. and days 3 and 2 i.v.).

Fully differentiated B cells (i.e. 8 days after boosting) do not fuse efficiently; the best time for fusion is 3 or 4 days after the last boosting. Myeloma cells are cultured 1–2 weeks before fusion to obtain cells in exponential growth and with high viability (Section 5.4.2.1). On the day of fusion, myeloma cells are flushed out from culture bottles and pelleted by low-speed centrifugation ($300 \times g$) for 10 min, pooled and diluted with saline, counted (Section 5.4.2.4), recentrifuged and taken up in saline to 10^7 cells/ml. Myeloma and spleen cells (prepared according to Section 5.4.2.4) are mixed with a $3 \times$ excess of the latter and centrifuged again. The supernatant is discarded, the pellet is loosened by tapping the tube, 1.0 ml of 40–45% PEG 4000 (Section 5.4.2.3) is added dropwise, mixed by gentle stirring with a pipet tip and centrifuged after 90s (6 min, $200 \times g$). The pellet is then taken up very slowly (critical! 2 ml first min, 4 ml second min, subsequently gradually 14 ml) with serum-free medium and allowed to stand for 5 min. The addition of 5% DMSO to the PEG solution decreases the effect of fast addition of PEG or media (Fazekas de St. Groth and Scheidegger, 1980). Cells are pelleted, and carefully taken up in HAT medium, by one of two methods described below (depending on the method of cloning), and left standing for 20 min. The initially fragile heterokaryons should not be subjected to pipetting.

5.4.3.2. Initial growth, screening, and cloning by limiting dilution
The most popular method for the production of clones, whenever the fraction of specific antibody-secreting hybrids is lower than 10^{-3}, is by limiting dilution.

Cells with a small fraction of heterokaryons obtained after fusion are taken up in 18 ml HAT medium (DMEM, containing FBS, HAT, glutamine, sodium pyruvate, 2-ME and antibiotics; Section 5.4.2.2) and added in aliquots of 50 µl to each of the wells of 96-well plates which received feeder cells the day before fusion (Section 5.4.2.4), so that the total volume in each well is 0.25 ml. This will give about 4 plates for each immunized mouse. Alternatively, 24-well (Costar) plates can be used (1 ml added). All cells but the heterokaryons (cells in which the multiple nuclei fuse during the first cell division) will die so that after 2 weeks the HAT medium can be replaced by HT medium (no aminopterin).

Screening and cloning should be attempted as soon as possible to avoid overgrowth by non-producers. The rapid loss of chromosomes after fusion frequently yields non-producing and producing variants from the same heterokaryon. As Goding (1980) pointed out, antibody production may take up 30–50% of the cellular activity and cells not producing antibody will divide more rapidly and overgrow the useful clones. The loss of chromosomes and the danger of overgrowth decreases with time, but recloning is nevertheless imperative.

A sensitive screening method is a sine qua non for successful hybridoma production and should be developed before starting the experiment. The first screening should take place 5 days after fusion, followed by other inspections every other day. EIA, particularly with POase are used for the screening of antibodies but it should be kept in mind that B lymphocytes contain APases and, much less, POase (in peroxisomes), which may interfere in the screening. The most suitable enzyme for these experiments is, therefore, BGase (though POase and urease are mostly quite satisfactory). Other methods, such as RIA (Nowinsky et al., 1979), the fluorescence-activated cell sorter (Ledbetter and Herzenberg, 1979), complement-mediated lysis, rosette formation (Reading, 1982), can also be used. From the original 10^8 cells only a few thousand hybridomas survive, of which a small fraction may produce specific antibody.

As soon as a positive culture is growing well ($1-5 \times 10^5$ hybridoma cells), its cells are cloned by limiting dilution. In a typical experiment an average of about 5 different clones could be expected to be present in the original well. In cloning by limiting dilution, cells are distributed over a number of wells at a dilution so that some wells should not show cellular growth. The fraction of wells without growth indicates the average number of clones per well and can be used to establish the fraction of wells with 1, 2, etc., clones. This follows the Poisson distribution

$$f(r) = \frac{a^r \cdot e^{-a}}{r!}$$

in which $f(r)$ is the fraction of wells with r (1, 2, etc.) clones, each derived from 1 viable cell, and a the average number of clones per well. The value of a is established by determining the fraction of wells without growth ($r = 0$), i.e. $f(0)$. If $r = 0$, then $a^r = 1$ and $r! = 1$; therefore $f(0) = e^{-a}$. If, e.g., 40% of the wells was negative, $0.4 = e^{-a}$ and $a = \ln 1/0.4 = 0.916$, i.e., when 40% of the wells contain no growing cells, there is an average of 0.916 clones over all wells. The a obtained can be used to calculate the fraction of wells having 1, 2, and 3 clones, which correspond to 0.367, 0.168, and 0.051, respectively, in this example. This shows that even with the high fraction of 40% negative wells, a large fraction of positive wells, $> 38\%$, has more than one clone. Recloning is thus necessary.

It is common practice to count the viable cells and to distribute over a series of plates at the rate of 1 cell/well, 3 cells/well, etc.

Evidently, the use of feeder cells (e.g., 1.5×10^6 thymocytes/ml) is imperative. After 10 days, one half of the medium is changed.

After about 4 weeks positive clones ($> 10^3$ cells) are transferred (in 0.5 ml medium) to cluster trays with larger wells (24-well tray, Costar 3524). Recloning of these cultures should yield at least 90% producing cultures. Clones are then expanded gradually (1:3), and antibody is recovered from the spent medium. The antibody concentration in the spent medium is about 2–50 µg/ml but much higher yields may be obtained by ascites production (Section 5.4.2.7), though a low percentage of unrelated proteins may then be present. At different suitable stages aliquots of the hybridomas should be frozen in liquid nitrogen (Section 5.4.2.8).

5.4.3.3. Selection and cloning of hybridomas on viscous medium

Many plates (up to several hundreds) may have to be used for the cloning of hybridomas by the limiting dilution technique. In a simpler method, selection and cloning is performed by a single step after fusion (Davis et al., 1982) using only about 40 Petri dishes (35 mm). This method is, therefore, particularly suitable for procedures with high yields of hybridomas.

Fusion is performed as in Section 5.4.3.1, and the cell pellet is taken up in 15 ml of Iscove's medium containing 53.3% FBS, 2.66% of HAT stock solution, 1.2×10^8 thymocytes and 2 mg LPS. To this, 25 ml of 0.2% (w/v) MC (Section 5.4.2.6) are added. The tube is then tipped several times and mixed for several seconds. Of this suspension 1 ml aliquots are distributed (with a syringe with an 18-gauge needle) into Petri dishes. Two of these dishes are placed in a 10 cm Petri dish, together with a third dish containing 1 ml distilled water and then placed in a 5% CO_2 incubator at 37°C.

From day 9 after fusion and every other day afterwards up to 4 weeks, the dishes are inspected for clearly visible colonies (not simple clumps of cell debris). A colony can be marked on the bottom of the dish with a fine felt-tip pen beneath the colony. Isolated colonies should be at least 0.5 mm in diameter. They are removed from the MC with sterile 10 µl capillary pipettes and transferred to 35-mm tissue culture dishes (Corning) containing 1 ml medium supplemented with 20% FBS and 1% HAT stock solution. The felt-tip marks should be left to prevent picking of the same clone as any remaining cell will grow back into a colony. The spent media of these new cultures are tested, after the cell density reaches 10^5–10^6 cells/ml, for the presence of antibody. About 60% of the colonies should reach this stage, but of those remaining nearly all develop further.

5.4.4. Production of monoclonal antibodies after in vitro immunization

Spleen cells are obtained from an unprimed BALB/c mouse (Section 5.4.2.4), washed and diluted to 20 ml with medium containing about 1 µg of immunogen per ml or 10^7 irradiated (2500 rad) or ethanol-fixed cells. Then, 10 ml of thymocyte-conditioned medium (Section 5.4.2.5) is quickly thawed and added to the spleen cell suspension which is mixed and left undisturbed for 5 days in a 75 cm^2 tissue culture flask in a 5% CO_2 atmosphere. After 5 days, when numerous blast cells are visible, the cells are ready for fusion with myeloma cells (line 653 is recommended). Fusion is performed as described in Section 5.4.3.1.

5.4.5. Some recurrent problems in the hybridoma technique

Hybridomas tend to lose chromosomes (Ringertz and Savage, 1976; Goding, 1980), and a significant number of initially positive clones may be ultimately lost. A failing but interesting clone may usually be saved by recloning, though this demands a large effort. To minimize these risks, it is necessary to prevent overgrowth in the wells or flasks, which tends to select for non-producing variants. Periodical recloning and keeping of frozen stocks are good preventive measures.

HAT solutions should be tested with myeloma cells (should not survive). Failing HAT solutions produce deleterious overgrowth by myeloma cells. On the other hand, no growth at all could be indicative of toxic effects (PEG, tissue culture plastic ware, etc.; Goding, 1980), the lack of proper feeder cells or a too high dilution rate of the culture during expansion.

Infections should not occur with good practices (vol. 8 in this series by Adams, 1980). The most common problem is caused by fungi, particularly if incubators with built-in fans have been contaminated. The use of antibiotics is widespread but could lead to antibiotic-resistant mycoplasmas (Rahman et al., 1967) or chromosome damage (Leonard and Botis, 1975).

Electron microscopy is a reliable way to detect mycoplasmas (Brown et al., 1974), but the mycoplasma stain (Hoechst 33258; Chen, 1976) is convenient.

CHAPTER 6

The nature and structure of antibodies

Antibodies belong to a structurally related family of glycoproteins called immunoglobulins (Ig). Though their essential basic structure is quite similar, they are heterogeneous with respect to function and physicochemical properties. This heterogeneity is important, not only for their purification and conjugation to enzymes, but also for the design of EIA or EIH.

6.1. Molecular structure of antibodies

6.1.1. Antibody classes and their constituent polypeptides

Antibodies are multichain proteins with an equal number of heavy chains (50–70 kDa) and light chains (about 25 kDa). Most Ig possess only the four-chain basic unit consisting of two identical light chain–heavy chain pairs linked by disulfide bridges and non-covalent inter-actions. The basic units are symmetrical, i.e. each half contains one light and one heavy chain, linked together by a disulfide bond, resulting in a Y-like structure. For some antibody classes (IgA and IgM), polymers of Ig with an extra chain (J chain) are encountered, whereas IgA in external secretions carries an additional polypeptide, the secretory component (SC).

Antibodies have a dual function: (i) recognition of the antigen; and, (ii) the activation, after antigen recognition, of a variety of biological functions to protect the host. The activation of these biological pathways depends on the different heavy chains and the Ig have, therefore, been classified according to the structure of these heavy chains. The heavy chains were designated with Greek letters and the Ig classified by adding the roman capital letter corresponding to the heavy chain name. According to the animal species, some classes can be subdivided into subclasses, which are then designated by the addition of a number (e.g., IgG1, IgG2, etc.). The two types of light chains (called κ and λ) are found in every Ig class. Interestingly, however, the ratio of κ : λ is constant in a species but different for the various animal species and for different subclasses (Schur, 1972). Table 6.1 compares some properties of the different Ig classes.

6.1.2. The domain structure of the heavy and light chains

Heavy and light chains are made up by a number of segments ('domains'), each of about 110 amino acids, which have striking sequence homologies (Edelman et al., 1969) and three-dimensional structures (Poljak et al., 1973). The light chains contain 2 domains, whereas the heavy chains have 3–5 domains depending on class (Fig. 6.1) or, for IgD, on the species (Blattner and Tucker, 1984). The peptide chain in each domain folds into two roughly parallel, though imperfect sheets (antiparallel β-pleated), linked by one, or sometimes two, essential intradomain disulfide bond(s). The interior between these two sheets is filled with hydrophobic amino acid side chains which occur at alternating positions and tend to be highly conserved among the Ig of the various species (Feinstein and Beale, 1977). The other residues in the domain have less overall homology and are probably responsible for the biological functions associated with the various domains, or for the secondary interaction with the neighbouring domains of the other chains. The particular compact structure of these domains render them quite resistant to proteases, a property often taken advantage of in EIA.

The amino-terminal domains of the light and heavy chains are both responsible for antigen recognition. The distal ends of these

TABLE 6.I

Human immunoglobulin classification[a]

Class	IgG	IgA	IgM	IgD	IgE
Heavy chain	γ	α	μ	δ	ε
Mass of heavy chain (kDa)	50	65	70	70	72.5
Light chain	κ or λ in all classes (mass 20–25 kDa)				
J-chains	−	+	+	−	−
Secretory component	−	+	rarely	−	−
Number of basic units	1	1,2	5	1	1
Valency for Ag binding	2	2,4	5(10)	2	2
% Carbohydrate	3	7	12	13	11
Approximate concentration in serum (g/l)	10	2	1	0.05	10^{-4}
Sedimentation coefficient (S)	7	9, 11	19	7	8
Mass (kDa)	150	160–400	900	185	200

IgG is involved in secondary response, placental transfer, and complement fixation. IgA is important for the immune response in respiratory and gastrointestinal tracts, body surfaces, colostrum, and isohemagglutinins. IgM is produced in primary response and in response to T-independent antigens. IgM is also a powerful agglutinin and is important for complement fixation. IgD is an early membrane receptor on lymphocytes. IgE plays a role in allergic responses.

[a] WHO designation: same Ig classes are found in other mammals but number of subclasses varies with species. IgA may be present as a monomer (serum) or dimer (with J and SC; primarily on body surfaces), whereas for some animals IgM may also occur as monomers, tetramers or hexamers.

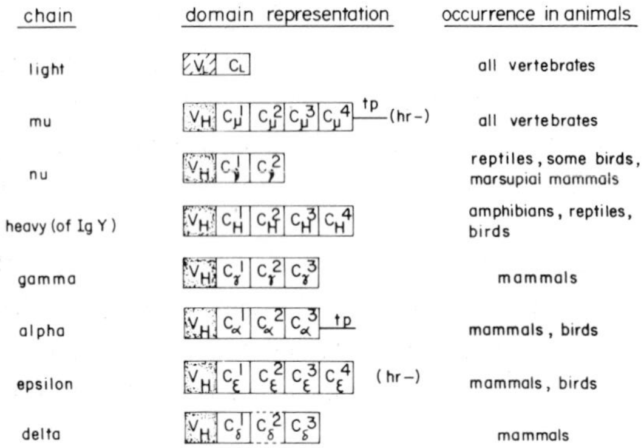

Fig. 6.1. The Ig chains and their domains. Domains are segments of polypeptide chains, consisting of about 110 amino acids, and have striking similarities in structure and sequence homologies. All chains have an amino-terminal variable domain (V) involved in the recognition of antigen. Some chains have an extra 'tail piece' (tp) or lack the hinge region (hr−) which confers structural flexibilities on the other heavy chains. Murine IgD, in contrast to human IgD, lack the $C_\delta 2$ domain pointing to an evolutionary divergence in the δ gene after the separation of the human from the rodent evolutionary lines (Blattner and Tucker, 1984).

so-called V-domains form a solvent-filled cleft (1.5×0.6 nm). The peptide segments surrounding this crevice are hypervariable in amino acid sequence (Wu and Kabat, 1970; Poljak et al., 1973), thus equipping the antibody with a surface complementary to the antigen ('key and lock' interaction). The peptide segments between these hypervariable regions are important for the V domain backbone structure ('framework residues') outside the antigen binding site. Hypervariable regions are also found outside the antigen-binding site. The other domains are called C (constant)-domains. Though the overall peptide folding of the V and C domains bears a strong resemblance, there is only about 30% homology in their amino acid sequence.

6.1.3. Disulfide bonds and the hinge region

The unusual stability of the Ig is due both to the compact globular structure of their domains and to the large number of stabilizing disulfide bonds (16–24 for human IgG of which 12 are intradomain). The S–S bonds between the polypeptide chains are not as deeply buried as those inside the domains and are more readily cleaved by 2-ME or dithiothreitol. Removal of the reducing agent and return to neutral pH reassociates the chains to native molecules, even if the SH groups are blocked chemically, demonstrating the strong secondary interactions of the neighbouring domains. The disulfide bonds link the heavy chains between the C_H1 and C_H2 domains (in the case of IgG, IgA, and IgD) or in the extraglobular portion of the domains (IgM) or in both (IgA). The light chains are mostly connected to the heavy chains, a notable exception is human IgA2(Am$^+$) where the two L chains are linked by S–S bonds. Depending on the class and subclass, the cysteine of the light chain (C-terminal or penultimate) connects to either a site of the C_H1 domain or of the hinge region. These sites are at either end of the domain but in close spatial proximity (Amzel et al., 1974). The hinge region has no obvious amino acid sequence homology with the C_H domains. This region contains cysteine residues which connect the two heavy chains and in some cases (e.g. human IgG1, mouse IgG1) also light and heavy chains. Another frequent feature of the hinge region is the many proline residues (up to about 1/3 of the total of its amino acids). These proline-rich sequences at the junction of the chains confer a certain lack of secondary structure and, hence, a high flexibility.

6.1.4. Proteolytic cleavage of immunoglobulins

Not surprisingly, the few cleavages caused by proteases in native Ig are often localized in this exposed hinge region. Treatment with papain cleaves the peptide chain at the N-terminal side of the hinge region resulting in two antigen-binding fragments (Fab), which are univalent, and a crystallizable fragment (Fc), containing most of the hinge region and the C-terminal domains (Fig. 6.2; Porter, 1959). Pepsin cleaves the peptide chains at the C-terminal side of the hinge

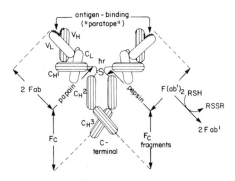

Fig. 6.2. Schematic representation of an Ig molecule (IgG). The heavy chains are shaded, and both the light and the heavy chains are shown as strings of domains. The hinge region (hr) is most exposed to proteolytic attack. Depending on protease (and origin of Ig), Fab or F(ab')$_2$ antigen-binding fragments are generated. F(ab')$_2$ can be further reduced.

region, yielding somewhat longer antigen-binding fragments, Fab', which are still connected by S–S bond(s) giving the bivalent fragment F(ab')$_2$. Mild reduction of the F(ab')$_2$ fragment yields two Fab' fragments with free SH groups. If Fab' fragments, prepared from antibodies with different specificities, are mixed and reoxidized, beside the original F(ab')$_2$ also hybrid molecules with different specificities at the two antigen-binding sites are obtained. The heavy chain piece in the constant portion of the Fab fragment, named Fd piece, and the N-terminal antigen-binding domains, named Fv, can also be obtained by digestion under controlled conditions (Inbar et al., 1972). Fragments analogous to the Fc, Fab, and F(ab')$_2$ of IgG can be obtained from IgM by other digestion procedures (reviewed by Metzger, 1970).

6.1.5. Additional polypeptides in polymeric forms of IgA and IgM

The polymeric forms of IgA and IgM contain another polypeptide, the J-chain, which has no homology with other Ig components but is important in the joining of the four-chain monomers. IgM of the lower vertebrates seem to lack the J-chain (Weinheimer et al., 1971). The J-chain is a relatively small protein (15 kDa) and rich in cysteine, aspartic acid and glutamic acid (Koshland, 1975). Both human and mouse J-chains have been sequenced (Mole et al., 1977; Cann et al., 1982). The J-chain joins two monomers by forming S–S bonds with the penultimate cysteine residues of one of the heavy chains of two monomeric subunits (Garcia Pardo et al., 1981).

Irrespective of the number of monomers, only one J-chain is found per polymer. In the case of IgM, the J-chain-containing dimer seems to serve as a nucleating unit to promote S–S binding among the other IgM monomers (Garcia Pardo et al., 1977). The plasma cell synthesizes both antibody and J-chain.

Monomeric IgA is found in the serum, whereas only the J-chain-containing dimers are capable of interacting with still another polypeptide, the so-called secretory component (SC; Koshland, 1975). Recently, Mostov et al. (1984) have shown that this SC bears structural resemblance to domains of other Ig; however, it is not synthesized in plasma cells, but in the mucosal epithelial cells of exocrine glands (intestinal, genito-urinary, respiratory, mammary mucosa, etc.). Plasma cells producing IgA are also abundant in these regions. The SC is a glycoprotein, the precursor (molecular weight of about 82000) of which acts as a receptor on mucosal epithelial cells for dimeric IgA (Mostov et al., 1984). A small transmembrane peptide is cleaved from the SC which becomes tightly coiled by strong non-covalent interactions around the Fc portion of both IgA molecules of the dimer (from one hinge region to the other) and seems to form S–S bonds with one of the two IgA molecules (Underdown et al., 1977).

SC has at least two important functions: (i) it transports the secretory IgA (sIgA) through the epithelium to the lumen, and (ii) it confers a greater resistance of the sIgA in the mucous secretions or colostrum against proteolytic attack. Sometimes, IgM with SC is found in patients with an IgA deficiency.

6.1.6. Evolution of immunoglobulins and their occurrence in vertebrates

The evolution of Ig occurred along the phylogenetic tree of the vertebrates (Kubo et al., 1973). All vertebrates seem to possess Ig (Nisonoff et al., 1975). A clear relation among the different classes of Ig in the diverse vertebrates is difficult to assess. Ig have not been shown conclusively in invertebrates (Marchalonis and Edelman, 1968).

Classification is difficult since Ig of different classes may still have some sequence homology and, hence, cross-react, or have similar biological functions but different physicochemical properties. For example, IgY of birds (Leslie and Clem, 1972) which in biological respect resembles mammalian IgG, is in physicochemical respects quite different (e.g. contains an extra domain in the heavy chain). Tentative conclusions which may be drawn are: (i) homologs of mammalian IgM seem to exist in all vertebrates; (ii) IgA is found in mammals and birds, IgE in mammals and, perhaps, birds; (iii) IgG is restricted to mammals only; and (iv) vertebrates other than mammalia may produce other Ig such as IgY and IgN (Fig. 6.1).

6.1.6.1. Avian antibodies

Relatively little is known about avian Ig. Best studied are those from domestic fowl. The predominant Ig is the IgY (5–7 mg/ml serum) which resembles in most of its functions the mammalian IgG: (i) a sedimentation coefficient of 7 S but a slightly higher molecular weight (170000); (ii) it is not adsorbed to DEAE-cellulose at low ionic strength; (iii) it is produced later in the immune response; (iv) digestion with papain or pepsin yields Fab and Fc fragments (Benedict and Yamaga, 1976). There are also some striking differences between IgY and mammalian IgG since IgY: (i) forms polymers at high salt concentrations (1.5 M NaCl) for some species (chicken); (ii) precipitates readily during dialysis against low ionic strength buffers; (iii) contains only λ light chains; (iv) contains heavy chains which have an extra domain, and show little homology with γ-chains; (v) has a higher carbohydrate content (5–6%). Reducing agents, often used to distinguish IgM (sensitive) from IgG (less sensitive) in mammalian sera, cannot be used for the same purpose for avian sera since IgY is quite sensitive to reductive dissociation at neutral or slightly alkaline pH (Kubo, 1970; Benedict and Yamaga, 1976).

The Ig found in egg yolk is IgY though IgA has also been reported to be present (Section 7.2).

Avian IgM is closely related to mammalian IgM. It cross-reacts strongly with human IgM (Mehta et al., 1972), also has a pentameric structure (Feinstein and Munn, 1969) and its J-chain cross-reacts with human J-chain (Kobayashi et al., 1973). Purified preparations of IgM often contain IgY due to the tendency of the latter to aggregate.

IgA-like molecules (Parry and Porter, 1978) are the major antibodies in bile and other secretions.

An additional class of Ig found in some birds (duck but not in chicken), is the IgN (5.7S) which has a mass of about 120 kDa (heavy chain, 40 kDa) and only two constant domains in the heavy chain (Kubo et al., 1973). It has little carbohydrate (less than 1%) and is sensitive to reducing agents. Its concentration in the serum is generally somewhat lower than that of the IgY.

6.1.6.2. Mammalian antibodies

The number of classes of Ig and their average relative concentrations varies from species to species (Table 6.2). Each class may have several subclasses; in man, mouse, rat, dog, and horse, IgG has 4 subclasses; 2 subclasses in the guinea pig, cow, and pig, and only one class in the rabbit and goat. For IgA several subclasses may also be found.

In general, IgM constitutes about 10% of the antibodies. Monomeric forms are occasionally found in low concentrations in serum. IgM is produced early in the immune response and reacts quite strongly with an antigen, despite its frequent low affinity, due to the avidity bonus (Section 8.5). The pentameric IgM is particularly sensitive to mild reduction by thiol reagents at neutral pH (splitting into monomers), thus loosing its high avidity. Such treatment can

TABLE 6.2

Mean concentrations of immunoglobulins (mg/ml) in some mammalian sera[a]

Species	IgM	IgG	IgA	IgD	IgE	Reference
Human	1.0	12.0	1.8	0.03	0.0003	Kyle et al., 1970
Cattle	2.6	18.9	0.5			Sawyer et al., 1973
	2.7	20.7	0.3			Williams et al., 1975
Dog	1.6	9.2	0.8			Reynolds and Johnson, 1970
Mouse	0.6	6.7	0.4			Molinari et al., 1974
Pig	3.15	18.3	1.44			Curtis and Bourne, 1971
Rat	0.6	16.5	0.13		0.02	McGhee et al., 1975
Horse	1.7	13.3	1.5			Ek, 1974

[a] Variations among different breeds are known to be significant.

be used to distinguish IgG from IgM (Deutsch and Morton, 1958).

IgG is the principal Ig in mammalian sera, particularly in older animals (80% of total Ig). This is due to a higher rate of synthesis and a longer half-life. The subclasses may be very different in their proteolytic sensitivities (probably due to hinge region differences): human IgG1 is quite resistant to pepsin, IgG2 and IgG4 are quite resistant to papain, whereas IgG3 and IgG1 are relatively sensitive (Wang and Fudenberg, 1972).

IgA constitutes 5–20% of the Ig in normal sera, and is primarily monomeric in serum. The most important form of IgA, the dimeric secretory form, is predominant in seromucous secretions (colostrum, tears, saliva, perspiration, sputum, feces, and vaginal and seminal fluid).

IgD and IgE, if present, are found in very low concentrations (less than 30 µg/ml).

6.1.6.3. Rheumatoid factors: a source of non-specificity in enzyme immunoassays   Most rheumatoid arthritis patients, but also patients with chronic inflammation or even healthy individuals, have rheumatoid factors (RF) in their serum or synovial fluid. Most RF are IgM, but some may be IgG or IgA, and react usually with the Fc of self-IgG molecules, but may also cross-react with IgG of other species (sometimes even stronger, Stone and Metzger, 1969).

These RF are often heterogeneous, but may become virtually monoclonal after a prolonged illness. It is not uncommon to find RF in hyperimmune sera. Their role is not clear, but they may clear the plasma of circulating immune complexes.

The anti-IgG nature of RF and the high detectability of EIA may be responsible for high background reactions in sandwich methods (Section 14.2.2) which, however, can be reduced to insignificant levels using different methods (Section 14.5.2).

6.2. Genetic variants of immunoglobulins

Studies on genetic variants of Ig have correctly predicted much of our current knowledge on the molecular biology of the synthesis of Ig and contributed much to our knowledge on the immunoregulatory circuits (Cantor and Boyse, 1977; Hofmann, 1980; Rosenthal, 1978; Taurog, 1981).

Ig themselves are also antigens, i.e. in a suitable host they will generate the production of antibodies. Three different levels of genetic variants can be recognized: (i) isotypes, which are determinants present in all individuals of the species and correspond to the various classes and subclasses of heavy and light chains; (ii) allotypes, which are present only in certain individuals of a population and, thus, will induce antibodies in individuals of the same species lacking this allotype; these variants are produced by allelic alternatives of isotypes in groups of individuals of the same species; and, (iii) idiotypes, which are determinants in the variable domains. Allotypically matched individuals of the same species will still have a number of idiotypic determinants related to the variable regions of the V domains. Idiotypes may exist with unique ('private') and shared ('public') structures (Ju et al., 1980).

6.3. Genetic basis of antibody diversity

Antibodies recognize antigens by their ability to stick to certain parts (epitopes) of the antigen by a variety of interactive forces. Since every antigen might have a unique, different surface, a virtually unlimited number of antibody structures is required. In the classical one-gene-one-polypeptide model, this would require an extremely large amount of genetic information. From the structure of Ig it was suggested that the constant and variable regions are encoded in two discontinuous stretches of DNA, with multiple copies for the V regions and single copies for the C regions (Dreyer and Bennett, 1965). This proved to be correct and gave a first clue as to how diversification is achieved and reduced the requirement for the amount of coding material.

The variable regions of light and heavy chains are encoded by 3 and 4 segments, respectively, each occurring in multiple different copies, and they are recombined at random in the somatic (body) cells (for reviews see Marcu, 1982; Leder, 1982; Tonegawa, 1983). The exact sites of some of these somatic recombinations are not uniform so that these segments are joined at different cross-over points which increases significantly the diversification of the V domain. The possibilities in combinational associations of V_H and V_L domains is a third important level for creating antibody diversification. The recombinations of the gene segments coding for the V region commit the lymphocyte and its progeniture to produce antibody of only that specificity. However, these lymphocytes retain the ability to switch the gene expression of the C_H regions so that the same V region may be attached to any of the C_H regions. The first antibodies produced by a lymphocyte are IgM, but after the so-called class switch, IgG, IgA, or IgE antibodies with the identical V domain appear. This class switching (in terminally differentiated plasma cells) is achieved by DNA reshuffling and by the final splicing of the hnRNA to the mature mRNA.

The diversity created by somatic recombination is supplemented in a remarkable way by somatic mutations. The variable region gene segments have been found to be highly unstable and mutations seem to occur at the rate of once per 10000 cells per generation (Leder, 1982). It was estimated that somatic recombinations and mutations of the germ line genes can generate about 18 billion different antibodies. Though a given lymphocyte is committed to the production of a certain antibody and displays this specificity in the form of surface IgM and IgD as a receptor, it requires the corresponding antigen for its activation. Simple thermodynamic laws (Section 8.4) rule that an antigen binds to the best fitting receptor among the billions of possible receptors which explains clonal selection. This interaction activates the cell which starts its proliferation and maturation to form a clone of antibody-producing B lymphocytes.

Unfortunately, the terminology used in this field does not correspond to the designations used for the antibody structure, e.g., the V genes do not correspond to the complete V domain and the J genes do not code for the J chains.

6.4. Synthesis of antibodies and clonal selection

The differentiation and maturation of a lymphocyte from a stem cell to an Ig producing plasma cell is summarized in Fig. 6.3. The combinational assortment of the gene segments coding for the heavy chain most probably occurs in rapidly dividing B cells in the B-cell-inducing microenvironment. In a following stage light chain gene segments recombine, which completes the selection of the various gene segments responsible for the specificity of the antibody produced by that particular cell. Surface receptors, consisting of sIgM and sIgD, are anchored in the membrane by extra hydrophobic sequences at their C-terminals. These small, metabolically quiescent, circulating B lymphocytes do not divide.

An immunogen reacting with the surface Ig thus selects the cell clone which will give rise to the antibody-producing and memory cells. Typically, the lymphocyte precursor cell is transformed by

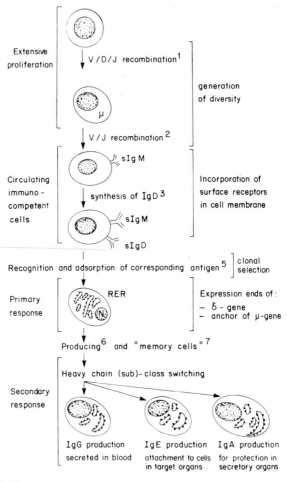

Fig. 6.3. Differentiation of a pre-B lymphocyte into antibody-producing plasma cells. The first stages are characterized by an extensive proliferation and generation of diversity, first of the heavy chain (1) and, subsequently, of the light chain (2), by shuffling of randomly chosen gene segments. The antibody specificity which is produced by a given cell is then displayed on its membrane, first by monomeric surface IgM and then also by IgD (3). The reaction of these receptors with the antigen (clonal selection) and interaction with other cells involved in immunoregulatory circuits (5) may result in a primary immune response. This is characterized by a strong development of the rough endoplasmatic reticulum (RER) in the producing cells

the immunogen into a large blast cell, which then proliferates into basophilic mononuclear cells and plasma cells. These plasma cells have a very extensive rough endoplasmic reticulum and are responsible for the production of IgM antibodies. The nature of stimuli responsible for class-switching is still surrounded by some uncertainties, but it seems that local influences are important.

←———

(6) but also by the production of memory cells (7). When these memory cells recognize a second infection, they differentiate further into IgG, IgE, IgA, or other memory cells. The specificity of the antibody may sometimes change due to point mutations.

CHAPTER 7

Purification of immunoglobulins and preparation of Fab fragments

Ig are a heterogeneous group of proteins, so that certain methods may lead to the overall enrichment in Ig but to the loss of the specific antibodies of interest, whereas other methods, which enrich for antibodies, tend to yield heterogeneous proteins with respect to both physicochemical properties and affinity. Although monoclonal antibodies are homogeneous in both respects, the optimal method for their purification may be unlike that for polyclonal antisera.

Ig are the most basic proteins in the serum, and have solubility properties unlike most other proteins. The sequential use of methods which separate proteins on the basis of different physicochemical properties is preferred, e.g. the classical fractionation with salts followed by ion-exchange chromatography. Purification of Ig by affinity chromatography, particularly with SpA, is becoming increasingly popular, due to high yield and simplicity. Among the theoretical advantages of pure antibodies in EIA are: (i) the amount of enzyme needed to label a given amount of antibody is reduced about 10-fold; (ii) background staining is minimized; and, (iii) larger amounts of antibodies can be immobilized on the solid phase, increasing considerably the detectability of the test (Section 8.5). A significant disadvantage is that antibodies purified by immunosorbents most often lack those with high affinity, which are essential for EIA.

7.1. Preparation of immunoglobulins from polyclonal sera

7.1.1. Selective precipitation of contaminating proteins

A large fraction of non-Ig proteins may be selectively removed with organic compounds such as Ethodine, Rivanol (Horejsi and Smetana, 1956; Gordon et al., 1962) or caprylic acid, CA (Steinbuch and Audran, 1969). CA (reagent grade, BDH) is suitable for the fractionation of large volumes of human, horse and rabbit sera and for monoclonal antibodies. The serum (100 ml) is diluted with 200 ml 60 mM acetate buffer, pH 4.0, yielding a final pH of 4.8. To this solution, 6.8 g CA are added dropwise with vigorous stirring, which is continued for 30 min at room temperature to prevent gelation. The precipitate is removed by centrifugation and washed with 200 ml 15 mM acetate buffer, pH 4.8. The pH of the combined supernatants which contain 90% pure IgG is raised to 5.7 with dilute NaOH and dialyzed against the buffer used for the batch-wise purification by ion-exchange (Section 7.1.3.2). The main contaminant in such preparations is IgA.

7.1.2. Salting-out procedures

7.1.2.1. Principles Precipitation by salting-out to remove non-specific proteins is highly effective, simple, cheap, avoids direct effects on the proteins, and concentrates the purified protein. It is often chosen as a first method if high purity is required.

The theoretical basis of these useful methods can be found in Cohn and Edsall (1943), Czok and Bücher (1961) and Dixon and Webb (1961). Contrary to widespread belief, the degree of saturation at which various proteins precipitate may vary widely with experimental conditions. The hydration of a large number of salt ions requires a considerable part of the solvent, thus lowering the solvation of the proteins and, consequently, inducing protein–protein interactions leading to precipitation. The salt concentration at which precipitation occurs is specific for each protein. Additional factors, such as pH, temperature and protein concentration, are also crucial for salting-out procedures and generally receive insufficient attention.

The relative solubility of a protein may vary considerably with pH, sometimes as much as 10-fold within one pH unit (Green, 1931). For most Ig the pH of precipitation should be their pI (generally between pH 7.0 and 8.0), but some proteins may precipitate better at a pH away from its pI (Section 3.1). Most proteins become less soluble at higher temperatures (e.g., change from 4°C to room temperature). The solubility of a protein first increases and then decreases with increasing salt concentrations. The factor of protein concentration is largely neglected (Dixon and Webb, 1961). Precipitation starts at a higher salt concentration in solutions with less protein. To minimize variation in these effects, serum should be diluted to obtain a final protein concentration of 2.5–3% prior to salting-out. A lower salt concentration should be used for a second precipitation if the precipitate is resuspended in a smaller volume than the original. Conditions for salting-out often make a compromise between high yield and degree of contamination.

7.1.2.2 Details of salting-out procedures Na_2SO_4 and $(NH_4)_2SO_4$ are the generally used salts for the precipitation of Ig. It has been customary to express the concentration of these salts in %, but with different meanings. The concentration of $(NH_4)_2SO_4$ is historically expressed as % of saturation, whereas for Na_2SO_4 this is given in % (w/v). Thus, 18% Na_2SO_4 equals 18 g salt/100 ml, whereas 18% $(NH_4)_2SO_4$ means 18% saturation (corresponding to 720 mM), which equals about 9.5 g/100 ml. The indication of molar concentrations is preferable to avoid confusion. Moreover, saturation is temperature-dependent, e.g. $(NH_4)_2SO_4$ saturation requires 700 and 765 g/l (3.9 and 4.1 M) at 0°C and room temperature, respectively. The solubility of Na_2SO_4 is both considerably lower and more temperature-dependent (5 times more soluble at 25°C than at 0°C).

A saturated $(NH_4)_2SO_4$ solution should be prepared carefully by adding 800 g $(NH_4)_2SO_4$ (without metal contaminants) to 1 l of distilled water at 35°C and stirred for 2 h at this temperature. The temperature is then lowered to 20°C or 4°C overnight, under stirring. The pH should be adjusted with diluted NH$_4$OH. However, the pH should not be measured directly in the saturated salt solution (essentially a 'dry' solution), since salt errors and junction potentials would cause considerable errors (more than 1 pH unit), but on small aliquots taken after each addition of NH$_4$OH, diluted about 20 times.

The addition of solid (NH$_4$)$_2$SO$_4$ or a saturated solution (density of about 1.245 g/ml) must be gradual under continuous stirring to avoid local high concentrations leading to precipitation of contaminants. The addition of a salt solution to the diluted serum is more gentle, but the use of solid salt may be necessary with large volumes of serum. The volume (v) of a concentrated salt solution ($c\%$) or the solid salt to be added to a solution, which is saturated for $i\%$, to obtain the final degree of saturation ($f\%$) can be calculated with the formulas:

$$v = \frac{f-i}{c-f} \times \text{initial volume} \quad \text{or,} \quad \frac{533(f-i)}{100-0.3f}. \text{g/l of solid salt}$$

For mammalian sera, excellent results are obtained with 33% (NH$_4$)$_2$SO$_4$, though both yield and contamination would be higher at 40% or 50%. The solution is stirred for 1 h if a salt solution is added or 3 h if solid salt is added, before centrifugation at low speed (15 min, 4000 × g). The pellet is redissolved in buffer of the same volume and reprecipitated. The precipitate is collected again by centrifugation, redissolved in the appropriate buffer and excess of salts removed by dialysis or by gel filtration through a Sephadex G-25 column (10 ml bed volume/ml sample). The complete removal of (NH$_4$)$_2$SO$_4$ may be verified with BaCl$_2$: the presence of (NH$_4$)$_2$SO$_4$ in the dialysate results in the precipitation of BaSO$_4$.

Alternatively, Na$_2$SO$_4$ is used by adding 18 g per 100 ml serum (equilibrated with phosphate buffer, pH 8.0, 0.1 ionic strength, by dialysis or by the addition of an equal volume of buffer). The precipitate obtained is collected by centrifugation and redissolved in buffer to 40% of the original volume. This suspension is clarified by centrifugation and Na_2SO_4 is added in the proportion of 12 g/100 ml. The precipitate is collected, dissolved and taken up in 20% of the original volume. The IgG thus obtained is fairly pure but can be further purified on DEAE-exchangers (Section 7.1.3).

If IgG is not further purified, lipoproteins can be eliminated by two successive dialysis cycles against water (12 h) and 50 mM sodium acetate (pH 5.0; 24 h), and centrifugation to remove the precipitate (Harboe and Ingild, 1983).

Reasonably pure chicken IgY can be rapidly prepared by precipitation with Na_2SO_4 at room temperature (solubility of Na_2SO_4 is too low at 4°C). An equal volume of 34% (w/v) Na_2SO_4 is added to the serum. The precipitate, collected by low-speed centrifugation, is washed twice with a volume of 17% Na_2SO_4 identical to that of the original serum. The precipitate is then dissolved in an equal volume of 60 mM Tris–HCl buffer, pH 8.0, and reprecipitated with 15 g Na_2SO_4/100 ml. The collected precipitate is washed and the pellet obtained is dissolved in the desired buffer.

7.1.3. Purification with ion-exchangers

7.1.3.1. Nature of ion-exchangers   The most often used ion-exchange adsorbents for the purification of Ig are weak anion-exchangers (diethylaminoethyl, DEAE), strong anion-exchangers (quaternary aminoethyl, QAE), and weak cation-exchangers (carboxymethyl, CM). The basic anion-exchangers interact with negatively charged proteins (i.e. at pH values above their p*I*), whereas the acidic cation-exchangers exchange their counterions (Na^+) for positively charged proteins. Some polar interactions and interaction by Van der Waals forces between the matrix and the macromolecules can also be expected (explaining differences observed between DEAE-Sephadex and DEAE-cellulose). The nature of the matrix also determines several important parameters, such as mechanical strength, flow characteristics, hydrophilicity, adsorbing capacity; higher porosity makes the interior of matrix more accessible. Details on cellulose ion-exchangers are in volume 2 of this series (Peterson, 1970). DE

52 (pre-swollen, DEAE-substituted; Whatman) is a widely used microgranular cellulose which consists of dense rod-like particles. High flow rates can be obtained with the recently developed bead-like particles, such as DEAE-Sephacel (Pharmacia) and DEAE-Servacel (Serva). Other, less frequently used anion-exchangers are DEAE-Sepharose CL-6B, DEAE-Sephadex A-50 and QAE-Sephadex A-50. Cationic exchangers are considerably less used than the basic exchangers for the purification of Ig.

In all these procedures, the choice and careful preparation of buffers are important. Cationic buffers, (Tris, imidazole, ethylenediamine, etc.) should be used with DEAE- and QAE-exchangers. Since such buffers carry the same charge as the ion-exchanger, they are not bound and will not cause local disturbances in pH or take part in the exchange process. Many examples exist in immunochemistry where good results were obtained without following this rule (e.g., phosphate buffer with DEAE-exchangers).

The ion-exchanger should be carefully equilibrated with the buffer. Initial equilibration is achieved with a concentrated buffer (0.2–1 M) but with the correct pH. The supernatant is decanted after settling of the exchanger and replaced by fresh buffer until the pH is stable. In the next step, the ionic strength, measured as the conductivity, is adjusted until it stabilizes (about 3–5 changes with 10 volumes of buffer). The slurry should be degassed before pouring, particularly if it has been moved from 4°C to room temperature. During packing, a relatively large pressure should be applied until the column bed height becomes constant (for DE 52: flow rate of 45 cm/h). The packed column is washed with buffer and the pH and conductivity of the effluent are checked.

7.1.3.2. Batch preparation of IgG using DEAE-cellulose   The batch preparation method (Baumstark et al., 1964; Perper et al., 1967; Reif, 1969) is suitable for rabbit IgG but less for human IgG. DE 52 is equilibrated with 10 mM phosphate buffer, pH 8.0. The wet cellulose (sucked 'dry' on a funnel) is weighed into a beaker in the proportion of 5 g wet cellulose for each ml of serum (optimal ratio). The serum, diluted with 3 volumes of distilled water, is added to the DEAE-cellulose (at 4°C). The slurry is incubated for 1 h and stirred every 10 min. The cellulose is filtered off on a Buchner funnel and washed with three half-volumes of the phosphate buffer. The yield of the combined filtrates should be about 70% (purity of about 96%).

7.1.3.3. DEAE chromatography   Two approaches are current: (i) adsorption of IgG at pH 8.0 followed by elution; or, (ii) adsorption of the contaminating proteins at neutral pH (or just below pH 7.0) while IgG passes unretained. It is good precaution to do a small-scale experiment before attempting purification of large quantities.

7.1.3.3.1. Fractionation of human serum with DEAE-cellulose. Serum (10 ml) is dialyzed against the starting buffer, 5 mM phosphate, pH 8.0, clarified by centrifugation, and applied to a DE 52 column (50 ml, 2.5×20 cm) equilibrated with the same buffer. IgG is eluted with phosphate buffer ($10 \times$ the column volume), using a linear gradient (10–300 mM). Three peaks emerge: the first, at about 20 mM phosphate, contains pure IgG with a yield of about 80%; IgM is desorbed at about 60 mM, whereas IgA is eluted at 100 to 150 mM (Rowe and Fahey, 1965). Using this technique, guinea pig IgG subclasses are obtained by a step-wise elution with phosphate buffers of decreasing pH and increasing ionic strength (Tracey et al., 1976). IgG2 is eluted at pH 8.0 with 5 mM phosphate buffer and IgG1 at pH 6.1 with 60 mM buffer. Mouse and rat IgG have also been purified on DEAE-cellulose (Capra et al., 1975; Bazin et al., 1974).

7.1.3.3.2. Selective removal of contaminating proteins with ion-ex-changers.   Rabbit IgG obtained by salt-fractionation is dialyzed against 17.5 mM phosphate buffer, pH 6.5 (Levy and Sober, 1960) and passed through a pre-equilibrated DE-52 or a DEAE-Sephacel column. All contaminants are retained, including a small fraction of electrophoretically fast-moving IgG (eluted at 200 mM phosphate, pH 8.0, if the column is not overloaded).

Alternatively, QAE-Sephadex A-50 may be rapidly equilibrated with ethylene-diamine (2.88 g/l)-acetic acid (73 ml of 1 M/l) buffer, pH 7.0, in a fume hood. The rabbit or human serum is diluted with an equal volume of the same buffer, and applied to the column. IgG passes through while other proteins are adsorbed. Contaminants may be desorbed with a buffer consisting of 435 ml 600 mM acetic acid and 130 ml 600 mM sodium acetate per litre (pH 4.0). Volume change of the ion-exchanger is avoided since the ionic strength of the buffer is maintained at 0.1 (Tijssen and Kurstak, 1974). The yield is 70–85% for the various sera with at least 90% purity if overloading is avoided. Not more than half the column volume of diluted serum should be applied.

7.1.4. Hydrophobic chromatography for purification of IgA

Since $(NH_4)_2SO_4$ requires much of the water available for the solvation of proteins, serum proteins may be fractionated on hydrophobic matrices. Doellgast and Plaut (1976) chromatographed sera in the presence of 1 M $(NH_4)_2SO_4$ on L-phenylalanyl-Sepharose. IgA is desorbed by lowering the salt concentration to about 20% (800 mM).

7.1.5. Purification of IgM by gel filtration

This technique is simple and gives high yields. A high resolution can be obtained with the upward flow, recycling method (Tijssen and Kurstak, 1974). Samples should be partially purified and concentrated by precipitation with 50% $(NH_4)_2SO_4$ and dialyzed against 500 mM of NaCl buffered with 50 mM Tris–HCl, pH 8.0, before gel filtration on Sephadex G-200 or Bio-Gel P-300.

7.1.6. Block electrophoresis on agarose

Zone electrophoresis is useful for the separation of electrophoretically distinct antibodies or proteins. It is easy and reproducible, but the sample size is limited. The technique presented here is essentially that of Jaton et al. (1979). Agarose (10 g) is dissolved in 2 l of 54 mM barbital buffer, pH 8.6, in a boiling water bath. The solution is then cooled to 50°C, poured into a Plexiglass box (40 × 40 × 1.5 cm) and allowed to gel overnight (covered with Saran wrap) at 4°C. A depth greater than 1 cm may lead to overheating during electrophoresis giving poorer results.

A trough of 1 cm wide is cut in the agarose perpendicular to the direction of electrophoresis at 20 cm from the anode (30 cm from the cathode). Generally, this trough is divided into 2 or 3 in-line troughs. The ends of the agarose block are connected with paper wicks over their full width, to the buffer compartments filled with 54 mM sodium barbital buffer which are, in turn, connected to the electrode compartments containing 200 mM phosphate buffer, pH 7.5. This electrode buffer can sustain more electrolysis without pH change and is cheaper. The connection between the buffer and electrode compartments is secured with U-tubes filled with agarose and buffer.

The serum dialyzed overnight against barbital buffer, is heated to 50°C and mixed with 1/7 volume 4% agarose dissolved and cooled to 50°C. This mixture is poured into the trough, allowed to set, and covered with 0.5% agarose solution at 50°C to level off the trough. A constant voltage of 600 V is applied for 50 h at 4°C. Albumin moves to the anode, followed by other proteins, whereas the Ig move to the cathode. The migration of albumin can be traced by the addition of 1/20 volume of 0.5% bromophenol blue to 1 ml serum. Excess dye moves slightly ahead of the albumin. Electrophoresis is stopped when the albumin is near the anode wick.

The Ig are recovered from 0.5 cm slices of the block cut perpendicular to the direction of electrophoresis. The slices are frozen in centrifuge tubes ($-20°C$), quickly thawed and the agarose is pelleted at $30000 \times g$ for 30 min. The pellets are washed 3 more times with 100 mM Tris–HCl buffer, pH 8.0, containing 500 mM NaCl. The protein content of the combined supernatants is measured by the Lowry method.

Several pure fractions of Ig are obtained. Yield is about 75%.

This method has also been applied successfully to the purification of IgE (Lehrer, 1979).

7.1.7. Isoelectric focusing (IEF) and isotachophoresis (ITP) of immunoglobulins

IEF is a high-resolution separation method and may be employed on an analytical scale (Williamson et al., 1973; Braun et al, 1979) or on a preparative scale (Radola, 1974; Schalch and Braun, 1979). It has, however, the drawback that proteins may precipitate during focusing due to the low ionic strength and the closeness to the pI. This can be overcome by the simple method of ITP.

IEF is rarely needed for EIA and the reader is referred to volume 12 of this series (Rhigetti, 1983) for technical details. In addition to the standard method, it is advisable, however, to add 2 M freshly de-ionized urea (Cramer and Braun, 1974) to the medium to disrupt aggregates of Ig (or antibody–antigen complexes) if hyperimmune sera are used, and to pre-purify the serum, e.g., by salt-precipitation.

ITP is based on the principle that ions are separated according to their different electrophoretic mobilities (Kohlrausch, 1897). Both large and small ionized molecules are stacked between the ion with the highest mobility ('leading ion') and the lowest mobility ('trailing ion'). This principle is also applied in discontinuous electrophoresis (Chapter 16). ITP has, therefore, the advantage over IEF that ionic strength can be regulated and that precipitation of Ig near their pI can be avoided (Ziegler and Köhler, 1979). The separation between two Ig molecules can be increased by spacer molecules (with mobilities intermediate of the two Ig). A drawback of this procedure is that side-by-side samples cannot be compared directly, since the separated proteins themselves contribute to the degree of spacing. Technical details can be found in Ziegler and Köhler (1976) and Barnstable et al. (1978).

7.1.8. Preparative ultracentrifugation

Density gradient centrifugation in 10–40% (w/v) sucrose in isotonic saline was an early method to separate IgG and IgM (McCall and Potter, 1973). This method is still used for the preparation of chicken IgM, for 16–18 h at 10°C at 35000 rpm (Beckman SW-39 rotor). IgM (19S) sediments close to the bottom but dilution may be significant.

7.1.9. Affinity chromatography of immunoglobulins or antibodies

7.1.9.1. Isolation of IgG and its subclasses with protein A-Sepharose (SpA-Sepharose)　　　SpA-Sepharose CL-4B is rapidly becoming a popular and simple tool in the purification of IgG and IgG subclasses. However, some subclasses of IgG interact very weakly with SpA (Kronvall et al, 1970; Table 7.1), whereas other Ig classes may sometimes also be adsorbed (Kronvall and Frommel, 1970; Harboe and Fölling, 1974; Inganäs et al., 1980). The capacity of SpA may vary with the species: adsorption of porcine IgG is only 70% of that of human IgG (Milon et al., 1978). SpA may be partially digested by proteases in the serum (Miller and Stone, 1978) and it is good practice to add protease-inhibitors (ε-aminocaproic acid) to the sample. Sometimes 20 mM NaN_3 is included in the buffer (Martin, 1982b).

　　7.1.9.1.1. Bulk desorption of IgG from protein A-Sepharose columns. SpA-Sepharose (1.5 g) is swollen in 10 mM phosphate-buffered saline (PBS), pH 8.0, at room temperature, to about 5 ml and poured into a small column (0.9×15 cm). This column may be stored with 0.1% NaN_3 at 4°C for long periods. The column is washed once with 100 mM sodium citrate buffer, pH 3.0, to elute any bound material, and then with PBS before use (3–4 volumes). Serum diluted with an equal volume of PBS is passed through the column at a rate of about 1 ml/3 min (capacity about 15 mg/ml). The absorbance of the effluent is monitored and buffer is passed until no more protein leaves the column. IgG is then eluted with 100 mM sodium

TABLE 7.1
Reactivity of protein A to immunoglobulins of different species[a]

Species	Binding[c]			References
	Strong	Weak	Unreactive	
Human[b]	*IgG1*,2,4		IgG3	Duhamel et al., 1979
Rhesus monkey	IgG, 3 sub-classes			Martin, 1982a
Rabbit	IgG			Goding, 1978
Cow	IgG1		IgG2	Goudswaard et al., 1978
Pig[b]	IgG			Milon et al., 1978
Sheep	IgG2		IgG1	Goudswaard et al., 1978
Goat	IgG2	IgG1		Delacroix and Vaerman, 1979; Duhamel et al., 1980
Dog[b]	IgG			Warr and Hart, 1979
Rat[b]	IgG1,2c	IgG2b	IgG2a	Rousseaux et al., 1981
Mouse	IgG2a,2b	*IgG1*		Ey et al., 1978
Hamster	IgG1	*IgG2*		Escribano et al., 1982
Guinea pig	IgG1,*2*			Martin, 1982b
Birds			IgY	Kronvall et al., 1974

[a] Italicized subclasses are the major components of IgG of the species.
[b] Other classes of Ig may also be bound.
[c] Strongly binding IgG elutes at pH < 6.0, weakly binding proteins elute at pH > 6.0.

citate buffer, pH 3.0–4.0, or with 0.58% acetic acid in 0.85% NaCl (Goding, 1976), or with 100 mM glycosyl tyrosine in 2% NaCl. A pH below 4.0 may increase significantly contamination with IgM (Vidal and Conde, 1980). The use of acidic elution buffers may be detrimental to Ig and 1 M Tris–HCl, pH 8.5, should be added immediately to the eluate. The column may be reused at least 50–100 times.

7.1.9.1.2. Stepwise gradient desorption of IgG subclasses from protein A-Sepharose.   Subclasses can often be isolated by this technique, though SpA has little affinity with some IgG subclasses (Table 7.1).

For the isolation of mouse IgG subclasses (Ey et al., 1978), the SpA-Sepharose column (Section 7.1.9.1.1) is equilibrated with 100 mM phosphate buffer, pH 8.0. The serum (5 ml) is diluted with 2 ml of the same buffer and the pH is adjusted to 8.1 with 1 M Tris–HCl buffer, pH 9.0. This sample is then applied to the column and washed with 30 ml of the pH 8.0 buffer. The effluent contains more than 80% of the IgM and IgA. IgG1 is then eluted with 30 ml 100 mM sodium citrate, pH 6.0. Most of the IgG2a (90%) is then eluted with a 100 mM citrate buffer, pH 5.5, and the rest at pH 4.5, but this risks some denaturation. Finally, IgG2b is eluted with 30 ml 100 mM citrate buffer, pH 3.5. The column is then regenerated and equilibrated as in Section 7.1.9.1.1.

With a similar approach, the two subclasses of hamster IgG can be obtained (Escribano et al., 1982). IgG2, which constitutes about 75% of the total, elutes at pH 6.0, whereas IgG1 elutes at pH 5.0.

Most of the goat IgG1 passes directly, even at pH 9.1, whereas IgG2 is eluted at pH 5.8–5.9 (Delacroix and Vaerman, 1979). In contrast, Duhamel et al. (1980) reported a somewhat stronger adsorption of goat IgG1 (elution at pH 6.7).

7.1.9.1.3. Continuous gradient desorption of IgG subclasses from protein A-Sepharose.   Guinea pig IgG have 2 subclasses with different SpA-binding properties (Forsgren, 1968) and can be separated by continuous gradient desorption from SpA-Sepharose (Martin, 1982b).

For the production of the gradient, the five buffers are prepared by adding 100 mM citric acid to 200 mM Na_2HPO_4 to obtain pH 6.5, 6.0, 5.5, 5.0, and 4.5. The pH gradient is generated by filling 5 chambers with 19 ml of each buffer, whereas a 6th chamber contains

100 mM citric acid, pH 2.1. The chambers are connected in order of increasing pH and each buffer is mixed with a magnetic bar. Serum (1 ml) is loaded on the column, previously equilibrated with a citrate–phosphate buffer, pH 7.3, and chased with 2 ml of this buffer. For elution, the chamber containing the pH 6.5 buffer is connected to the column. IgG1 is eluted at pH 4.7 and IgG2 at pH 4.3. These peaks are too close for efficient stepwise elution.

A similar method is used for rhesus monkey IgG with the two peaks resolved at pH 4.8 and 4.4 (Martin, 1982a). The IgG found in the pH 4.8 fraction can be further resolved into two components on DEAE-cellulose. Fractionation of human IgG shows similar problems (Duhamel et al., 1979): IgG3 is not bound by SpA-Sepharose, IgG2 elutes at pH 4.3 and IgG1 at pH 3.9, whereas IgG4 is found in both peaks. Van Kamp (1979) noted that about 30% of the IgA (both subclasses) and some IgM are also bound to SpA. Nevertheless, SpA can be used to obtain IgG3 (Patrick and Virella, 1978) by first purifying total IgG by the classical method (Sections 7.1.2. and 7.1.3.3) followed by chromatography on SpA. Pure IgG3 passes directly. It is necessary to include ε-aminocaproic acid (200 mM) in the serum and all buffers to prevent proteolytic degradation of the IgG3.

7.1.9.2. Immunosorbents for the purification of antibodies and removal of cross-reactivity   Immunosorbents can be used for the specific isolation of antibodies or of antigens, or for the removal of contaminants from a preparation. Obviously, the purity obtained depends on the purity of the corresponding immunoreactant. Antibody obtained with this method is physicochemically heterogeneous, unless it is subjected to further fractionation. Unfortunately, the success in eluting the antibodies with the highest affinity, critical for EIA (Section 8.6), is quite often limited.

Immunosorbents may be prepared with many different matrices, such as polyacrylamide, agarose, dextran, cellulose, or by cross-linking the antigens which requires an ample supply of the antigen (Table 7.2). Spacers (mostly hexyl) are often used to prevent steric interference between the matrix and the antigen. Sepharose 4B is

TABLE 7.2
Some examples of activated matrices for the preparation of immunosorbents

Derivatization of matrix	Group involved in binding	Antigen
CNBr-activation	amino	protein, polynucleotide, coenzyme, steroid, etc.
Periodate-activation	amino	idem
Carboxyhexyl (+CDI)[a]	amino	idem
Aminohexyl (+CDI)	carboxyl	protein
Thiopropyl	thiol	protein
	mercurated base	polynucleotide
N-hydroxysuccinimide ester	amino	protein, hapten

[a] CDI is carbodiimide.

a widely used matrix; however, when disruptive eluents (guanidine–HCl, urea) are used for the elution of antibodies, it should be replaced by the covalently cross-linked Sepharose CL-4B. The capacity of cross-linked adsorbents is usually lower, since the interior of the beads is less accessible.

7.1.9.2.1. Activation of matrices with vicinal glycols using periodate and coupling of antigens. Matrices with vicinal glycols (agarose, Sepharose, Sephadex) may be oxidized with $NaIO_4$ which produces aldehyde groups on the beads. These aldehydes may form Schiff's bases with free amino groups of proteins which can subsequently be stabilized by reduction. The method presented here for cellulose is modified from that of Ferrua et al. (1979).

Microcrystalline cellulose (1 g) is washed with distilled water and oxidized in 40 ml 100 mM $NaHCO_3$ containing 60 mM $NaIO_4$ in the dark for 2 h at room temperature in a closed container. This activated matrix is quickly washed on a sintered glass filter with 100 mM sodium carbonate buffer, pH 9.0, to remove by-products. For conjugation, the cellulose is suspended in 40 ml of the pH 9 buffer containing 10^{-7} M antigen or antibody and stirred overnight at room temperature, followed by two additions (30 min incubation each) of 1/20 volume of a 0.1 mM NaOH solution, containing 10 mg/ml NaBH$_4$ (freshly prepared). The solid phase is then extensively washed with 0.5 mM NaHCO$_3$, 100 mM sodium acetate buffer, pH 4.0, PBS, and 0.05% Tween 20 in PBS (to prevent non-specific binding). Sephacryl can be used instead of cellulose, but agarose or Sephadex are less useful (Section 13.5.1).

7.1.9.2.2. Activation of Sepharose with cyanogen bromide and linking of antigen. Though CNBr-activated Sepharose 4B is commercially available, it is quite simple to prepare (Livingston, 1974). With this convenient matrix, antigens (or antibodies) containing free amino groups are immobilized in a controlled manner, and often with a multi-point attachment, producing a more stable adsorbent. The pH of the Sepharose suspension (0.33 g/ml, washed with distilled water) is raised to 11.2 (controlled with pH meter) with 3 N NaOH with continuous gentle stirring. The poisonous, solid CNBr is added to a pre-weighed stoppered tube in a fume hood, weighed and dissolved in distilled water to a concentrated solution. CNBr is added to the Sepharose to a final concentration of 33 mg/ml, in a fume hood, while constantly adjusting the rapidly falling pH by the intermittent addition of 3 N NaOH until the pH ceases falling (after about 6–10 min). The activated Sepharose is washed with 20–40 volumes of ice-cold water.

Commercial CNBr-activated Sepharose should be washed on a sintered glass filter with 1 mM HCl (200 ml/g) and, just before use, with the coupling buffer (100 mM NaHCO$_3$, pH 8.2, containing 500 mM NaCl).

Antigen is equilibrated with the coupling buffer and gently mixed with the gel for 3 h at room temperature or overnight at 4°C. The Sepharose/protein ratio (w/w) should be about 30, whereas for small haptens this ratio may be 600. Since 3.5 ml Sepharose 4B contains about 1 g dry material, about 10 mg protein per ml of gel should be used. After this incubation the concentration of protein in the supernatant is determined to establish the extent of coupling. The remaining active groups are blocked by the addition of 1 M ethanolamine or 200 mM glycine and the gel is washed with the pH 4.0 and pH 8.0 buffers alternately and then with the buffer used for immunosorption. This immunosorbent is stable for at least 6 months at 4°C in the presence of 100 mM NaN$_3$. In the preparation of immunosorbents: (i) hydrolysis of the activated gel at the high pH used for its activation can be avoided by washing the gel in a buffer of lower pH as soon as titration with NaOH is stopped; (ii) the activated gel in the coupling buffer should be used immediately; (iii) buffers with amino groups, such as Tris, should be avoided during coupling since they will block the coupling sites; (iv) stirring should be very gentle; and, (v) protein–protein interactions are minimized by using 500 mM NaCl in the buffer. Molecules which may not be bound directly to CNBr-activated Sepharose can be first conjugated to a protein, which is then coupled to the activated Sepharose (Axén et al., 1967).

7.1.9.2.3. Preparation of immunosorbents with small antigens or haptens.   It is generally advantageous to link haptens or other small ligands to the matrix through a spacer, in order to prevent interference by the matrix with the hapten–antibody interaction. AH-Sepharose is prepared by the CNBr method (Section 7.1.9.2.2) by linking covalently of 1,6-diaminohexane (6–10 μmoles for each ml) to the activated Sepharose. CH-Sepharose is prepared in a similar manner using 6-aminohexanoic acid (10–14 μmoles incorporated per ml swollen gel). These derivatized Sepharoses are also commercially available.

Before coupling the ligand to the appropriate CH- or AH-Sepharose, the gel is washed with 500 mM NaCl (5 ml gel is about 1 g), and diluted with two volumes. The ligand is dissolved in water (or mixtures of water and organic solvent) and the pH is adjusted to 4.5 with HCl. A 50-fold molar excess of *N*-ethyl-*N*-(3-dimethylaminopropyl) carbodiimide hydrochloride (10 mg/ml gel) dissolved in water at pH 4.5 and a 5-fold molar excess of ligand, both with respect to the side-arms, are mixed with the gel suspension and incubated overnight with gentle mixing. Tris, phosphate or acidic buffers may compete with the hapten for coupling and should be avoided. It is usually necessary to re-adjust the pH to about 5 after 1 h with dilute NaOH (check with pH paper to prevent damage of the electrodes). After coupling, the gel should be washed with the same mixture used for the solubilization of the hapten. The gel can be stored in a slightly acidic buffer containing 1 M NaCl.

7.1.9.2.4. Immunoaffinity chromatography with N-hydroxysuccinimide (NHS)-derivatized agarose. NHS ester-derivatized cross-linked agarose couples with high efficiency all ligands containing a primary amino group. NHS is displaced from the spacers and a stable amide bond is formed (Section 11.2.3.2.1.1). NHS-affinity supports with different spacer arms (15 µmoles NHS per ml packed gel) are commercially available from Bio-Rad. Affi-Gel 10 is recommended for neutral or basic proteins (p*I* 6.5 or higher, e.g., IgG) and Affi-gel 15 for acidic proteins. They may bind 20–30 mg of protein per ml of gel and have been used for the purification of antibodies or antigens (Maze and Gray, 1980; Brooks and Feldbush, 1981; Knudsen et al., 1981; and Naito and Ueda, 1981).

The gel to be coupled is suspended uniformly, transferred to a sintered glass funnel and washed with 3 volumes of iso-propanol and 3 volumes of cold distilled water (less than 20 min). The cold ligand solution (0.5–1 volume) in 100 mM $NaHCO_3$ is mixed gently with the gel for 1 h at room temperature. This is followed by an incubation (1 h) with ethanolamine–HCl buffer, pH 8.0. The gel is washed and ready for use. Ligands not soluble in water may be used in methanol, ethanol, acetone or DMF.

7.1.9.2.5. Preparation of immunosorbents by cross-linking antigens. Antigens can be directly cross-linked (e.g., with GA; Avrameas and Ternynck, 1969) rendering them highly insoluble while retaining their antibody-binding capacity. The major disadvantage of this method is the amount of antigens required.

A 2.5% solution of GA is added in a ratio of 0.5 ml per 100 mg protein. The proteins should be at a concentration of about 20 mg/ml, in 200 mM sodium acetate buffer, pH 5.0, or in 100 mM phosphate buffer, pH 7.4. The gel, which forms almost immediately, is kept for 3 h at room temperature, homogenized with a Potter homogenizer in 200 mM phosphate buffer, pH 7.4 (20–40 mg of gel/ml), washed and centrifuged (6000 × g for 15 min) until the undiluted supernatant is free of UV-absorbing material (indicating the complete removal of free proteins which interfere with the immunosorbent). Before use, the gel should be washed with the buffer used for elution and re-equilibrated to neutrality. Proteins with few amino groups, e.g. POase, may not be cross-linked by this method but often can be polymerized in the presence of a carrier protein.

7.1.9.2.6. Isolation of specific antibodies on immunosorbents.
For every particular antigen–antibody system the maximum binding of antibody per ml of gel and the optimum conditions (ionic strength, pH, temperature, solvent conditions) for the elution of the antibodies should be determined in a systematic way in pilot studies.

The column is washed with 500 mM phosphate buffer, pH 7.4, containing 100 mM NaCl, and antibodies are adsorbed in the same buffer. Best results are obtained (Eveleigh and Levy, 1977) by using a relative low ligand concentration (5 mg/ml) and 0.5% Tween 80 to eliminate non-specific interactions.

Whole antiserum or physicochemically purified Ig is mixed with the immunosorbent in 100 mM phosphate buffer, pH 7.4 at 4°C overnight. Adsorbed antibodies are eluted batchwise, after washing of the adsorbent until the optical density of the supernatant is less than 0.05 at 280 nm. Alternatively, the immunosorbent may be packed in a column after removal of the fine particles (Avrameas and Ternynck, 1969).

Best dissociation conditions vary with the antibodies (Section 8.2). Most techniques depend on the deformation of the interacting surfaces of the antibody and antigen, obtained with chaotropic ions (3.5 M potassium thiocyanate in 100 mM phosphate buffer, pH 6.6), organic acids with low surface tension (propionic acid, acetic acid, Section 8.2), denaturants (8 M urea, 7 M guanidine-HCl), and pH extremes (100 mM glycine-HCl, pH 2.5).

In a systematic study (O'Sullivan et al., 1979) the most useful eluents were 100 mM NaCl-HCl, pH 2.0, for protein antigens or 7 M guanidine-HCl, pH 2.0, for small hydrophobic molecules (haptens). Conditions which are effective in the desorption of antibodies may, however, irreversibly denature both desorbed material and the ligand (Kristiansen, 1976). Organic solvents (10% dioxane) may often help desorption (Andersson et al., 1979).

The eluted antibodies and the immunosorbent should be neutralized at once and denaturants should be immediately removed to minimize permanent denaturation.

7.1.10. Purification of immunoglobulins from hemolyzed sera and removal of lipoproteins

Hemolysis of plasma drastically reduces the yield and purity of Ig. Carter and Boyd (1979) developed a simple method based on precipitation with PEG (Polson et al., 1964). This method is better suited than precipitation with $(NH_4)_2SO_4$ or chromatography on DEAE-cellulose. The hemolyzed serum is diluted with an equal volume of 60 mM potassium phosphate buffer, pH 7.0, incubated overnight at 4°C and centrifuged at $27000 \times g$. PEG 6000 (50% PEG solution, prepared as in Section 5.4.2.3) is added dropwise to a final concentration of 13% (w/v) while stirring vigorously for 1 h. After another 30 min, the precipitate is collected by centrifugation ($27000 \times g$ for 30 min; room temperature) and dissolved in the potassium phosphate buffer (double of original plasma volume). Precipitation with 13% PEG is repeated to remove all residual hemoglobin and albumin. The pellet is dissolved in 30 mM potassium acetate, pH 4.6 (adjusted with HCl). The α-globulins and fibrinogen are precipitated with 10% PEG and removed by centrifugation. The pH of the supernatant is raised to 5.8 with 2 N NaOH. Ig are precipitated again with 13% PEG, centrifuged after 30 min of stirring and the pellet is taken up in 60 mM potassium phosphate buffer, pH 7.0 containing 0.85% NaCl. The Ig are obtained in concentrated form. PEG may be removed from the purified proteins by chromatography on DEAE-cellulose in conditions where all Ig are bound (Section 7.1.3.3.1) or by ethanol precipitation. For the latter, the solution is clarified by centrifugation, cooled to $-8°C$ and precooled ethanol ($-8°C$) is added to 25% (v/v). The precipitate consists of Ig.

A simple method to remove lipoprotein from sera (Tijssen and ˈrstak, 1974) consists of the addition of Aerosil 380 (Degussa), n-ionic detergent, to the serum (2%, w/v) and stirring the mixture ˈ for 4 h at room temperature. The precipitate is removed ʋy centrifugation ($12000 \times g$ for 30 min).

7.2. Purification of Ig Y from egg yolk

Jensenius et al. (1981) reported two methods which circumvent many of the earlier problems for the isolation of IgY. The yolk, of which 50% is non-aqueous, is separated from the egg white and its membrane is cut open. The yolk (20 ml) is diluted with 80 ml TBS (10 mM Tris–HCl buffer, pH 7.4, and 140 mM NaCl), and may be stored for several months in the cold in the presence of 0.1% NaN$_3$. Any precipitate formed is removed by centrifugation and 6.0 ml 10% (w/v) dextran sulphate (Pharmacia) in TBS is added, under mixing. Excess of dextran sulphate is precipitated with 15 ml 1 M CaCl$_2$. The precipitate is extracted with 50 ml TBS to recover any protein carried with the precipitate. IgY is then recovered from the combined supernatants by the method given in Section 7.1.2.2.

An alternative, simple method, with somewhat lower yield, is based on the aggregation of yolk lipid at neutral pH and low ionic strength. The yolk is diluted with 9 volumes of water and the pH is adjusted to 7.0 with 100 mM NaOH. After freezing and thawing, lipids are removed by centrifugation and IgY further purified from the supernatant as in Section 7.1.2.2.

7.3. Purification of monoclonal antibodies

The same methods described for the purification of polyclonal antisera may be employed though conditions may be stricter, e.g. salt concentration, pH, etc. Properties of a monoclonal antibody may, however, be very different from the average encountered in polyclonal antisera. For example, a mouse IgG2a, which normally elutes from SpA between pH 5.5 and 6.0 may elute at a very different pH. Stability and solubility are often more restricted for monoclonal antibodies, particularly elution at low pH may be deleterious and precipitation at the pI may occur. Whereas for a polyclonal antiserum the loss of a particular antibody, due to the lack of stability in the purification conditions, may be almost inapparent, the same conditions may be disastrous for a given monoclonal antibody. An alternative is the use of DEAE Affi-Gel Blue or Blue Sepharose CL-6B for chromatography (Bruck et al., 1982). These supports are prepared by attaching Cibacron Blue F3G-A to a matrix (Böhme et al., 1972) which may be cross-linked Sepharose 6B (Pharmacia) or DEAE Bio-Gel A (Bio-Rad). The latter yields higher purity, though a slightly lower recovery. The DEAE Affi-Gel Blue also removes proteolytic activities.

The method described here is essentially that of Bruck et al. (1982). Ascitic fluid is centrifuged to remove cells ($1000 \times g$ for 5 min) and debris ($100000 \times g$ for 30 min) and dialyzed against 20 mM Tris–HCl buffer, pH 7.2, and centrifuged again at $100000 \times g$ for 15 min. The DEAE Affi-Gel Blue column (7 ml) is equilibrated with the Tris–HCl buffer. The complete procedure is carried out at 4°C. The ascitic fluid is applied to the column without exceeding the ratio of 1 ml/5 ml of gel, and the column is washed with about 25 ml Tris buffer. Transferrin is eluted with 20 ml of Tris buffer containing 25 mM NaCl. The monoclonal antibody is collected after 20 ml Tris buffer containing 50 mM NaCl is added. Albumin is eluted at about 80 mM NaCl. The main contaminant in the Ig fraction is transferrin. Yield is around 80%. The column may be regenerated by passing 3 bed volumes of 6 M guanidine-HCl or 8 M urea, followed by 5 volumes of 500 mM NaCl and 5 volumes of Tris buffer.

This method is less suitable for the purification of unprocessed polyclonal mammalian sera, due to the high ratio of albumin to Ig. A useful alternative for monoclonal antibodies is the caprylic acid method (Section 7.1.1).

7.4. Assessment of the purity and quantity of immunoglobulins

A particular property of mammalian IgG is that their absorbance at 278 nm is about 2.5–3.0 higher than at 251 nm, in contrast to other serum proteins where this ratio is about 1–1.5 (in neutral buffers). Measurements at these two wavelengths may, therefore, indicate the fractions which contain IgG and their approximate degree of purity. The actual A_{278}/A_{251} ratio may vary for individual antibody clones. At the same time, the absorbance at 278 nm is an indication of the IgG concentration: if the optical pathway is 1 cm, a 1% solution (10 mg/ml) has an absorbance of $13.5 \pm 10\%$ (Little and Donahue, 1967).

The SDS–PAGE method of Laemmli (1970) is convenient to verify the purity of the Ig, particularly with the very sensitive silver staining method (Section 16.1.1). It is good practice to analyse both unreduced and reduced (with 2-ME) samples.

7.5. Preparation of Fab fragments

In some situations, Fab fragments (Section 14.4.2) are preferred over the complete Ig or are even essential for EIA.

Fab fragments produce a lower background in sandwich assays, decrease non-specific adsorption of rheumatoid factors and restrict specificity of the antibodies. Since the conjugated anti-Ig generally recognizes the Fc fragment only, in an EIA both Fab and IgG from the same serum can be used in different layers without interference. Fab fragments have also advantages in EIH since they penetrate better the tissues and eliminate non-specific adsorption by Fc receptors if present. The major disadvantage of Fab fragments is a loss of avidity (Section 8.5).

Ig often are conveniently cleaved into Fab and Fc fragments due to sensitivity of their hinge regions to proteolytic attack. Enzymes most often employed are pepsin or papain (see Fig. 6.3). Various Ig and even their subclasses differ greatly in their sensitivity to proteolytic digestion. The inability, in most cases, of the enzymes to degrade Ig at multiple sites is thought to be due to the unique conformation of Ig (Section 6.1.4). Incubation periods of different IgG with various proteases are given in Table 7.3.

7.5.1. Standard proteolytic cleavage methods

7.5.1.1. Papain

Papain (2 × crystallized; Sigma) is dissolved

TABLE 7.3
Incubation periods (in hours) required for digestion of IgG

IgG	Papain	Pepsin	Trypsin
Human			
IgG1	4	24	48–72
IgG2	48[a]	6	48–72
IgG3	4	1	48–72
IgG4	24[a]	2	47–72
Rabbit	24[b]	20	—
Mouse			
IgG1	27	12[c]	—
IgG2a	4	4–8[c]	—
IgG2b	4	—[c]	—
IgG3	—	15 min[c]	—
Bovine	48[a]	—	—
Sheep	48[a]	48[a]	1
Horse	48[a]	—	—

[a] Rather resistant.
[b] Subpopulations are quite resistant.
[c] IgG1 should be digested at pH 4.2; IgG of the other subclasses at higher pH (4.5); however, some F(ab')$_2$ will be digested; IgG2b is completely degraded in 15–30 min (no immunologic reactivity left).

(10 mg/ml) in 200 mM sodium phosphate buffer, pH 7.4, containing 2 mM EDTA and 10 mM cysteine. Enzyme solution is added to the protein in the same buffer (1 mg/100 mg protein) and gently shaken for 4–48 h at 37°C. The reaction is stopped by adding iodo-acetic acid (recrystallized from ether prior to use) to 10 mM. The digest is then dialyzed against the appropriate buffer. Ig classes other than IgG are generally much more sensitive to papain, leading to the inactivation of Fab so that shorter incubation periods are required (Stanworth and Turner, 1973).

For the digestion of mouse monoclonal IgG, pilot experiments are required since a given monoclonal antibody may react differently than polyclonal IgG. IgG2 antibodies are very sensitive to papain, whereas IgG1 is quite resistant. Papain is pre-activated with 50 mM cysteine in 100 mM acetate buffer, pH 5.5, in the presence of 3 mM EDTA for 30 min at 37°C and passed through a Sephadex G-25 column, pre-equilibrated with acetate buffer containing EDTA, to remove the cysteine. The digestion of IgG1 is then performed without cysteine (i.e. 100 mM acetate, pH 5.5, and 3 mM EDTA) at an IgG1/activated enzyme ratio of 20, for 27 h at 37°C. A new fresh aliquot of activated papain is added after 18 h (papain should always be inactivated after the digestion). At this point it is useful to separate F(ab')$_2$ from Fc by chromatography on DEAE-Sephacel. The digest equilibrated with 5 mM Tris–HCl buffer, pH 7.5, is applied to the ion-exchanger equilibrated with the same buffer. Fc is adsorbed whereas F(ab')$_2$ passes freely. Fab' is subsequently prepared from F(ab')$_2$ by reduction with 10 mM cysteine for 1 h at 37°C. Reoxidation is usually very slow. Non-activated papain produces a mixture of F(ab')$_2$ and Fab' (Parham et al., 1982).

7.5.1.2. Pepsin   Pepsin (2 × crystallized; Worthington) is dis-solved (10 mg/ml) in 200 mM sodium acetate buffer, pH 4.7, and added to the protein in the same buffer (protein/enzyme ratio of 100) for 1–48 h at 37°C. For the digestion of mouse IgG2a, it is necessary to use more enzyme (ratio of 33) during 48 h (Lamoyi and Nisonoff, 1983). IgG3 is digested only for 15 min, whereas

IgG1 is digested at a lower pH (4.2) for about 12 h. Human IgM and IgG are incubated for 24 h. The reaction is stopped by raising the pH to 7.5 with 1 M Tris.

Digestion of mouse, rabbit or human IgG with pepsin yields $F(ab')_2$ fragments (Fig. 6.3) which can be reduced to Fab' fragments. The sample is dialyzed against 550 mM Tris–HCl buffer, pH 7.8, degassed in vacuum; 2-ME is added to 10 mM and incubated for 1 h at 37°C. Subsequently, the pH is lowered to 6.5 and 10 mM N-ethylmaleimide is added to alkylate free thiol groups (if not used for conjugation). The temperature is lowered to 0°C and the Fab' solution dialyzed against the appropriate buffer.

Fc is digested to smaller fragments due to the partial disruption of the three-dimensional structure at the pH used.

7.5.1.3. Trypsin   Trypsin yields the same type of fragments as papain. These fragments are, therefore, designated as Fab(t) and Fc(t). Trypsin is the best protease for sheep IgG whereas rabbit IgG is resistant (Davies et al., 1978).

Porcine trypsin (crystallized, type IX; Sigma) with an activity of about 12000 BAEE units/mg protein is dissolved at a concentration of 2 mg/ml in 100 mM Tris–HCl buffer, pH 7.8, containing 20 mM $CaCl_2$ and added to the Ig at a ratio of 200 (protein/enzyme). For sheep IgG, 1 h of incubation at 37°C suffices to obtain complete digestion, whereas for human IgG a double concentration of enzyme and addition of fresh trypsin at several intervals during a 2-h incubation is advised. Human IgM requires an 18-h incubation. Mouse IgM which has a different arrangement of disulfide bonds than human IgM (Milstein et al., 1975) is digested under slightly different conditions (Matthew and Reichardt, 1982) and yields 200 kDa fragments. The buffer contains 50 mM Tris–HCl, pH 8.0, 150 mM NaCl and 20 mM $CaCl_2$ (ratio IgM/trypsin is 100). After digestion for 5 h at 37°C, 10 mM 2-ME is added and the reaction is stopped (see below). Free SH groups are blocked with 60 mM iodoacetamide at room temperature for 10 min. Iodoacetamide (stored in dark) should be recrystallized from distilled water to remove iodine (yellow color). Digestion with trypsin is stopped by the addition of 1 mM phenyl methylsulphonyl fluoride or 0.1 mg/ml soybean trypsin inhibitor.

7.5.2. Purification of Fab and Fab′ fragments

Fab and Fab′ fragments may be purified by the various methods given in Section 7.1. The most popular techniques are chromatography on CM- or DEAE-cellulose, gel filtration (Tijssen and Kurstak, 1974) and affinity chromatography.

DEAE ion-exchangers in 5 mM sodium phosphate buffer, pH 8.0, will either let the Fab pass or retain it lightly, so that the first protein to be desorbed by increasing the NaCl concentration in the buffer will be Fab.

SpA-Sepharose can also be convenient for the purification of the Fab fragment of IgG. Since this adsorbent retains Fc fragments and complete IgG, the Fab fraction can be recovered free of complete antibody.

Purity of the fragments is best checked with SDS–PAGE (Section 16.1.1).

Kinetics and nature of antibody–antigen interactions

The crucial step in immunoassays is the specific recognition of the antigen by the antibody. An understanding of the physicochemical and mathematical basis of this interaction and the way it is influenced by external factors is of paramount significance for the quality of the immunoassays.

8.1. Physicochemical basis of antibody–antigen interaction

The repulsive and attractive forces involved in antibody–antigen interactions are the same as for other non-covalent protein–protein interactions. Four types of forces promote binding: (i) electrostatic interactions; (ii) dispersion forces; (iii) hydrogen bonds; and, (iv) hydrophobic interactions. A lack of complementarity (steric factor) between the antigen and antibody binding sites is important among the repulsive forces and prevents a close approach of the two molecules necessary for the weak, attractive forces to be effective. The dependence of this repulsive force on distance has been estimated as ranging from the inverse 12th power to the inverse 9th power for various molecules (Lifson, 1972). Due to the virtually unlimited variety in the composition of the paratope, numerous different physical forces, as well as complementarities of shape, are possible, resulting in a wide range of affinities and cross-reactivity strengths.

Hydrophobic interactions are a major driving force for the antibody–antigen reaction and are based on repulsion of water by non-polar groups rather than on attraction of molecules (Tanford, 1978). The water molecules squeezed from the binding site gain entropy. The change of the microenvironment between the two surfaces in close apposition decreases the local dielectric constant and enhances the tightness of electrostatic or ionic binding, since water molecules no longer compete with the latter.

Attractive interactions between non-polar residues of the antibody and the antigen are due to dispersion forces (transient mutual perturbation in electron clouds between two residues results in oscillating dipoles). This interactive force decreases with the inverse 7th power of the intermolecular distance until a certain minimum distance (the so-called van der Waals contact distance of about 0.3 to 0.4 nm). Two important characteristics of these forces are that they act, for practical purposes, over small distances only, and their additivity, i.e., the force between two large sites equals the sum of all interactions. A single van der Waals bond accounts for a decrease of only about 4 kJ/mol, which is just slightly more than the average thermal energy of molecules at room temperature (2.5 kJ/mol).

Electrostatic interactions are usually not dominant in antibody–antigen complexes (Karush, 1962; Nisonoff et al., 1975). These forces are inversely proportional to the second power of the intermolecular distance and to the dielectric constant which decreases drastically when water molecules are squeezed out. Therefore, complementarity around the bond, which determines the degree of water elimination, is directly related to the energy gain. The level of ionization depends on the pH of the immediate environment. Hydrogen bonding is primarily exothermic and thus driven to completion by reduced temperatures (Le Chatelier's principle). Consequently, antigen–antibody interactions for which hydrogen bonding is important are more stable at lower temperatures ('cold antibodies').

Several conclusions may be drawn from these considerations. A high affinity of the antibody for the antigen is given by a multitude of weak interactions which require a close fit. The release of energy of 4 kJ/mol of a typical van der Waals bond results in a 5-fold increase in affinity. The high degree of complementarity required to avoid strong repulsive forces and to obtain many (weak) interactions forms, therefore, the basis of antibody discrimination. Electrostatic interactions increase significantly the affinity (about 100 to 10000 times for one bond) but are relatively more effective at longer distances, since their decrease is proportional only to the square root of the distance. Thus, non-specific interactions of antibodies with other macromolecules are often electrostatic.

An effective method, still very rarely used in EIA (Sections 14.5.2 and 17.3.4.3.2.2), is to reduce these non-specific interactions by increasing the ionic strength of the medium. Charges taking part in non-specific interactions are then shielded by the ions present. The chemical nature of a small hapten may, in contrast to that of large antigens, suggest the type of interaction it will form with its corresponding antibody (Freedman et al., 1968; Nisonoff et al., 1975). This can be taken into consideration to optimize the antibody–antigen reaction.

As expected, the reaction of the hapten with the antibody has a stabilizing effect on the latter, since the N-terminals of the chains are no longer separated by a cleft, as in the free antibody, but held together by the hapten (Zavodsky et al., 1981).

8.2. Influence of pH, ionic strength, temperature, and organic solvents on the stability of the antigen–antibody complex

It is difficult to predict a priori the optimum conditions for antigen–antibody interactions (or dissociation of the antigen–antibody complex) since the forces holding these complexes together are quite heterogeneous. Particularly ionic antibody–ligand interactions vary considerably with pH and are severely disrupted outside the pH 6–8 range (Hughes-Jones et al., 1964). For example, the binding of p-aminoazobenzoate by its antibody decreases by lowering the pH from 7 to 4 or by increasing the ionic strength from 0.1 to 1 (Eisen, 1980).

Chaotropic ions (SCN$^-$, I$^-$, Br$^-$ and Cl$^-$) distort, particularly at higher concentrations, the three-dimensional structure leading to disruption of the antibody–antigen interacting surfaces (Dandliker et al., 1967; Edgington, 1971).

Organic solvents may also disrupt interactions and are sometimes used to elute 'warm antibodies' (Chan-Shu and Blair, 1979). Organic acids of low surface tension (propionic acid, acetic acid) disrupt van der Waals bonds and dissociate antibody–antigen complexes quite efficiently.

Temperature influences are strong on 'cold antibodies' which may be eluted from the complexes at 37°C (Weiner, 1957). In other cases, the rate of complex formation is increased at 37°C (Tijssen et al., 1982). The standard use of 37°C in EIA may, therefore, not be universally suited. In fact, increasing the temperature to 37°C may just be a habit of serologists, since only precipitation, agglutination and complement fixation are accelerated none of which being essential in EIA. For homogeneous, monoclonal antibodies a more pronounced optimum in ionic conditions and temperature can be expected than for polyclonal antisera for which the use of a pH near neutrality and an ionic strength of 0.15 is nearly always safe.

The stability of the various domains of Ig is, despite their structural resemblance, quite often dissimilar. Fab fragments and light chains resist conformational changes down to pH 2.0, whereas the conformation of the Fc portion deteriorates below pH 3.9 (Abaturov et al., 1969; Day, 1972). This property can be used to excellent advantage in EIA (Chapter 13).

8.3. Measurement of the affinity of antibodies

Affinity determines the detectability (increases with affinity) and the specificity (increases with greater differences in affinity of antibodies for specific and non-specific antigen). This pivotal element of EIA must be understood for meaningful assay designs. Affinity can be expressed both in terms of reaction kinetics and thermodynamics.

The equilibrium between antibody (Ab), antigen (Ag) and immune complexes (Ab–Ag) may be expressed as:

$$\text{Ab} + \text{Ag} \underset{k_d}{\overset{k_a}{\rightleftharpoons}} \text{Ab–Ag} \tag{1}$$

where k_a and k_d represent the association and dissociation rate constants. The equilibrium (affinity) constant, K, may be established by measuring the respective concentrations at equilibrium, according to the law of mass action:

$$k_a[\text{Ab}][\text{Ag}] = k_d[\text{Ab–Ag}] \quad \text{and} \tag{2}$$

$$K = \frac{k_a}{k_d} = \frac{[\text{Ab–Ag}]}{[\text{Ab}][\text{Ag}]} \tag{3}$$

Thermodynamically, the affinity constant K is determined by the change of the total free energy during the complex formation in standard conditions, i.e., at steady-state concentrations of 1 M according to the expression:

$$\Delta F^0 = -RT \ln K \tag{4}$$

where R is the gas constant (8.3 J/mol·degree) and T the absolute temperature. Thus, a release of 40 kJ/mole at room temperature (293 K) corresponds to an affinity constant of $1.35 \times 10^7 \text{ M}^{-1}$. The presence of a single charged group, which typically increases the standard free energy by 15 kJ/mole, increases the affinity more than 400 times. Such groups are, therefore, often the immunodominant residues in the determinant.

If, (i) the total concentration of antibody is M and the valence of the antibody n (the concentration of antibody binding sites being nM); and, (ii) r represents the molar ratio of bound hapten/antibody, then:

$$r = \frac{[\text{Ag}]_{\text{bound}}}{[\text{Ab}]_{\text{total}}} = \frac{[\text{Ag}]_{\text{bound}}}{M} \quad \text{or} \quad [\text{Ag}]_{\text{bound}} = rM \tag{5}$$

since [free antibody sites] = [total sites] − [occupied sites]:

$$[Ab]_{sites} = nM - rM = M(n-r) \qquad (6)$$

Let the concentration of free hapten be c, then according to eqs. 3, 5, and 6:

$$K = \frac{[Ab\text{–}Ag]}{[Ab][Ag]} = \frac{[Ag]_{bound}}{[Ab]_{sites}[Ag]} = \frac{rM}{M(n-r)c} \text{ or } \frac{r}{c} = nK - rK \quad (7)$$

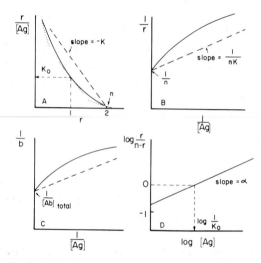

Fig. 8.1. Scatchard (A), Langmuir (B and C) and Sips (D) forms of the Law of Mass Action for antibody–antigen interactions. The abbreviations and the derivation of the equations are given in Section 8.3. Polyclonal sera yield curved lines in A, B and C, whereas the interrupted lines represent homogeneous interaction. In the Scatchard (1949) plot, three of the different populations of antibodies are indicated by dotted lines: low affinity (K is small) at $r = 2$, intermediate ('average') affinity, K_0 at $r = 1$ and high affinity at small r. The Langmuir (1918) adsorption isotherm can be graphically presented if the total amount of antibody is known (B) or not (C). In the latter case b represents bound antibody (Ab_{bound}) and n/r in eq. 9 is substituted by Ab_{total}/Ab_{bound} to obtain:

$$\frac{1}{b} = \frac{1}{[Ab]_{total} \cdot K \cdot [Ag]} + \frac{1}{[Ab]_{total}}$$

The value for n, however, cannot be obtained from this plot. The Sips (1949) equation (eq. 11) takes the heterogeneity of the polyclonal antiserum into consideration (heterogeneity index is α).

Plotting r/c against r yields the Scatchard plot, which is a straight line for monoclonal antibodies, but a curved line with polyclonal antisera (Fig. 8.1). This curvature with multivalent acceptors and divalent ligands is not necessarily due to population heterogeneity (Calvert et al., 1979). In order to characterize the affinity of polyclonal sera, a so-called intrinsic affinity constant, K_o, is determined which is the affinity measured when half the antibody binding sites are filled. In this case, [Ab–Ag] = [Ab]$_{total}$ for divalent antibodies ($n = 2$) and monovalent antigens ($r = 1$ and $K_o = 1/c$) i.e. the intrinsic affinity constant can be defined as the reciprocal of the free hapten concentration at equilibrium when half the binding sites of the divalent antibody are occupied. IgM, in contrast, has a theoretical valence of 10, but in practice this is mostly 5, so that $K_o = 1/4c$.

The Langmuir plot (Fig. 8.1) is a variant of the Scatchard plot and can be derived from eq. 7:

$$\frac{1}{r} = \frac{1}{n} \cdot \frac{1}{K} \cdot \frac{1}{c} + \frac{1}{n} \tag{8}$$

Not surprisingly, this plot suffers from the same shortcomings as the Scatchard plot with polyclonal sera which are heterogeneous with respect to affinities. It is, therefore, difficult to obtain precisely the total amount of antibody present.

A method used frequently to express heterogeneity of the antibody population of a serum is the Sips plot. From eq. 7 (cf. eqs. 14–16) it follows that:

$$\frac{r}{n} = \frac{cK}{1 + cK} \tag{9}$$

According to a derivation by Sips (1949) which is mathematically complex, this may be rewritten, in case of normal distribution of affinities as:

$$\frac{r}{n} = \frac{cK^\alpha}{1 + cK^\alpha} \tag{10}$$

where α is the so-called heterogeneity index of the various affinities (between 0 and 1, 1 for monoclonal antibodies). After rearrangement, eq. 10 becomes:

$$\log \frac{r}{n-r} = \alpha \, (\log K + \log c) \tag{11}$$

The Sips graphic representation is then obtained by plotting log $r/(n-r)$ against log c (Fig. 8.1). The intrinsic affinity constant $K_o = 1/c$ is obtained when log $r/(n-r) = 0$, and the heterogeneity index equals the slope. An inherent drawback of this procedure is the mathematical insensitivity of a double log plot. Assuming normal distribution (with peak at K_o), 75% of the affinities would be scattered over a range between 0.16 K_o and 6 K_o (Nisonoff et al., 1975).

Gaussian or Sipsian distribution functions do not describe accurately polyclonal sera (Siskind, 1973) which may show skewed, bimodal or even discontinuous distributions. A partial solution to this problem is the analysis of a restricted region of the binding curve, but this does not allow an assessment of heterogeneity. Steensgaard et al. (1980) used a computer model for the simulation of the antibody–antigen interaction (using the Weibull distribution discussed in the annex of their paper) and found that antigenic valence may have a considerable influence, making it impossible to distinguish between the effects of affinity heterogeneity and of complex formation. Table 8.1 gives some recent approaches to determine the binding constant.

8.4. Kinetics of antibody–antigen interactions

Temperature-jump relaxation and the stopped-flow methods are suitable to follow the concentration changes over extremely short time intervals. Such studies have indicated that immune reaction kinetics resemble other biological systems in which ligands are bound to proteins (Weber, 1975) in that the binding strength of small molecules is largely dictated by the k_d constant. The association rate constants k_a, are very similar for various antibody–antigen systems, i.e., for

TABLE 8.1
Determination of affinities and their ranking

Ranking of affinities
The method of van Heyningen et al. (1983), employed earlier with success by Odell et al. (1969), is analogous to Michaelis–Menten kinetics (Section 9; Fig. 9.1). A rectangular hyperbola is obtained by replacing enzyme activity by antigen-antibody complex concentration, the V_{max} by the maximum complex concentration, the K_m by the affinity constant and [S] by the antibody concentration. Labeled antigen concentration is kept constant while the antibody concentrations are varied. Maximum binding is observed at high antibody concentrations and 50% binding is indicative of the affinity. The lower the antibody concentration to achieve 50% binding, the higher the avidity. This method is useful for monoclonal antibodies.

Relative antibody affinities (avidities)
Quantitative immunoelectrophoresis (Birkmeyer et al., 1981) and reverse quantitative immunoelectrophoresis (Birkmeyer et al., 1982) allow the determination of average affinity of different antibody populations for an antigen. Plots of rocket area vs. the amount of antibody applied yield straight lines, the slope of which is indicative of affinity (steeper if the affinity is higher). Actual values of K_a are not obtained. Relative avidity indices can also be obtained with the test of Farr (1958) (Griswold and Nelson, 1984).

Classical methods
In these methods (e.g., Ehrlich et al., 1982) antibody concentrations are, in contrast to the ranking method, kept constant (methods in Section 8.3).

many haptens around 10^7–10^8, which are only slightly below the diffusion rate and depend directly on, but cannot be faster than, the diffusion-controlled encounter of an antigen with its antibody. The initial rate for protein antigens can be about 100 times lower, due to their slower diffusion. In contrast, k_d can vary from around 10^{-4} for high affinity antibodies to 10^3 for low-affinity antibodies, depending on the closeness of fit (Steward, 1977). The half-life ($t_{1/2}$) of the interaction is directly related to k_d since the rate of dissociation can be expressed as:

$$\frac{d[Ab-Ag]}{dt} = -k_d[Ab-Ag] \quad \text{or} \quad \frac{d[Ab-Ag]}{[Ab-Ag]} = -k_d \cdot dt \qquad (12)$$

which after integration yields:

$$-\ln \frac{[Ab-Ag]_t}{[Ab-Ag]_{t(0)}} = k_d[t - t(0)] \quad \text{or} \quad \ln 0.5 = k_d \cdot t_{1/2} \tag{13}$$

Therefore, $t_{1/2} = 0.693/k_d$ and for a high-affinity antibody ($K = 10^9$ M^{-1} with a typical k_a of 2×10^7 M^{-1} sec^{-1}), the k_d would be 0.02 sec^{-1} (from eq. 3) and the half-life 35 sec (eq. 13). For a low-affinity antibody ($K = 10^5$ M^{-1}) the half-life would be about 0.003 sec.

8.5. Concept of avidity and its importance in enzyme immunoassays

The terms affinity and avidity are frequently confused in the immunological literature. Affinity is a thermodynamic measurement of the strength of the non-covalent interaction between one site of the antibody and of the antigen. In contrast, avidity is an operational term expresssing the ability of an antiserum to bind antigens and depends, therefore, not only on affinity but also on multivalency and other non-specific factors. The half-life of an antibody–antigen interaction is, in general, short and results in a continuous association–dissociation process during which antibody and antigen may become separated. However, in case of multivalency, the multiple bonds do not separate synchronously, making it less likely that the complex becomes separated (Fig. 8.2). It is common that the multivalent IgM has an avidity of 10^2–10^4 times higher than the affinity of the isolated sites (its Fab fragments).

Avidity may also be an important characteristic of polyclonal antisera, since they generally contain antibodies against all determinants of a given antigen. These subpopulations of antibodies contribute to avidity, which would not be obtained with monoclonal antibodies reacting with unique antigenic determinants (Fig. 8.2). Mixing of monoclonal antibodies against two or more different determinants on the same antigen may result in an affinity bonus (Ehrlich et al., 1982). This 'bonus effect' (avidity) decreases with increasing affinity constants.

I - Polyclonal antibodies :

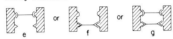

II - Monoclonal antibody :

III - Mixing monoclonal antibodies :

IV - Multiple identical determinants on antigen :

Fig. 8.2. Concept of avidity. Antigens with, e.g., 2 epitopes react with different antibodies of a polyclonal antiserum (I, a and b). However, half-life may often be rather short (few seconds or a fraction of this; Section 8.4) resulting in a continuous dissociation–association process. A second antibody (I, c) on the same antigen keeps the complex intact since dissociation from the two antibodies will not occur at exactly the same moment. This affinity bonus is not obtained with monoclonal antibodies (II), unless two appropriately chosen monoclonal antibodies are mixed (III; mixture of monoclonal antibodies to different epitopes does not necessarily lead to an affinity bonus, e.g. if epitopes are located on opposite sites of the antigen) or if multiple epitopes are present on the antigen (IV).

TABLE 8.2

Influence of antibody affinity on determination of hapten concentration by a solid-phase EIA[a]

Days after last boost	Affinity constant ($\times 10^{-6}$)			Standard EIA (μg/ml)	Amplified EIA (μg/ml)
	$K_{25\%}$	$K_{75\%}$	$K_{50\%}$		
10	22	0.55	2.56	trace	45
20	33	0.43	2.9	3.85	102
40	312	9.5	78.6	16.5	132
56[b]	340	30.5	109	3575	7051

[a] Results from Butler et al. (1978). Values for the EIA are based on a standard rat–anti DNP pool (= 0.82 mg/ml) which was measured by the quantitative precipitin assay. Amplified EIA is an EIA test in which immunologically conjugated enzyme is used (see Section 14.2.1.3).

[b] The animal was boosted again at day 49.

The importance of affinity in heterogeneous (solid-phase) EIA is widely underestimated and is best illustrated by an example (Table 8.2) with antisera from the same animal but taken at different intervals (reflecting affinity maturation).

The quantity of antibody which can be attached to the wall of a well of a microtitre plate is limited by the surface of the well and the fraction of antibodies present in the immunoglobulin preparation. Assuming a maximum adsorption of 1.5 ng/mm^2 and an average molecular weight of 150000 (IgG), the maximum attainable concentration of IgG attached to the wall is about 10^{-7} M using monoclonal antibodies, but for affinity-purified antibodies, hyperimmune antisera and postinfection sera, typically 3, 10, and 100 times less would be present, respectively. The fraction of antigen bound by the solid-phase antibody can be calculated with the law of mass action (eq. 3):

$$\frac{[Ab]}{[Ab-Ag]} = \frac{1}{K[Ag]} \tag{14}$$

By adding $[Ab-Ag]/[Ab-Ag]$ and $K[Ag]/K[Ag]$ to the left and right term, respectively, the following expression is obtained:

$$\frac{[Ab-Ag] + [Ab]}{[Ab-Ag]} = \frac{1 + K[Ag]}{K[Ag]} \tag{15}$$

Since $[Ab] + [Ab-Ag] = [Ab]_{total}$, the fraction of antibody sites occupied (b) can be expressed as:

$$b = \frac{[Ab-Ag]}{[Ab]_{total}} = \frac{K[Ag]}{1 + K[Ag]} \tag{16}$$

From eq. 16, which has the form of a Langmuir adsorption isotherm, the amount of bound antigen can be calculated. For simplicity, in the following example all molecules are considered monovalent. The concentration of antigen required to reach a certain degree of saturation of the antibodies (if $K = 10^7$ M^{-1}) can be calculated: if total antibody concentration is 10^{-7} M, at 80% saturation [Ab–Ag] $= 0.8 \times 10^{-7}$ M and [Ab] $= 0.2 \times 10^{-7}$. These values can be substituted into eq. 16 and yield $[Ag] = 4.0 \times 10^{-7}$ M. The total concentration of antigen required is, therefore, 4.8×10^{-7} M. It is evident from Table 8.3 that a large excess of antigen is required to obtain a reasonable saturation of the antibody if $K[Ab]_{total} < 1$.

Removing free antigen during the washing steps dissociates the Ab–Ag complex in order to re-establish the equilibrium as dictated by the K value. This will affect both sides of eq. 16. Calculations of the amount of antigen remaining bound after each washing (assuming that equilibrium had been reached each time) for antibodies with different K values (sites initially saturated for 50, and 95%, respectively) are represented in Fig. 8.3. In each subsequent washing step, b changes since $[Ab]$ increases.

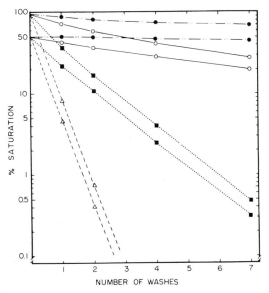

Fig. 8.3. The effect of washes on the dissociation of immune complexes for antibodies with different affinities and with different initial saturations (Table 8.3). The antibody (immobilized on the solid phase) concentration is 10^{-7} M (fairly typical for microtitre plates). Low affinities result in rapid dissociation and the activity measured is more representative for affinity than initial antigen concentration. With high affinities, however, activities are representative for concentrations. $K = 10^9 (-\cdots-), 10^8 (-), 10^7 (\cdots\cdots), 10^6 \, M^{-1} (---)$.

TABLE 8.3

The concentration of antigen required to saturate antibody immobilized in a well of a microtitre plate (10^{-7} M) and the dependence on the K of the reaction (concentrations in M $\times 10^7$)

Saturation level (%)	[Ab–Ag]	[Ag]	[Ag]$_{total}$ required if		
			$K = 10^6$	$K = 10^7$	$K = 10^8$
50	0.5	0.5	10.5	1.5	0.6
80	0.8	0.2	40.8	4.8	1.2
90	0.9	0.1	90.0	9.9	1.8
95	0.95	0.05	190.95	19.95	2.85

Two important conclusions can be drawn from Table 8.3 and Fig. 8.3: (i) the affinity of the antibody influences strongly the initial antigen adsorption and the stability of the complex during the washings; antibodies with a K lower than the reciprocal of their concentration yield poor results; (ii) an increasingly larger excess of antigen is required to saturate antibodies to higher levels (as indicated by the percentage of complex remaining). For low-affinity antibodies, the response in EIA is determined predominantly by the avidity for low-affinity antibodies, whereas at high avidity responses reflect more the antigen concentration in the initial incubation step. The assumption that equilibrium is reached during each washing is generally not the case, particularly with high-affinity antibodies. However, the considerable elution of low-affinity antibodies is compounded by their short half-life and, consequently, equilibrium is attained faster for lower-affinity antibodies. It is, therefore, imperative to use high-affinity antibodies in solid-phase EIA or EIH.

Cross-reacting antigens (or antibodies) with lower affinities, elute more rapidly through repeated washings than the specific antigen (or antibody). Successive washings can, therefore, be beneficial for the elimination of cross-reacting immunoreactants.

8.6. Cross-reactivity, specificity and multispecificity in immunoassays

Immunoassays demonstrated a fundamental ambiguity in the concepts of cross-reactivity, or its complement, specificity, with important consequences. Antibodies having the ability to bind structurally related epitopes are named polyfunctional antibodies (Richards et al., 1975). The strength of their fit is restricted to an increasingly limited number of haptens. Ig produced by myeloma clones were tested with panels of haptens (Varga et al., 1974) and a relatively high percentage of these proteins showed an affinity, though often low, for randomly chosen haptens. Polyfunctional antibodies have been reported on numerous occasions (e.g., Streefkerk et al., 1979). The term multispecificity is used for antibodies with reactivity towards structurally very different antigens. The first concept of cross-reactivity can be based on the binding of structurally different determinants by the same antibody. The second concept of cross-reactivity involved the existence of common epitope(s) on different antigens.

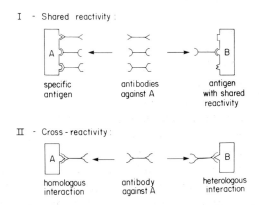

Fig. 8.4. Concepts of shared (I) and cross-reactivity (II). Two antigens (A and B) may have one or more identical epitopes and a subpopulation of antibodies from a polyclonal antiserum will react equally with both antigens (shared reactivity). If monoclonal antibodies against the common epitope were used, it would not be possible to distinguish A and B. In cross-reactivity, antibodies reactive with the homologous antigen are also reactive with different epitopes (generally less fit thus lower affinity).

In contrast to the first, this cross-reactivity is not based on differences in affinity and the term 'shared reactivity' should be used. These two phenomena are schematically represented in Fig. 8.4.

A common experimental design in immunoassays is the displacement of a labeled antigen from the complex by increasing the concentration of competing non-labeled antigen. Such displacement curves reveal the difference in cross-reactivity and shared reactivity (also called cross-reactivity in the literature), as illustrated in Fig. 8.5. Cross-reactivity with non-specific molecules is almost always of lower affinity. The labeled specific ligand is, therefore, displaced only with high concentrations of the competitor, though the displacement curve is similar to that of the specific antigen. The dose of the competitor yielding 50% displacement is roughly inversely proportional to the binding affinities, though several corrections have been made to assess more accurately this relationship (Cheng and Prusoff, 1973; Munson and Rodbard, 1980). In contrast, antigens with shared reactivity compete only for the antibodies reacting with the common epitope (one of three antibodies in Fig. 8.4,I) and, therefore, lower

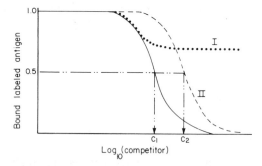

Fig. 8.5. Effect of antigens with shared (I) or cross-reactivity (II) on the displacement of labeled, bound antigen from the immune complex. Non-labeled specific antigen will displace 50% of the label at a concentration of C_1. A cross-reacting antigen generally has a lower affinity and a higher concentration (C_2) is required to displace 50% of the labeled antigen. In contrast, antigen with shared reactivity will have the same affinity for a subpopulation of the antibodies and displace the labeled antigen in the immune complex at the same concentrations as the specific non-labeled antigen but only to a certain limit (I) (i.e., only for antibodies for the common epitope).

the bound labeled antigen to a certain level. Berzofsky and Schechter (1981) developed a mathematical method to analyze such binding curves.

The concept of specificity is complementary to the concept of cross-reactivity and can also be subdivided into two types. Specificity, in the sense of opposing cross-reactivity, is determined by the ratio of the respective affinity constants. An antibody is considered highly specific when the ratio of its affinity constant for the specific and cross-reacting antigen is 1000; a 10-fold difference is not considered specific. A polyclonal antiserum may be highly specific, without being uniform for all subpopulations of antibodies. The spectra of affinities of the various antibodies generated may be quite different and each may have various degrees of cross-reactivity with other antigens (different from the immunogen). These cross-reacting antigens are different for the various antibodies so that the combined cross-reactivity is diluted out. This phenomenon confers thus a high specificity to a polyclonal antiserum, but the effects of this 'specificity bonus' are lost by the cloning in the hybridoma production. On the other hand, problems with shared reactivity can generally be avoided with monoclonal antibodies by the judicious selection against the appropriate epitope.

8.7. Kinetics of enzyme immunoassay

8.7.1. Kinetics of AM-type enzyme immunoassays

Modulation of the activity response by competing, unlabeled immunoreactants may be achieved by two approaches: (i) the labeled and unlabeled ligand compete simultaneously for the available binding sites of the antibodies (equilibrium techniques); and, (ii) the unlabeled ligand (test or calibration sample) is reacted first with the available binding sites and the number of occupied binding sites is estimated by the subsequent addition of the labeled reactant (sequential saturation). These methods are conceptually different and it is necessary to outline their theoretical differences in order to demonstrate the rationale of their applicability. Many of the homogeneous AM-type EIA techniques are based on sequential saturation.

8.7.1.1. Equilibrium techniques in saturation analysis   These techniques rely on the partial saturation of the antibody (Ab) (or other binding agent) by the test substance (H) and on its competition with the labeled substance (L, indicator) for the available sites.

The reaction is expressed as:

$$
\begin{array}{c}
K_{\mathrm{H}} \\
\mathrm{H} + \mathrm{Ab} \rightleftharpoons \mathrm{Ab\text{-}H} \\
+ \\
\mathrm{L} \\
\updownarrow\ K_{\mathrm{L}} \\
\mathrm{Ab\text{-}L}
\end{array}
$$

in which the affinity constants K_{H} and K_{L} (in M^{-1}) can be expressed as $K_{\mathrm{H}} = k_{\mathrm{a,1}}/k_{\mathrm{d,1}}$ and $K_{\mathrm{L}} = k_{\mathrm{a,2}}/k_{\mathrm{d,2}}$, i.e., as the ratios of the corresponding association and dissociation rate constants. For this reaction two differential equations can be written:

$$\frac{d[\mathrm{Ab\text{-}H}]}{dt} = k_{\mathrm{a,1}}[\mathrm{Ab}][\mathrm{H}] - k_{\mathrm{d,1}}[\mathrm{Ab\text{-}H}] \qquad (17)$$

and

$$\frac{d[\mathrm{Ab\text{-}L}]}{dt} = k_{\mathrm{a,2}}[\mathrm{Ab}][\mathrm{L}] - k_{\mathrm{d,2}}[\mathrm{Ab\text{-}L}] \qquad (18)$$

and the total concentrations of the antibody (*ab*), hapten (*h*) and labeled hapten (*l*), respectively, can be expressed with the conservation equations:

$$ab = [\mathrm{Ab}] + [\mathrm{Ab\text{-}H}] + [\mathrm{Ab\text{-}L}] \qquad (19)$$
$$h = [\mathrm{H}] + [\mathrm{Ab\text{-}H}] \qquad (20)$$
$$l = [\mathrm{L}] + [\mathrm{Ab\text{-}L}] \qquad (21)$$

in the units of $1/K$ (thus dimensions of ab, h, and l are M).

When $K_H = K_L$ the equilibrium reaction is defined by the simple quadratic equation (Ekins et al., 1968):

$$R^2 + R(1 + K \cdot h + K \cdot l - K \cdot ab) - K \cdot ab = 0 \qquad (22)$$

whereas in the case when $K_H \neq K_L$, this equation becomes:

$$R^2 + R(1 + K_L \cdot l - K_L \cdot ab) - K_L \cdot ab + \frac{R \cdot h \cdot K_H (R + 1)}{R(K_H/K_L) + 1} = 0 \qquad (23)$$

where R corresponds to the fraction of bound labeled ligand over free labeled ligand. Considering the simple case when $K_H = K_L$, 3 essentially different immunoassays were set up in classical RIA, though these may not be optimal (Section 15.4):

(i) a trace of labeled ligand i.e. $l \rightarrow 0$ is used and the concentration of $ab = 0.5/K$. From eq. 22 it can be calculated that this gives $R = 0.5$ (i.e., 33% bound/66% free). These were the conditions of the original RIA devised by Yalow and Berson (1959). Assays run under such conditions give the steepest dose-response curves (high sensitivity) but suffer from poor precision, leading to a much poorer detectability than theoretically possible. This method also requires the knowledge of the affinity constant to obtain the correct antibody concentration;

(ii) the concentrations are chosen as $l = 4/K$ and $ab = 3/K$, so that regardless of the value of the affinity constant, R is always 1 (Ekins et al., 1968). The labeled ligand is used at a higher concentration than in the first method; and,

(iii) a rather high concentration of antibody is used ($ab \approx 50/K$) with a slight but obligatory excess of labeled ligand ($\approx 1.5 \times ab$). This method has less detectability than the other two, but does not require as strongly, as the other methods, antibodies of high affinity due to the excess used.

Thus, in (i) the addition of H may increase saturation from about

0 to 100%, in (ii) from 66 to 100%, whereas in (iii) antibody is nearly always saturated for at least 95%. These differences in saturation levels have important implications for the dose-response curves. The changing of $l/(l+h)$, due to the addition of H, has no influence on the binding capacity in the third system, but the two other methods behave as if the binding capacity increases. The l measured is then inversely proportional to the extent by which l exceeds saturation level or binding capacity.

8.7.1.2. Sequential saturation analysis   The sequential saturation reaction can be formulated as:

$$H + Ab_0 \underset{}{\overset{K_H}{\rightleftharpoons}} Ab\text{--}H \tag{24}$$

followed by:

$$L + Ab_1 \underset{}{\overset{K_L}{\rightleftharpoons}} Ab\text{--}L \tag{25}$$

where Ab_0 is the original molar concentration of antibodies and Ab_1 is the antibody remaining free after reaction with H. Thus,

$$[Ab_1] = [Ab_0] - [Ab\text{--}H] \tag{26}$$

However, the Ab–H complex is not stable (Section 8.4), and a high-affinity of the antibody for H in the first step is desirable. Otherwise, L replaces H in the Ab–H complexes and the results resemble those of equilibrium techniques.

Theoretically an infinite incubation period would be needed to reach perfect equilibrium in the first step (incubation with H). However, in practice, conditions are chosen so as to shorten this period to reach near-perfect equilibrium. The association and dissociation constants ($k_{a,1}$ and $k_{d,1}$) are usually not known, but according to the law of mass action the higher the Ab and H concentrations, the faster Ab–H is formed. The concentration of H, however, should not exceed that of Ab. In the commercial kits (Section 14.3), the concentrations are sometimes so high that the few seconds between the sequential pipetting steps are sufficient for maximal complex formation. In the second step L is added until a sufficient amount is bound for a suitable response. However, the added L becomes immediately diluted with unbound H. During the formation of Ab–L, also some Ab–H dissociates and the free Ab reassociates with L or H depending on their relative concentrations (the dissociation rate is independent of the concentration (monomolecular process)):

$$\frac{[\text{Ab–H}]}{[\text{Ab–L}]} \neq \frac{[\text{H}]}{[\text{L}]} \quad \text{or} \quad \frac{l}{h+l} \neq \frac{ab-l}{ab-h+ab-l} \tag{27}$$

Thus, there are two processes: (i) additional binding of L or H to Ab; and, (ii) exchange of H by L or free H. If the incubation period of the second step is longer than needed to obtain quasi-equilibrium, total [Ab–L] + [Ab–H] will not change, but the ratio [Ab–L]/[Ab–H] increases. On the other hand, termination of the second incubation period before near-equilibrium is reached may markedly increase the experimental error. A computer-based analysis of a series of differential equations has been published by Rodbard et al. (1971).

A portentous aspect of the sequential saturation technique is that in contrast to equilibrium techniques greatly differing affinities (e.g., due to enzyme-labeling) become much less important. A higher affinity in one of the two steps behaves as if greater excess of the reactant had been added. This results in a steeper slope (higher sensitivity) but a shorter range. Disadvantages of this sequential technique are the limited dose range, the necessity of the exact timing of the second incubation period, the poor precision obtained at low concentrations (i.e., in terms of $1/K$) and lower specificity.

8.7.1.3. Interrelationships of commonly used mathematical methods to describe AM-type immunoassays   To detect the presence of a substance and determine its quantity, immunoassays are generally performed simultaneously on test and calibration samples. The latter serve for the construction of a standard curve. An unambiguous standard curve cannot be obtained from a few points, but with

$$Y = \frac{(h_r + l)V_f}{ab \cdot V_{ab}} + \frac{K^{-1}V_i}{ab\,V_{ab}}\left(\frac{Y}{Y-1}\right) + \frac{I}{ab\,V_{ab}} \cdot H_x$$

Basic equation (Fernandez et al , 1983)

omitting first term   omitting second term

$$Y = \frac{K^{-1}V_i}{ab\,V_{ab}}\left(\frac{Y}{Y-1}\right) + \frac{I}{ab\,V_{ab}} \cdot H_x \qquad Y = \frac{(h_r + l)V_f}{ab\,V_{ab}} + \frac{I}{ab\,V_{ab}} \cdot H_x$$

$$R = \frac{ab_{dil}}{\dfrac{h}{1+R} + \dfrac{l}{K}} \qquad\qquad \frac{B_0}{B} = \frac{i}{i_0} + 1$$

Equation of Hales and Randle (1963)

or

$$R^{-1} = \frac{h}{ab_{dil}(1+R)} + \frac{I}{K\,ab_{dil}} \qquad\qquad logit\,\frac{B}{B_0} = a - ln\,H_x$$

Equations of Ekins et al.(1968)   logit - log plot of Rodbard et al.(1968)

Fig. 8.6. Relationships of the various mathematical models used in immunoassays to the basic general equation as derived by Fernandez et al. (1983). Those used in EIA are discussed in detail in Chapter 15. Y is the ratio total activity/bound activity, h_r and l the concentration of unlabeled and labeled ligand (undiluted), respectively, V_l the volume of undiluted labeled ligand added to the mixture and V_{ab} the volume of undiluted binder added; ab the concentration of binding sites (undiluted) and ab_{dil} the concentration in the incubation mixture. V_i is the total volume of the incubation mixture, H_x the mass of ligand in the incubation mixture. R is the bound/free ratio, h the concentration of unlabeled ligand in the incubation mixture, i the concentration of the standard or unknown, i_0 the concentration of ligand contributed by the label, B bound label and B_0 bound label at zero standard concentration; a is a constant.

many standards the method becomes costly and time-consuming. To obviate these problems, theoretical and semi-empirical equations have been developed (Yalow and Berson, 1959; Hales and Randle, 1963; Ekins et al., 1968; Rodbard et al., 1968). The algebraic equivalency of these methods has not yet been investigated in depth. However, the key parameters, such as slope and intercept are stressed more in one approach than in another (Fig. 8.6; Fernandez et al., 1983). Though the theory of these methods has been developed for RIA, it equally applies to EIA and these data reduction methods are discussed in Sections 15.2.5 and 15.3. Generally it is easier to modify the experimental conditions of the assay to fit the theoretical model than to find an algorithm to fit the data, as pointed out by Rodbard (cited in Shaw et al., 1977).

The differential equations describing the reactions involved in AM-type immunoassays are rather complicated for regression analysis. They were modified by the simplification procedures of Naus et al. (1977) and Wellington (1980). These rather complex mathematical procedures serve mostly as an aid in assay development.

8.7.2. Kinetics of AA-type enzyme immunoassays

For each different AA-type EIA particular mathematical models can be devised to describe their kinetics. Such models provide a basis for the optimization of the assay conditions and the evaluation of side effects. The particular EIA discussed here (from Rodbard and Feldman, 1978) is the widely used sandwich assay (Fig. 2.5(1),also Section 14.2.2.1).

In this assay, the Ab is immobilized on the solid phase and the calibration or test sample, containing H, is added to form immobilized immune complexes, according to:

$$\text{Ab} + \text{H} \underset{k_{d,1}}{\overset{k_{a,1}}{\rightleftharpoons}} \text{Ab–H} \tag{28}$$

This incubation is followed by another washing and an incubation with enzyme-labeled antibody (Ab·E):

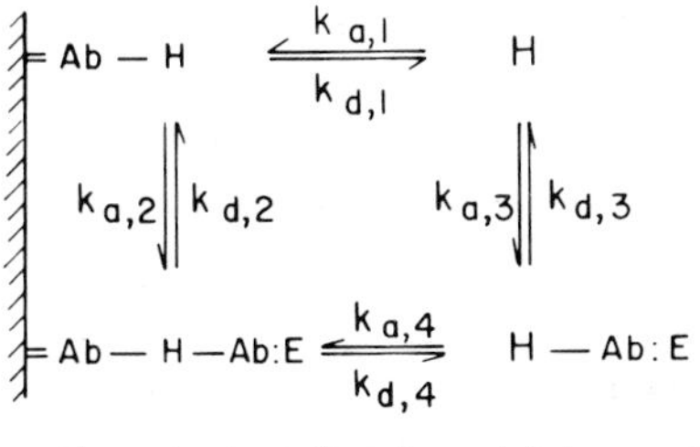

Fig. 8.7. Schemes of most important reactions in an AA-type sandwich EIA, assuming that antibodies are homogeneous with respect to affinity (monovalency of the immunoreactants is assumed).

$$Ab-H + Ab\cdot E \underset{k_{d,2}}{\overset{k_{a,2}}{\rightleftharpoons}} Ab-H-Ab\cdot E \tag{29}$$

Free Ab·E is removed by washing and the enzyme activity of the Ab–H–Ab·E complex is measured. However, this representation does not take into account the reversibility of the reactions (Section 8.4). At least two additional reactions should be considered (Fig. 8.7):

$$H + Ab\cdot E \underset{k_{d,3}}{\overset{k_{a,3}}{\rightleftharpoons}} H-Ab\cdot E \tag{30}$$

and the reaction of this complex with solid-phase Ab:

$$Ab + H-Ab\cdot E \underset{k_{d,4}}{\overset{k_{a,4}}{\rightleftharpoons}} Ab-H-Ab\cdot E \tag{31}$$

without considering other possible reactions, such as the formation of Ab–H–Ab or Ab·E–H–Ab·E and assuming that the solid-phase antibody is irreversibly immobilized. These side reactions may deteriorate the precision, sensitivity and detectability of the assay. The extent of this deterioration depends on the relative rate constants (affinity), as discussed in Section 8.4, and on the reaction time, buffer conditions and temperature (Section 8.2), as well as on the concentration of the reagents.

This reaction scheme can be described by a set of differential equations:

$$\frac{d[Ab-H-Ab]\cdot E]}{dt} = k_{a,2}[Ab-H][Ab\cdot E] + k_{a,4}[H-Ab\cdot E][Ab] -$$

$$(k_{d,2} + k_{d,4})[Ab-H-Ab\cdot E] \tag{32}$$

$$\frac{d[Ab-H]}{dt} = k_{a,1}[H][Ab] + k_{d,2}[Ab-H-Ab\cdot E] - k_{d,1}[Ab-H] -$$

$$k_{a,2}[Ab-H][Ab\cdot E] \tag{33}$$

$$\frac{d[H-Ab\cdot E]}{dt} = k_{a,3}[H][Ab.E] + k_{d,4}[[Ab-H-Ab\cdot E] -$$

$$k_{d,3}[H-Ab\cdot E] - k_{a,4}[H-Ab\cdot E][Ab] \tag{34}$$

whereas the statements of conservation of mass for the three reactants are:

$$h = [H] + [Ab–H] + [H–Ab·E] + [Ab–H–Ab·E] \qquad (35)$$
$$ab = [Ab] + [Ab–H] + [Ab–H–Ab·E] \qquad (36)$$
$$ab·e = [Ab·E] + [H–Ab·E] + [Ab–H–Ab·E] \qquad (37)$$

Evidently, the incubation period of H with the immobilized antibody should be sufficiently long to reach near-equilibrium, otherwise the assay is not used at its full potential. The ratio of bound/free antigen ($R = [Ab–H]/[H]$) can be described by eq. 22 by replacing K by K_1 which corresponds to $k_{a,1}/k_{d,1}$:

$$R^2 + R(1 + K_1·h - K_1·ab) - K_1·ab = 0 \qquad (38)$$

from eq. 38 and $R = [Ab–H]/[H]$ it can be deduced that before addition of Ab·E (when $h = [H] + [Ab–H]$):

$$[Ab–H]_o = \frac{R}{1 + R} \times h \qquad (39)$$

which describes the concentration of the immobilized immune complex ($[Ab–H]_o$) before washing, whereas the original concentration of the immobilized free antibody $[Ab]_o$, is:

$$[Ab]_o = ab - [Ab–H]_o \qquad (40)$$

Assuming a completely effective washing without dissociation of the complex, the initial free antigen concentration, $[H]_o$, at the start of the incubation with Ab·E is zero. Rodbard and Feldman (1978) solved eqs. 32–37 simultaneously, using numerical methods, with the computer system developed by Reece and Knott (1973) and confirmed the intuitive expectations that this assay performs best if the reactions are irreversible (or have high affinities) and that the side-reactions diminish the precision and detectability of the assay. The formation of the complex was found to be a monotonic increasing function of dose for any specified reaction time. Thus, the side-reactions described by eqs. 30 and 31 do not seem to be responsible for the 'high-dose hook' effect (a lower activity at increasing antigen concentrations beyond a certain limit, Section 13.2.1).

In order to extend these mathematical models to provide a theoretical basis for the high-dose hook effect, Rodbard et al. (1978) considered two mechanisms: (i) heterogeneity of the antibodies immobilized on the solid phase; and, (ii) incomplete washing after the first reaction. If two different antibodies are immobilized, Ab_A and Ab_B, they both react with the antigen, according to the equations:

$$Ab_A + H \underset{k_{d,5}}{\overset{k_{a,5}}{\rightleftharpoons}} Ab_A\text{–}H \tag{41}$$

and,

$$Ab_B + H \underset{k_{d,6}}{\overset{k_{a,6}}{\rightleftharpoons}} Ab_B\text{–}H \tag{42}$$

The complexes formed, after washing, react with Ab·E

$$Ab_A\text{–}H + Ab\cdot E \underset{k_{d,7}}{\overset{k_{a,7}}{\rightleftharpoons}} Ab_A\text{–}H\text{–}Ab\cdot E \quad \text{and,} \tag{43}$$

$$Ab_B\text{–}H + Ab\cdot E \underset{k_{d,8}}{\overset{k_{a,8}}{\rightleftharpoons}} Ab_B\text{–}H\text{–}Ab\cdot E \tag{44}$$

Some of the most important side-reactions are:

$$Ab\cdot E + H \underset{k_{d,9}}{\overset{k_{a,9}}{\rightleftharpoons}} H\text{–}Ab\cdot E \tag{45}$$

$$Ab\text{–}H\text{–}Ab\cdot E \underset{k_{d,10}}{\overset{k_{a,10}}{\rightleftharpoons}} Ab_A + H\text{–}Ab\cdot E \tag{46}$$

$$Ab_B\text{–}H\text{–}Ab\cdot E \underset{k_{d,11}}{\overset{k_{a,11}}{\rightleftharpoons}} Ab_B + H\text{–}Ab\cdot E \tag{47}$$

These reactions can be represented in a simple diagram (Fig. 8.8) in which 12 of the 14 rate constants are independent. As in Fig. 8.7 monovalency is assumed for simplicity. Differential equations

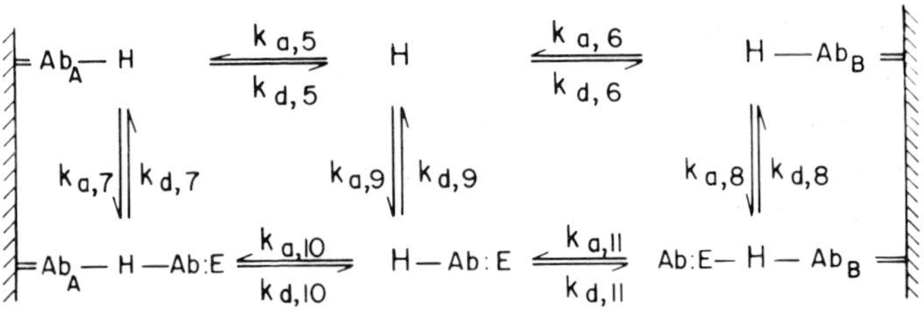

Fig. 8.8. Reactions between antigen (H), antibody–enzyme conjugate (Ab:E) and two immobilized species, Ab_A and Ab_B, which differ with respect to affinity to the antigen (Section 8.7.2).

and statements of conservation of mass for all these reactions can be derived easily. The response variable for activity, y, is directly proportional to $[Ab_A–H–Ab·E]$ and $[Ab_B–H–Ab·E]$. Numerical integration of the differential equations with a computer simulate the high-dose hook effect and show that a heterogeneous antiserum containing Ab_A and Ab_B may produce this hook effect if one of the two antibodies has a low affinity (Rodbard et al., 1978). Moreover, it may also occur if washing is incomplete after the first incubation with the antigen. Too low Ab·E concentrations may also result in a high-dose hook effect (Ryal et al., 1982).

Although these studies clearly indicate that effective washings are important to prevent the hook effect, the extent of dissociation of the Ab–H–Ab·E complex also increases (Section 8.5). Therefore, the elimination of the hook effect may be at the cost of detectability.

CHAPTER 9

The nature of enzyme activity in immunoassays

The accuracy of the EIA is affected by all parameters which influence the action of the enzyme, and a meaningful test cannot be developed without a real understanding of the effects the test design may have on the enzyme activity.

The primary interest in EIA is not in the mechanism of enzyme action. It is, nevertheless, essential to understand the elementary nature of enzyme reaction and of the effect of external factors, such as pH, temperature, ionic strength, other molecules and the solid-phase, on enzymic activity. For an optimal assay it is necessary to know: (i) the stoichiometric details of the reaction; (ii) the molecule(s) which should be present or avoided; (iii) the kinetic dependence of the reaction on these molecules; (iv) the optimization of experimental conditions; and, (v) the accurate monitoring of the enzyme activity. Knowledge of the kinetic behaviour makes it possible to estimate the quantity of the immunoreactant present and to compare EIA to other assays.

9.1. Elementary principles of enzyme kinetics

9.1.1. Overview of the nature of enzyme catalysis

The popularity of enzymes in immunoassays is due to their enormous catalytic power and their high specificity for the substrate. Enzymes do not alter reaction equilibria, but accelerate the forward and reverse reaction. The substrate to product transformation proceeds through unstable (transition) intermediates which have a higher energy content than either the initial substrate or the final product. The difference in the energy content in the transition and substrate state is called the Gibbs free energy of activation. If it is high, only a few molecules will have a momentous energy content sufficiently high to pass this activation barrier. A rise in temperature can increase the proportion of substrate molecules with enough energy to pass this barrier. The increase in the reaction constant is proportional to the collision rate and can be expressed with the Arrhenius formula:

$$k = Z \cdot e^{-A/T} \tag{1}$$

where k is the reaction rate (proportionality factor), Z the collision frequency, A a constant and T the absolute temperature. By multiplying A with the gas constant, R, the activation energy present per mole is obtained which is designated as α. The term $e^{-\alpha/RT}$ represents the fraction of molecules having sufficient energy for product formation.

Enzymes combine with their specific substrate in such a way that the activation energy α is decreased to a lower value of α_1. For example, for the decomposition of H_2O_2 without catalysis, the activation energy is 70 kJ/mol, whereas with the catalase (an enzyme with a very high turnover number) this becomes 7 kJ/mol. Since $R = 8.314$ J/mol·K, from eq. (1) it follows that the acceleration by the enzyme is:

$$\frac{k'}{k} = e^{(\alpha-\alpha_1)/RT} = e^{63/2.5} = 8.8 \times 10^{10} \tag{2}$$

Some enzymes have group specificity, i.e. they act on different but closely related substrates, whereas others have absolute specificity.

Though the active site occupies a relatively small portion of the complete enzyme, the other parts of the enzyme may have significant influences on the activity. This phenomenon has a direct bearing

on EIA where regions outside the catalytic site are modified by
or for the conjugation. Details of enzyme kinetics can be found
in the review by Cornish-Bowden (1979).

9.1.2. Single-substrate enzyme-catalyzed reactions

It is useful to have a high substrate (S) and a lower product (P)
concentration (usually $[P] = 0$) before the start of the enzymic reaction since the presence of P affects the reaction negatively. The
initial conversion speed (v_0) can easily be specified at the beginning
of the reaction: (i) the concentration of all reactants are known
at this point; (ii) loss of enzymic activity has not yet occurred;
and, (iii) the backward reaction (inhibition by P) is negligible since
the P concentration is very small (Michaelis and Menten, 1913).
This rate is easier and more accurately determined by the appearance
of P rather than by the disappearance of S which is very large
at the beginning.

In general chemistry the dependence of v_0 on the initial S (S_0)
concentration can be measured by varying $[S]_0$ while keeping other
variables constant. Graphical analysis (Fig.9.1) of such single-react-
ant reactions can be very useful. For single-substrate enzymes and
multi-substrate enzymes (provided that all S concentrations but one
are constant), graphical expressions differ from those for ordinary
chemical reactions, namely rectangular hyperbolae (Fig. 9.1; Michaelis
and Menten, 1913). This can be explained by the involvement of
at least two enzyme parameters in the binding of S to the enzyme
molecule, forming a complex (ES; central axiom of enzyme kinetics)
which then proceeds to the liberation of P and free enzyme:

$$E + S \underset{k_{-1}}{\overset{k_1}{\rightleftharpoons}} ES \underset{k_{-2}}{\overset{k_2}{\rightleftharpoons}} E + P \tag{3}$$

An enzyme molecule is not working faster at higher $[S]_0$, but a
larger number of enzyme molecules will be involved reflecting a
higher conversion rate v_0. At a certain limit (Fig.9.1) virtually no

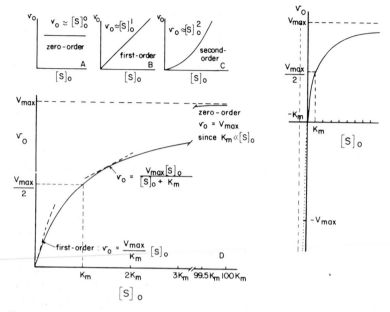

Fig. 9.1. Relation of reaction speed (v) to substrate concentration ([S]) in the absence (A, B, C) and presence of enzyme (D, E). The Michaelis constant, K_m, is the substrate concentration at which half the maximum reaction speed is obtained. To saturate the enzyme completely with substrate, close to $100 \times K_m$ is required (D). When the dependence of the rate of enzyme-catalyzed reaction on the substrate concentration can be described by a rectangular hyperbola (E), the reaction is said to obey classical or Michaelis–Menten kinetics.

enzyme molecule is unemployed and increasing $[S]_0$ does not result in a higher v_0: the reaction is of zero-order. Almost all initial enzyme (E_0) is then present as ES and the maximum v_0 (V_{max}) thus obtained is, therefore, only limited by and related to the speed of the release of P from the enzyme complex which is determined by k_2 or k_{cat}, according to:

$$V_{max} = k_2 \cdot [ES] = k_2[E]_0 = k_{cat} \cdot [E]_0 \qquad (4)$$

where k_{cat} is the catalytic constant, i.e. the rate constant of the limiting step in the reaction. Michaelis and Menten considered only the formation of ES and assumed that the formation of P from ES was too slow to disturb this equilibrium, an assumption which has quite often been shown to be correct. With simple algebra the following is obtained:

$$v_0 = \frac{V_{max} \cdot [S]_0}{[S]_0 + K_S} = \frac{k_{cat} \cdot [E]_0 \cdot [S]_0}{[S]_0 + K_S} \tag{5}$$

in which K_S is the dissociation constant of the complex (k_{-1}/k_1) and has the same dimensions as [S]. In this expression, V_{max} is indicative of the maximum conversion rate of reactants by a given amount of enzyme and K_S is indicative of the affinity of the enzyme for S. A low K_S value indicates a high affinity: Briggs and Haldane (1925) modified this equation by introducing a generally more valid approach, that of the steady state, by considering also the equilibrium of ES with E + P in eq. (3). They argued that [E] and [ES] are negligible compared to [S] and [P] and that, therefore, the rate of change of [ES] would be negligible with the change of [S] and [P], except during the first instants of the reaction when ES is being formed. Kinetic studies of fast reactions, performed in the first fraction of a second, using stopped or continuous flow techniques or temperature jump-relaxation procedures, have demonstrated that this assumption was indeed correct for most enzyme-catalyzed reactions. Briggs and Haldane in their more rigorous derivation, but with equally simple algebra, obtained the so-called Michaelis–Menten equation:

$$v_0 = \frac{V_{max} \cdot [S]_0}{[S]_0 + K_m} \tag{6}$$

in which K_m is the Michaelis constant and can be expressed as:

$$K_m = \frac{k_{-1} + k_2}{k_1} = \frac{k_{-1}}{k_1} + \frac{k_2}{k_1} = K_S + \frac{k_2}{k_1} \tag{7}$$

The equilibrium expression by Michaelis and Menten is, therefore, a special case of the more general steady-state assumption, namely if $k_1 \gg k_2$, $K_S = K_m$. It is evident from eq. 5 or 6 that if $[S]_0 = K_S$ or $[S]_0 = K_m$, the enzyme reaction proceeds at half of its maximum rate. V_{max} varies with the amount of enzyme present, whereas K_m is independent of the enzyme concentration but characteristic of the system investigated. Steady-state kinetics are applicable to many enzyme-catalyzed reactions and the constants V_{max} and K_m can be determined. K_m and V_{max} may be affected by the presence of certain substances or by reaction conditions. It is, in practice, most reliable to work in conditions of high $[S]_0$ so that nearly all enzyme is saturated. Integration of the relationships obtained produces an estimation of the reaction time or maximum possible rate of conversion of S. Integration of the Michaelis–Menten equation demonstrates a more prolonged linear steady-state phase at high saturation of E with S (other factors being constant), because of the smaller importance of the amount of S used compared to the total $[S]$. At high $[S]_0$, $[S]_0 + K_m \approx [S]_0$ and thus $v_0 \approx V_{max}$ or $k_2 \cdot [E]_0$. The time required for one round of catalysis is thus $1/k_2$. Though very high $[S]_0$ would seem ideal, several other factors have to be considered: (i) possibility of inhibition by S (e.g., H_2O_2 inhibits POase); (ii) cost and availability of S; and, (iii) solubility of S which is often limiting since high concentrations are required for complete saturation (e.g., $100 \times K_m$).

In the cases where S is not in excess, the reverse direction of enzyme action (i.e., P → S) will decrease appreciably the net rate of P formation. It follows from eq. 3 that:

$$v_{net} = k_2 \cdot [ES] - k_{-2}[E][P] \tag{8}$$

or

$$v_{net} = \frac{V_{max,f} \cdot \dfrac{[S]}{K_{m,s}} - V_{max,b} \cdot \dfrac{[P]}{K_{m,P}}}{1 + \dfrac{[S]}{K_{m,S}} + \dfrac{[P]}{K_{m,P}}} \tag{9}$$

in which $V_{max,f} = k_2[E]_0$ and $V_{max,b} = k_{-1}[E]_0$,

$$K_{m,S} = \frac{k_{-1} + k_2}{k_1} \quad \text{and} \quad K_{m,P} = \frac{k_{-1} + k_2}{k_{-2}} \qquad (10)$$

Therefore,

$$\frac{V_{max,f}}{V_{max,b}} = \frac{k_2}{k_{-1}} \quad \text{and} \quad \frac{K_{m,S}}{K_{m,P}} = \frac{k_{-2}}{k_1} \qquad (11)$$

At equilibrium, the Haldane equation applies:

$$K_{eq} = \frac{k_1}{k_{-1}} \times \frac{k_2}{k_{-2}} = \frac{V_{max,f}}{V_{max,b}} \times \frac{K_{m,P}}{K_{m,S}} \qquad (12)$$

Many enzyme reactions have more than one intermediate for which King and Altman (1956) devised a method, based on matrix algebra, by establishing the rate equation of a given enzymic reaction simply by inspecting all complexes and the reactions between them.

9.1.3. Kinetics of multisubstrate reactions

Enzymes may act simultaneously on more than one S. Theoretically, the hydrolytic enzymes belong to this class, however, in practice they may be considered as monosubstrate users due to the excess of water present.

The mechanism by which multisubstrate, non-allosteric enzymes react can be divided into two major groups: (i) sequential mechanisms, in which all reactants combine with the enzyme before the reaction occurs, and, (ii) a mechanism called ping-pong by Cleland (1970), in which release of some of the P occurs before all S have combined with the enzyme.

The sequential mechanisms can be subdivided in those which have a compulsory order and those which have a random order of S binding. These mechanisms are often described with the popular shorthand notation given by Cleland (1963), in which uni, bi, ter, etc. denote the number of S and P species. The K_m values of the various reactants are concentration values at which half of the maximum velocity is obtained when all other S are at infinite concentrations and no P or inhibitors are present. Many bi- and multireactant mechanisms obey the Michaelis–Menten equation at constant concentrations of all but one of the reactants. For a general overview of this large subject the reader is referred to Alberty (1953), King and Altman (1956), Dalziel (1957) and Cleland (1970).

A number of multimeric enzymes do not obey the classic Michaelis–Menten kinetics, since the value of their kinetic properties, K_m and k_{cat}, depend on the specific binding of small molecules called effectors. Such regulatory enzymes have, in addition to the catalytic sites, regulatory sites which bind effectors and alter so the properties of the catalytic site. If these effectors are the same as S, they are called homotropic or allosteric (Monod et al., 1963).

Homotropic effectors enhance the binding of subsequent S molecules, i.e. they exhibit a cooperative S binding, resulting in a sigmoid relationship between v and [S].

Heterotropic effectors may act on either K_m or k_{cat} (thus V_{max}). Lowering the K_m of the reaction translates in an activating effect; inhibition effectors raise the K_m. The allosteric transitions of the subunits may be concerted (Monod et al., 1965) or sequential (Koshland et al., 1966). The sigmoidal response allows a much more sensitive control of the reaction rate than by reactions which follow the classical Michaelis–Menten kinetics. In the latter, the ratio of S concentrations to increase the reaction rate from 10% to 90% of V_{max} is 81, but is much less for the sigmoidal response curve. These sigmoidal curves can be described by the Hill equation originally derived for the oxygen–hemoglobin system (Fig. 9.2).

9.1.4. Methods to determine the parameters of the Michaelis–Menten equation

Fig. 9.1. shows the relation between the initial reaction velocity and the initial S concentration, and its dependence on the parameters, V_{max} and K_m. V_{max} is reached only at very high S concentrations and it is difficult to locate the correct asymptotes of this curve,

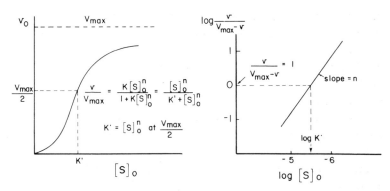

Fig. 9.2. Graphical representation of the Hill equation (left). The exponent n can be determined directly from the slope of the curve relating $\log v/(V_{max}-v)$ and $\log [S]_o$ (right, numerical values serve as an example).

corresponding to K_m. An alternative to this method is to fit an integrated form of the Michaelis–Menten equation to the progress curve:

$$V_{max} \cdot t = K_m \cdot \ln \frac{[S]_0}{[S]_t} + [S]_0 - [S]_t = K_m \cdot \ln \frac{[S]_0}{[S]_t} + [P] \qquad (13)$$

where $[S]_0$ is the initial substrate concentration and $[S]_t$ its concentration after time t. This equation may be rewritten as:

$$\frac{1}{t} \ln \frac{[S]_0}{[S]_t} = -\frac{1}{K_m} \cdot \frac{[P]}{t} + \frac{V_{max}}{K_m} \qquad (14)$$

This is an equation for a straight line, where

$$y = t^{-1} \ln [S]_0/[S]_t \qquad \text{and} \quad x = [P]/t \qquad (15)$$

Thus K_m and V_{max} are determined from the slope and the intercept of the straight line by measuring the concentration of the S used (or P produced) several times during the reaction. The usefulness of this approach has been shown repeatedly (e.g. Duggleby and Morrison, 1978). Systematic errors may change the value of K_m

but scarcely its linearity (Newman et al., 1974) and small errors in the estimation of [S] or [P] lead to large variations in K_m and V_{max}.

Another method to obtain estimates for K_m and V_{max} is the rearrangement of the Michaelis–Menten equation to a linear form. The estimation for the initial velocities, v_0, from progress curves is not a particularly reliable method. A better way to estimate v_0 is by the integrated Michaelis–Menten equation (Cornish-Bowden, 1975). Nevertheless, the graphical methods are popular among enzymologists. The three most common linear transformations of the Michaelis–Menten equation are the Lineweaver–Burk plot of $1/v_0$ vs. $1/[S]$ (sometimes called the double-reciprocal plot), the Eadie–Hofstee plot, i.e. v_0 vs. $v_0/[S]$, and the Hanes plot, i.e., $[S]/v_0$ vs. $[S]$ (Fig. 9.3).

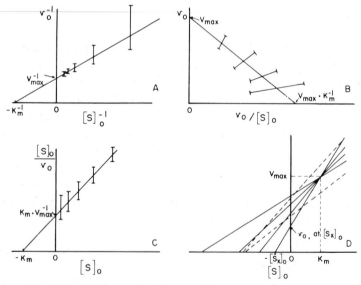

Fig. 9.3. Determination of the parameters of the Michaelis–Menten equation (K_m and V_{max}) by the Lineweaver–Burk (A), Eadie–Hofstee (B), Hanes (C), and direct linear (D) plots. The error bars in A, B and C represent a variation of 5% of V_{max} and show the large effect small errors at low [S] may have on the estimates. Outlying lines obtained in the direct linear plot (D) are easily recognized, at least if a large fraction of the lines do converge in the same intersection.

To obtain these plots the initial velocity is measured against several S concentrations.

Despite their appealing simplicity, these methods have serious limitations. The Lineweaver–Burk and Hanes plots are unreliable, e.g., the variation of the variance almost certainly results in an incorrect weighting, whereas in the Eadie–Hofstee plot v_0 is present in both variables. The direct linear plot of Eisenthal and Cornish-Bowden (1974), for which the Michaelis–Menten equation is rearranged to relate V_{max} to K_m, i.e., $V_{max} = v_0 + v_0 \cdot K_m/[S]$ is very simple but is mathematically equivalent to the Lineweaver–Burk and Hanes plots (Atkins and Nimmo, 1980). However, this direct plot does not require calculations and is based on non-parametric statistics using median rather than mean values (Fig. 9.3).

9.1.5. Inhibition of enzymes

In textbooks dealing with enzyme kinetics, it is customary to distinguish four types of reversible inhibitions: (i) competitive; (ii) non-competitive; (iii) uncompetitive; and, (iv) mixed inhibition. Competitive inhibition, e.g., given by the product which retains an affinity for the active site, is very common. Non-competitive inhibition, however, is very rarely encountered, if at all. Uncompetitive inhibition, i.e. where the inhibitor binds to the enzyme–substrate complex but not to the free enzyme, occurs also quite often, as does the mixed inhibition, which is a combination of competitive and uncompetitive inhibitions. The simple Michaelis–Menten equation can still be used, but with a modified V_{max} or K_m, i.e.:

$$v_0 = \frac{V'_{max} \cdot [S]_0}{[S]_0 + K'_m} \tag{16}$$

The values for V'_{max} and K'_m are given in Table 9.1, but can be derived with simple algebra (see Cornish-Bowden, 1979).

Competitive inhibition can be overcome by high concentrations of substrate. V_{max} does not change in this type of inhibition, in contrast to K_m which increases:

TABLE 9.1
Change of Michaelis–Menten parameters by inhibition

Type of inhibition	V'/V_{max}	K'_m/K_m
Competitive	1	$(1 + [I]/K_I)$
Uncompetitive	$(1 + [I]/K_i)^{-1}$	$(1 + [I]/K_i)^{-1}$
Mixed	$(1 + [I]/K_i)^{-1}$	$(1 + [I]/K_I) \cdot (1 + [I]/K_i)^{-1}$
Non-competitive	$(1 + [I]/K_i)^{-1}$	1

$$
\begin{array}{c}
+ \ I \overset{K_I}{\rightleftharpoons} EI \\
E \\
+ \ S \underset{K_S}{\rightleftharpoons} ES
\end{array}
\qquad (17)
$$

The influence the competitive inhibitor has on the Michaelis–Menten plot and on its double reciprocal linear transformation, as well as the evaluation of K_I is given in Fig.9.3. An example of the practical importance of competitive inhibition in EIA will be discussed in Section 10.1.3.5.

In uncompetitive inhibition both V_{max} and K_m are decreased by the same factor (Table 9.1) so that $V'_{max}/K'_m = V_{max}/K_m$ and the slope in the Lineweaver–Burk plot is not changed. However, the values are shifted to produce parallel lines. In practice, primary plots are first established at different concentrations of inhibitor and the apparent parameters V'_{max} and K'_m are replotted against [I]. For statistical reliability, the same cautions are warranted as for the transformations discussed in Section 9.1.4. An example of uncompetitive inhibition is, in some cases, substrate inhibition. The Michaelis–Menten equation can then be simplified, since [S] = [I], and expressed as:

$$
v_0 = \frac{V_{max} \cdot [S]_0}{[S]_0(1 + \{[S]_0/K_i\} + K_m)} = \frac{V_{max}}{1 + [S]_0/K_i} \quad \text{(if } [S]_0 \gg K_m) \quad (18)
$$

In mixed inhibition, two K values can be distinguished, one for the competitive factor K_I, and one for the uncompetitive factor K_i (Table 9.1).

9.2. Practical details of enzyme catalysis and inhibition

9.2.1. Effects of pH, buffer composition and temperature on reaction rates of enzymes

Influence of H^+, which exists in solution as H_3O^+, on enzyme catalysis can be very complex and traced to the stability of the enzyme, changes in its conformation, protonation of sensitive groups (amino groups, histidine), association state of free enzyme, effects on enzyme–substrate interactions, chemical changes in ES, etc.

The rate of an enzyme-catalyzed reaction as a function of pH generally yields a bell-shaped curve. Some enzymes are very sensitive to small changes in pH (lysozyme), whereas others (POase) are relatively insensitive (within 1–2 pH units near their optima). Enzymes with similar activities but from different origin may have very different optima. APase from *Escherichia coli* is optimally active at a pH of about 8, whereas APase from calf intestine is most active around pH 10 and the activity of these enzymes decreases strongly outside their optima. Nevertheless, the *E. coli* enzyme is often assayed at the pH optimum of the intestinal enzyme. The optimum substrate concentrations may also be pH dependent for some enzymes (Chapter 10).

Temperature effects can be either negative or positive on the K_m or the k_{cat} of the reaction but can only be negative on the enzyme (denaturation). If $K_m = K_S$, K_m may be determined at various temperatures. The k_{cat} can be established directly from the Arrhenius equation (eq. 1):

$$\ln k_{cat} = \ln Z - \frac{\alpha}{RT} \tag{19}$$

plotting $\ln k_{cat}$ vs. $1/T$ yields a straight line with a slope of $-\alpha/R$.

An increase of 1°C in the temperature may enhance the reaction rate by more than 10% until the optimum. Thereafter the enzyme is inactivated. The standard temperature for the measurement of enzyme activity is 30°C, though 25°C or 37°C have also been used. The pH optimum for an enzyme may shift with the temperature: APase has an pH optimum of 10.3, 10.1 and 9.9 at 25, 30, and 37°C, respectively.

The preferred temperature for POase is around 15°C; though it may initially be more active at a somewhat higher temperature, it is relatively faster inactivated. The addition of a non-ionic detergent delays this inactivation and higher temperatures may be used (Section 10.1.1.4.2).

Buffers may influence the kinetic properties of enzymes in a number of ways. For example, certain enzymes may require the presence of divalent ions with some buffers, but not with others (e.g. APase, Section 10.1.3.4); some enzymes may be inhibited by certain buffers, such as APase by phosphate buffers. The ionic strength may also be important to obtain optimal experimental conditions and the nature of the buffer may affect enzyme conformation and activity in various ways (e.g., changing surface tension, dielectric constant).

9.2.2. Effects of solid-phase immobilization on the activity or inhibition of the enzyme

The effects immobilization of the enzyme has on its activity have been neglected in EIA. Fortunately, a large body of information is now available based on studies on immobilized enzymes (Trevan, 1980; Sharma et al., 1982). The immediate vicinity of a solid-phase may profoundly affect the activity of the enzyme. The first noticeable effects are the partitioning of the substrate between the fluid phase and the charged-polymer solid-phase, due to the charges of ionic species, and the limitation of diffusion of the solute to the solid-phase due to an unstirred layer of about 1 μm (i.e., more than 100 times the diameter of an average protein).

A negatively charged polyanion as solid-phase attracts protons which change considerably the pH in this microenvironment. The widely used polystyrene has a negative ζ potential. The actual conditions for the enzyme are different from those in the fluid phase and the composition of the medium has to be adjusted. The requirement of a shift of 1 or more pH units to obtain maximum activity on the solid phase is common (Goldstein, 1972; Weetall, 1973). The concentration of H_3O^+ ions at neutral or alkaline pH is much lower than the substrate concentration and an enzyme liberating or complexing protons profoundly affects the pH in the microenvironment. It is common to observe curved Lineweaver–Burk plots under these conditions.

Immobilization of the enzyme may also have direct effects on its catalytic ability in that conformational changes may lead to partial inactivation which affects the Michaelis–Menten parameters. Allosteric enzymes may, moreover, loose their ability to undergo allosteric activation. Steric restrictions may also be responsible for lower activities of immobilized enzymes by preventing or hindering the access of the substrate or effectors. On the other hand the stability or activity of enzymes on a solid phase is often better than in the fluid phase, probably due to the local high concentration of enzyme. Certain solid phases may, however, directly inactivate the enzyme, such as polystyrene for horseradish POase (Berkowitz and Webert, 1981).

Inhibitors may behave differently with immobilized enzymes: depending on the ionic characteristics of the inhibitor and of the polymer, inhibition may be higher or lower than for the corresponding free enzyme in solution. Polymers may repel like-charged and attract oppositely-charged inhibitors. Severe limitation of diffusion may modify the effects of an inhibitor. A high concentration of substrate (no diffusion limitation) results in a degree of inhibition similar to that obtained with free enzyme in solution. With product inhibition, the lack of rapid diffusion may inhibit the enzyme more than in the liquid phase. This may be serious in EIA using APase. On the other hand, substrate inhibition, such as for POase by H_2O_2, may be lowered by a restricted diffusion (see Section 10.1.1.3). Changes in the substrate or in the polymer may have profound effects on partitioning.

Substrate concentration in solid-phase EIA is often higher than for the same system in solution, to counteract diffusion limitation. Diffusion effects are more pronounced with enzymes with high intrinsic activities.

These profound effects on enzyme activity necessitate the adjustment of the experimental conditions for optimal results in EIA. It is not correct to establish optimum conditions in the liquid phase and to expect that the same conditions yield optimal results with the enzyme immobilized on a polystyrene microplate. Chemical modification of the support to immobilize one of the immunoreactants may also have pronounced effects. Unfortunately, such important and essential features have been ignored for various EIA.

The K_m, as measured in the fluid phase, is different (K'_m) from that in the solid phase. The reaction velocity is affected by both the uneven distribution of the enzyme, which requires the diffusion of the substrate from the interior of the fluid phase to the solid phase and an electrical effect, i.e. a gradient of electrical potential, grad φ, generated by charge differences between the solid phase and the interior of the fluid phase (Hornby et al., 1968). The substrate transport due to the electrical effect is proportional to the negative gradient of the electrical potential ($-$ grad φ), the concentration of substrate in the interior of the fluid phase $[S]_0$ and the valence of the substrate (z). On the other hand, transport of the substrate by thermal diffusion is related by D to the substrate concentration gradient. At the steady state the net substrate transport is limiting and the reaction rate becomes v_{net} which can then be expressed as:

$$v_{net} = \frac{V_{max} \cdot [S]_0}{[S]_0 + (K_m + \dfrac{x \cdot V_{max}}{D}) \left(\dfrac{RT}{RT - z \cdot x \cdot F \cdot \text{grad } \varphi} \right)} \qquad (20)$$

in which x is the distance from the solid phase, D the diffusion constant of the substrate, R the gas constant, T the absolute temperature and F the Faraday constant. Eq. (20) differs from the Michaelis–Menten equation (eq. 6) only by the Michaelis–Menten constant. The second term of the product replacing the K_m becomes 1 if either z or grad φ is zero, so that only the diffusion term remains, whereas the second term is >1 if z and grad φ have the same sign.

Some important conclusions can be drawn for solid-phase EIA: (i) the higher the diffusion constant of the substrate, the lower the increase in K_m of the reaction, resulting in an increased reaction rate; and, (ii) the accumulation or depletion of ionic species (e.g., protons) influences the reaction rate. Therefore, extreme care should be taken to agitate equally each reaction vessel. This is often more difficult with coated tube assays than with microtitre plates. Shaking of plates during the enzyme reaction may be advantageous.

Not surprisingly, enzymes with large V_{max} values are affected more by an increase in K_m than enzymes with small V_{max} values, since the latter cause relatively smaller substrate differences between the solid and fluid phase.

9.2.3. Measurement of enzyme activity

9.2.3.1. Purity and activity of enzyme   Enzyme reactions depend on the various parameters discussed previously, and a rigorous adherence to the principles is required to obtain optimal results.

The purity of the enzyme is reflected by its specificity for a panel of substrates. Many preparations may contain 'contaminating' activities and the number of crystallizations indicated for commercial preparations is a poor criterion for purity. The absence of proteases is important to maintain maximum stability of the preparations. Contaminating microorganisms very often produce proteases; however, the addition of preservatives may interfere with enzyme activity. For example, POase is extremely sensitive to both contaminating bacteria and NaN_3. Sometimes, enzymes can be stabilized by the addition of substrate homologues.

Lyophilized enzymes usually contain residual water, which is not considered an impurity, but it should be taken into account when preparing the enzyme solution. Quite often, freeze-dried POase contains 10–20% water. This depends on the conditions of drying and storage of the enzyme, as well as on the extent of its hygroscopic nature. Highly diluted enzyme solutons are not very stable. Lyophilized enzymes should be stored in the cold in dry containers which should not be opened before equilibration at room temperature. Coenzymes should also be stored in the cold and protected from light. The water used in the assays should be doubly distilled recently (POase is extremely sensitive to impure water). Commercial distilled water often contains reducing agents. NADH and NADPH are acid labile ($<$pH 7.5), whereas NAD^+ and $NADP^+$ are alkali labile. Glassware cleaned by surface-active detergents is often alkali and should be rinsed with dilute HCl and distilled water.

9.2.3.2. Determination of enzyme activity with a coupled enzyme reaction   Sometimes an indicator reaction is necessary to establish the amount of P formed in the catalytic process, such as in:

$$S \overset{E_1}{\rightleftharpoons} P \overset{E_2}{\rightleftharpoons} P'$$

If the decrease in S or the increase in P cannot be established, a second enzyme, E_2, may be introduced into the system to produce P′ which is measurable. E_2, which transforms P into P′, is faced with low initial P concentration. At a given moment, however, a steady state is obtained, i.e. the two reaction rates become equal.

It has been noted (Section 9.1.2), that in the conditions where [S] $\ll K_m$:

$$v_0 = \frac{V_{max}}{K_m} \cdot [S] = a_1[S] \tag{21}$$

or in the present case where P is converted into P′:

$$v_2 = \frac{V_{max,2}}{K_{m,2}} = a_2[P] \tag{22}$$

i.e., at very low intermediate [P] the enzyme reactions behave as uncatalyzed reactions, and in the steady state, $V_{max,1} = V_{max,2}$, is obtained. The only free variable in this equation is $V_{max,2}$, which can be made larger by increasing the quantity of E_2, since according to eq. (4), $V_{max,2} = k_{cat} \cdot [E_2]$.

The purpose of the test is that E_1 in the first step should be measured accurately. Therefore, $a_2 \gg a_1$, should be obeyed. A rough calculation shows that a_2 should be $> 100 a_1$. The greater a_2/a_1 the shorter the lag time.

Instead of a succeeding indicator reaction, it is also possible to have preceeding indicator reaction(s). This approach is useful when the substrate for the reaction to be measured is unstable.

Coupled enzymes may prove particularly promising for a new design of EIA, the proximal linkage of EIA (Section 2.5.2).

9.2.3.3. Determination of low metabolic concentrations with enzymatic cycling   In some cases where small amounts of substrate have to be measured, it may be advantageous to use a cycle of reactions (Passoneau and Lowry, 1974). This method has been applied successfully in EIA by Harper and Orengo (1981; Section 14.6.1).

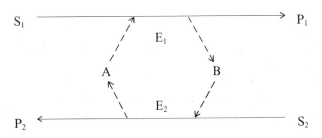

With an increase of S_1 and S_2, small quantities of A and B (much less than their respective K_m concentrations) may be measured through the production of P_1 or P_2. If both enzymes have high activities, a small quantity of A can result in a large quantity of products. If the concentration of the substance (A) to be measured is lower than the K_m, product formation is proportional to the quantity of A generated.

9.2.3.4. Photometric determination of enzyme activity   Most
quantitative estimations in EIA are performed by photometric or
fluorimetric methods. Generally, the concentration of enzyme is sufficiently low to prevent a significant change in [S], while [P] is measured.
Measurements are based on absorbance (*A*) or fluorescence (*F*) of
P:

$$v = \frac{dP}{dt} = \frac{A}{t} \quad \text{or} \quad \frac{F}{t} \tag{23}$$

Progress curves are usually not established in solid-phase EIA; instead, end-point transformation of S → P is measured after a standard
time and plotted against standard curves. From the Lambert–Beer
law:

$$A \text{ (or } F) = abc \tag{24}$$

in which *a* is the extinction coefficient of the product (cm^2/μmole),
b the optical pathway, and *c* the concentration of the product (μmole/
ml); *c* is expressed as:

$$c = \frac{A}{ab} \quad (\mu\text{mole/ml}) \tag{25}$$

The activity in the assay mixture is then:

$$\frac{c}{t} = \frac{A}{t} \cdot \frac{1}{ab} \quad (\mu\text{mole/ml} \cdot \text{min}) \tag{26}$$

and the activity in the sample of which a volume *v* has been transferred to the assay mixture with volume *V* is:

$$\frac{c}{t} = \frac{A}{t} \cdot \frac{1}{ab} \cdot \frac{V}{v} \quad (\mu\text{mole/ml} \cdot \text{min or U/ml}) \tag{27}$$

and 1 U (international unit) of enzyme activity is defined as transforming 1 μmole of substrate per min. Activity can also be expressed
as (MW is molecular weight of substrate):

$$\frac{c}{t} = \frac{A}{t} \cdot \frac{1}{ab} \cdot \frac{V \cdot MW}{v} \quad (\mu g/ml \cdot min)$$

The specific activity of the enzyme, i.e. activity per mg ($c_e =$ concentration of enzyme in mg/ml), is then:

$$\frac{c}{t} = \frac{A}{t} \cdot \frac{1}{abc_e} \cdot \frac{V}{v} \quad (U/mg)$$

The turnover number, TN, is defined as:

$$\frac{[\text{substrate}]_{\text{converted}}}{[\text{enzyme}] \times \text{time} \times \text{number of active sites/molecule}}$$

Since specific enzyme activity relates to mole of substrate produced per mg of enzyme, it should be multiplied by a factor $10^3 \times MW$ (enzyme)$/10^6$ to obtain the TN (if enzyme is not multimeric).

CHAPTER 10

Properties and preparation of enzymes used in enzyme-immunoassays

No enzyme fulfills all the criteria for an ideal label in EIA (Table 10.1) and a compromise has to be made.

In solid-phase EIA, the influence the solid phase has on the enzyme (Section 9.2.2) should be minimal. Conjugation should be easy and the conjugates should be active and stable. These are undoubtedly major factors for the frequency of the selection of horseradish peroxidase (POase) or β-galactosidase (BGase). Alkaline phosphatase (APase), which is difficult to conjugate in defined form (extensive polym-

TABLE 10.1

Properties which make an enzyme ideal for EIA

- High turnover number.

- Low K_m for substrate, but a high K_m for product.

- High K_i or K_I.

- Stable upon storage (in free or conjugated form).

- Purity, ease of preparation, and low cost of enzyme.

- Easily detectable activity.

- Absence of endogenous enzyme or interfering substances in the sample.

- Compatibility with the assay conditions (pH, ionic strength, buffer composition, etc.).

erization), is, nevertheless, widely used due to the absence of endogenous enzyme in plant tissues, high stability, and to the technically undemanding preparation of very stable conjugates.

Homogeneous, AM assays pose different requirements. Here, the enzyme should be easily conjugated near the active site without altering its activity. The reaction of hapten- or antigen-labeled enzyme with antibody should affect strongly the enzyme activity, e.g., through steric inhibition of the substrate at the catalytic site. The requirements for optimal ionic conditions and temperature for both enzyme activity and antigen–antibody interaction should be compatible.

EIH poses another set of requirements: (i) the enzyme should be small to avoid problems of penetration into the fixed cell; (ii) the substrate should be soluble and the product insoluble, so that the product is deposited near the enzyme.

The enzymes used in EIH or EIA are listed in Table 10.2.

10.1. Enzymes used in activity amplification assays

EIA based on visual titration require clear-cut endpoints. Both horseradish POase and urease produce easily detectable products, whereas the products of APase or BGase are less strongly colored.

The relative costs of the enzymes for EIH or EIA should not be ignored. For example, BGase is about 26 times more expensive per mg than POase and at least 150 times more expensive than POase prepared according to Section 10.1.1.2. Moreover, for 1:1 conjugates about 10 times more (in mg) BGase is needed than POase due to the molecular weight, increasing the relative cost of BGase by about 10 times. However, BGase is more efficiently conjugated than POase which lowers its relative cost to about 200 and is, under certain conditions, capable of detecting smaller amounts of antigen than POase and shows less problems with background staining by endogenous enzyme. If background staining poses problems, APase, the usual alternative of POase, is only slightly less costly than BGase, but conjugation methods for APase and its detectability are far

TABLE 10.2
Enzymes used in EIA

Activity amplification assays	Activity modulation assays[a]	Immunohistochemistry
Peroxidase[b]	β-galactosidase[b]	peroxidase[b]
β-Galactosidase[b]	lysozyme[c]	alkaline phosphatase[b]
Alkaline phosphatase[b]	malate dehydrogenase[c]	(microperoxidase)[d]
Urease[b]	glucose-6-phosphate dehydrogenase[c]	cytochrome *c*
Glucose oxidase[b]	ribonuclease[c]	glucose oxidase[b]
Glucoamylase		
Carbonic anhydrase		
Acetylcholinesterase		

[a] The enzymes used in the AA-assays can also be used for solid-phase AM-assays.
[b] Described in detail in Section 10.1.1 through Section 10.1.5.
[c] Described in detail in Section 10.2.1 through Section 10.2.4.
[d] Described in detail in Section 10.3.1.

inferior. A comparison of the relative costs for each enzyme, considering the best chemical conjugation method and their detectabilities, is given in Table 10.3. It is evident that the frequently used APase is quite expensive indeed, though its use on a small scale is not prohibitive. In general, commercial conjugates are several-fold more expensive than those prepared in the laboratory.

10.1.1. Horseradish peroxidase (POase)

10.1.1.1. Physicochemical properties of peroxidase   POase (hydrogen-peroxide oxidoreductase, EC 1.11.1.7) is the most widely used enzyme in EIA and EIH. Its physicochemical properties are given in Table 10.4. Typical POases are hemoproteins and transfer

TABLE 10.3

Relative costs of various commercial enzymes for AA-type EIA for the preparation of monoconjugates and their relative detectabilities (all values are relative to peroxidase)

Enzyme cat. No.[a]	Relative price/mg	Relative molecular weight	Relative conjugation efficiency	Relative costs	Relative detectabilities	
	(a)	(b)	(c)	(a·b/c)	col.[b]	flu.[b]
POase 108090	1.00	1.00	1.00	1.00	1.00	1.00
APase 567744	34.24	1.92	0.10	650	400	2.00 (0.20)
BGase 567779	25.82	10.57	1.33	200	40 (4)	0.04 (0.004)
GOase 105139	0.91	3.47	1.00	3.15		10.0 (1.00)
Urease 174882	1.34	10.91	0.10	146		
MPOase (8) M4757	45.45	0.034	0.50	3.09[c]		
MPOase (9) M9635	22.72	0.037	0.50	1.68[c]		
MPOase (11) M6751	2.59	0.042	0.50	0.22[c]		

[a] Boehringer catalogue 1982–1983 for enzymes, Sigma catalogue 1983 for MPOases (MPOase 8, 9, or 11 are heme octapeptide, nonapeptide or undecapeptide, respectively).

[b] Results reported by Ishikawa et al. (1983); best are underlined (lowest figure), e.g., the colorimetric (col.) assay using POase allows the detection of 400 times less antigen than with APase. Results were obtained after 10 min (detectability after 100 min, if changed with respect to POase, between brackets). After 10 min, the fluorimetric (flu.) assay for POase had a 5-fold increased detectability over the colorimetric assay, and increased 50 times after 100 min (down to 0.5 amol in this assay). Substrates used: POase, OPD; APase, p-NPP; BGase, o-nitrophenyl-β-D-galactoside; for fluorometric assays: POase and GOase, p-hydroxyphenylacetic acid; APase, 4-methylumbelliferyl phosphate; and BGase, 4-methylumbelliferyl-β-D-galactoside.

[c] Several MPOases (e.g., 20/IgG) should be conjugated to obtain satisfactory results.

TABLE 10.4
Physicochemical properties of horseradish peroxidase

Mass (daltons)	44000[a]
Molecular composition	polypeptide: 308 amino acids[a], 33890 daltons[a]
	protohematin IX and calcium: 700 daltons[b]
	carbohydrate (calculated): 9535 daltons[a]
	carbohydrate composition (residues)
	fucose 10[c], 6[d], 8[e]
	xylose 9[c], 7[d], 8[e]
	mannose 34[c], 18[d], 24[e]
	glucosamine 47[c], 17[d], 8[e]
	disulfide bridges: 4[a]
Stokes radius	3 nm[f]
Isoelectric point (C isozyme):	POase: 8.7–9.0[a,g]
	apoprotein: 6.8[a]
Spectral optima	prosthetic group ('Soret band'): 403 nm[h]
	apoprotein: 275 nm[h]
Extinction coefficient	22.5
(1%; 403 nm; 1 cm):	

References: a, Welinder, 1979; b, Haschke and Friedhoff, 1978; c, Clarke and Shannon, 1976; d, Haschke (cited by Welinder, 1979); e, Phelps et al., 1971; f, Ishikawa et al., 1980b; g, Delincée, 1977; h, Saunders et al., 1964.

hydrogen from hydrogen donors (H-donors) (DH) to H_2O_2:

$$HOOH + 2DH \xrightarrow{\text{POase}} 2H_2O + 2D$$

POases often occur as multiple isozymes and are widely distributed, particularly in plants (Theorell, 1942; Shannon et al., 1966). They appear to catalyze the same reaction, but differ markedly in physico-chemical and kinetic properties (Shannon et al., 1966; Kay et al., 1967). It is very likely that the different iso-POases serve specialized, albeit unknown biological functions. Three main types of POases have been identified: (i) the acidic (probably cell-wall-associated) POases with a very high carbohydrate content (Mazza et al., 1973; Welinder, 1979); (ii) POases with a pI around neutrality (or slightly basic) with a somewhat lower sugar content; and, (iii) very basic

POases ($pI > 11$) of low sugar content (Paul and Stigbrand, 1970). A further microheterogeneity has been noted (Section 11.2.3.1.1). Among the POases used in EIA, the 'C' isozyme of horseradish (*Armoracia rusticana*) dominates to a large extent. However, commercial pure POase contains, beside the C isozyme, other isozymes with much lower activities.

The components of the POase molecule can be represented (Saunders et al., 1964) as:

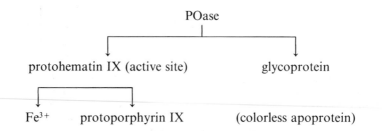

The six co-ordination positions of iron are occupied by the nitrogen atoms of porphyrin, by the protein (probably through histidine; Haschke and Friedhoff, 1978) and by the substrate. The complete amino acid sequence of POase-C has been established (Welinder, 1979). The apoprotein specifies and amplifies the inherent properties of the prosthetic group (Saunders et al., 1964).

The covalent structure of POase-C (Fig. 10.1; Welinder, 1979) consists of 2 compact domains, between which the hemin group is sandwiched. Carbohydrates are attached to the polypeptide at 8 different sites, particularly in the C-terminal half of the molecule at Asp–X–Ser sequences. The native enzyme has very few net charges ($+2$ at pH 7), no free α-amino groups, and only two titratable histidines (Welinder, 1979). The 6 lysines seem to be shielded by the carbohydrate shell.

A widely used practice of suppliers and investigators is to give the so-called *RZ* (Reinheits Zahl) number which is the ratio (often around 3.0) of the absorbance at 403 nm (Soret band) and 275 nm. This value, however, is not a real measure of purity. In fact,

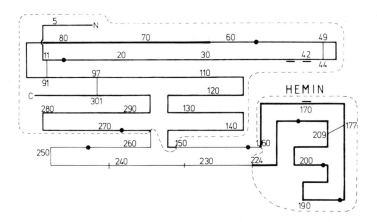

Fig. 10.1. Planar view of structure of horseradish POase (Welinder, 1979). There are 4 disulfide bridges (11–91, 44–49, 97–301, and 177–209). The 2 domains are encircled. The iron-coordinated histidines are at positions 42 and 170 in the active site. Full circles indicate the sites of carbohydrate attachment (Courtesy of author and *European Journal of Biochemistry*).

different isozymes of POase differ in *RZ* values, ranging between 4.19 and 3.15 (Kay et al., 1967) or lower, though the exact range is still disputed and may vary according to the origin of the POase. 'Pure' commercial POase with an *RZ* of 3.0 contains several isozymes, the major component (isozyme C) has the highest activity and an *RZ* of around 3.50 (Tijssen and Kurstak, 1984) and can be isolated easily.

10.1.1.2. Purification of horseradish peroxidase   POase is much more sensitive than APase to contaminants. Water deionized with polystyrene resins is often toxic to POase; in fact, POase is inactivated by polystyrene plates (or cuvettes) in solid-phase EIA if Tween 20 is omitted (Berkowitz and Webert, 1981). POase is also very sensitive to the presence of bacteria or bacteriostatic agents (NaN_3) and is inactivated by oxygen (degassing recommended), hypochlorous acid and aromatic chlorocarbons often found in laboratory water.

The rather expensive POase is usually purchased rather than purified. The method presented here is exceedingly simple, fast, may decrease the cost sometimes more than 10 times, and yields a preparation of very high activity since isozymes with low activities are eliminated. This method starts with a low-priced crude extract (RZ of 1.0) which is dissolved in 2.5 mM sodium phosphate buffer, pH 8.0. A DEAE–Sepharose column is equilibrated with the same buffer and the POase solution is applied (up to 5 mg protein per ml gel). Impurities and less active isozymes are retained whereas pure POase passes directly (Table 10.5), and is collected by monitoring the eluate (at 401 nm or visually). This POase preparation has higher RZ values (3.20–3.30) and higher activities than the commercial 'pure' preparations, though RZ values will be slightly higher if 'pure' commercial POase is purified by this method.

POase can also be purified by affinity chromatography on a Con

TABLE 10.5

Purification of peroxidase by a single step on DEAE-Sepharose[a]

Prepara-tion	Frac-tion	Concentra-tion of elu-tion buffer[b] (mM)	RZ[c]	Recovery in % at:		% of total activity recovered	Specific activity[e] (%)
				275 nm	403 nm		
Crude	1	2.5	3.21	26.1	73.0	89.40[d]	111.5
	2	20	3.35	5.2	15.3	4.37	27.0
	3	350	0.36	27.5	8.7	3.25	3.8
'Pure'	1	2.5	3.50	78.3	95.6	96.4[d]	124.0
	2	20	[f]	0.7	1.5	N.D.[g]	N.D.
	3	350	0.27	9.8	0.8	N.D.	N.D.

[a] 7 ml DEAE–Sepharose, equilibrated with 2.5 mM sodium phosphate buffer, pH 8.0. Applied quantities: crude extract (type II POase from Sigma) and 'pure' POase (type VI from Sigma), 52 and 30 optical density units at 403 nm, respectively. Data from Tijssen and Kurstak, 1984.
[b] Sodium phosphate buffer, pH 8.0.
[c] Optical density ratio at 403 and 275 nm.
[d] Total recovery for crude POase: 97% for 'pure' POase: 97.9%.
[e] Relative to commercial 'pure' enzyme.
[f] Not enough for reliable measurements.
[g] N.D. = not done.

A–Sepharose column followed by gel filtration. This method, however, is not recommended, since it is time consuming, expensive, applicable to small amounts (which become diluted) and does not remove the less active isozymes (Table 10.5).

POase may also be isolated directly from horseradish roots (Shannon et al., 1966). Roots are cut into small cubes, homogenized in a minimal volume of 100 mM K_2HPO_4 in a Waring blender, and the homogenate is filtered through a cheese cloth. $(NH_4)_2SO_4$ is added to 1.4 M, the precipitate is removed by centrifugation, and the $(NH_4)_2SO_4$ concentration is raised to 3.6 M (taking volume increase into account). The precipitate formed during stirring overnight is collected by centrifugation, redissolved in a minimal volume of 50 mM Tris–HCl buffer, pH 7.0, and dialyzed against this buffer. The precipitate which may appear is removed by centrifugation and virtually 100% of the POase activity is recovered in the supernatant. This POase is then further purified by gel filtration on Sephadex G-100 followed by ion-exchange chromatography as described above.

10.1.1.3. Catalytic properties of horseradish peroxidase   The reaction scheme in Fig. 10.2, supported by many studies (e.g., Chance,

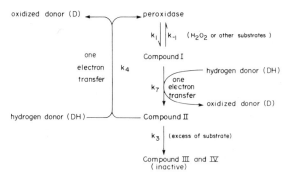

Fig. 10.2. Scheme of catalysis by POase. POase combines with H_2O_2 (substrate) to form component I and is reduced in two successive steps by a H-donor to the original state. Generally, the appearance of oxidized donor is measured. An excess of H_2O_2 will inactivate enzyme (compound III and IV). The activation energy for k_1 is 9 kJ·mole^{-1} (Marklund et al., 1974).

1952; Yamazaki, 1971), dictates the correct experimental conditions for POase assays: POase is divalently oxidized by peroxide to Compound I, which is, in turn, reduced to the initial state by 2 successive univalent interactions with H-donors. Compound II is the one-electron oxidized, intermediate form. Some H-donors, e.g. o-dianisidine, produce a direct, two-electron transfer reduction (Claiborne and Fridovich, 1979a). Nitrogenous compounds (nucleophilic catalysts: pyridine, imidazole), may stimulate this transfer (Claiborne and Fridovich, 1979b).

An excess of substrate inactivates the enzyme by forming compound III (red) or IV (emerald green). This substrate inhibition is very substantial in some of the current EIA procedures using POase (Tijssen et al., 1982).

Specific formation of Compound I can be obtained only with certain peroxides but many substances can serve as H-donors. Whether a K_m can be obtained is a matter of controversy (Pütter, 1974). POases from different origins or their isozymes may have quite different activities toward a certain donor (Maehly, 1954).

The k_4 rate constants vary largely (Table 10.6). In general, k_7 is about 50–100 times greater than k_4, thus k_4 represents the donor limiting step and k_1 the substrate limiting step. The rate of substrate utilization is expressed as (Chance and Maehly, 1955):

$$-\frac{d[S]}{dt} = \frac{d[P]}{dt} = \frac{[E]}{\dfrac{1}{k_1[H_2O_2]} + \dfrac{1}{k_4[DH]}} \qquad (1)$$

The C isozyme reacts faster with the aromatic amines, whereas the acidic isozymes react much faster with acidic donors (Marklund et al., 1974).

Cyanide or sulphide reversibly inhibits POase at concentrations of 10^{-5} to 10^{-6} M (Saunders et al., 1964). Cyanide inhibits all POases and has been used to identify 'true' POase activity. Fluoride, azide, or hydroxylamine inhibits only at concentrations higher than 10^{-3} M. Dithionite reduces ferri-POase to ferro-POase which then

TABLE 10.6

Rate constants of horseradish peroxidase type C (pH of assay mixture in brackets)[a]

Rate constant	Substrate or donor	Wavelength (nm)	$M^{-1}sec^{-1}(\times 10^{-4})$ according to	
			Marklund et al., 1974	Chance, 1949
k_1	hydrogen peroxide		1200 (4.5) 1400 (7.0) 1300 (9.0)	400 (4.7)
	methylhydroperoxide		130 (7.0)	150 (4.7)
	ethylhydroperoxide		400 (7.0)	360 (4.7)
	propylhydroperoxide		480 (7.0)	
	p-nitroperoxybenzoic acid		3700 (4.5)	
k_4	1,2-dihydroxybenzene (= catechol)	387	29 (7.0) 28 (4.5)	200 (7.0)
	1,3-dihydroxybenzene (= resorcinol)	282	22 (7.0) 17 (4.5)	30 (7.0)
	1.4-dihydroxybenzene (= hydroquinone)	288	590 (7.0) 21 (4.5)	300 (7.0)
	1,2,3-trihydroxybenzene (= pyrogallol)			30 (6.7)
	o-phenylenediamine (= o-diaminobenzene)	445		5000 (7.0)
	o-methoxyphenol (= guaiacol)	470	52 (7.0) 23 (4.5)	25 (6.7)
	coniferol	262	890 (7.0) 280 (4.5)	
	leucomalachite green	600	10 (4.5)	30 (4.7)
	benzidine	278	4300 (7.0) 4900 (4.5)	
	ascorbic acid	427	0.05 (7.0) 1.4 (4.5)	2 (7.0)

[a] Buffers: pH 9.0: 10 mM Tris-HCl.
  pH 6.7 and 7.0: 10 mM sodium phosphate.
  pH 4.5 and 4.7: 10 mM sodium acetate.

combines with carbon monoxide. The enzyme is irreversibly inhibited by hydroxymethylhydrogenperoxide (Marklund, 1973).

10.1.1.4. Hydrogen donors: tools for the determination of POase activity in enzyme immunoassays   Almost without exception, POase activity is measured indirectly by the rate of transformation of the hydrogen donor. It is also possible to measure residual substrate, which offers the possibility to separate POase activity from contaminating activities (Maehly, 1954).

The kinetic features of POase in solid-phase assays may be masked by diffusion or partitioning phenomena (Section 9.2.2). Most probably, an incorrect H_2O_2 concentration is the most important single factor in interassay variations and enzyme inactivation.

Like with other enzymes, POase activity depends on the temperature. Without non-ionic detergents, the highest activity is attained at 15°C. At higher temperatures a higher initial rate is followed, after about 10 min, by an inactivation which is stronger for free POase than for immobilized POase. Tween 20 and Triton X-100 delay POase inactivation (Porstmann et al., 1981), depending on the nature of the H-donor (e.g., pronounced for *o*-dianisidine).

H-donors should have the following properties to be suitable for EIA: (i) negligible oxidation rate in the absence of enzyme; (ii) the product should not undergo secondary reactions unless yielding another single product with a rate constant much faster than k_4; (iii) much slower reaction rate between the donor and enzyme than k_1; (iv) little pH dependence of the oxidation reactions; (v) oxidation of donor must produce a stable change in a physical property, in a single form, which can be quantitated, e.g., spectrophotometrically; (vi) both the reduced and the oxidized states of the donor should be sufficiently soluble in the case of EIA, whereas in EIH the oxidized donor should be highly insoluble; and, (vii) the donor should not be toxic.

The rate of product formation depends on two rate constants, k_1 and k_4, which can be described after conversion of eq. 1 as:

$$\frac{d[P]}{dt} = \frac{k_1 \cdot k_4 \cdot [E][H_2O_2][DH]}{k_4 \cdot [DH] + k_1 \cdot [H_2O_2]} \tag{2}$$

Any sound activity determination should depend on one rate constant only. This is the case if:

$$k_1[H_2O_2] \ll k_4[DH] \text{ then } d[P]/dt = k_1[H_2O_2][E] \quad \text{or} \qquad (3)$$

$$k_1[H_2O_2] \gg k_4[DH] \text{ then } d[P]/dt = k_4[DH][E] \qquad (4)$$

In the latter case, i.e. if the enzyme activity is measured in terms of k_4, then $[E \cdot H_2O_2]$ must approach $[E_o]$. These conditions can be established in parallel experiments; in an example, conditions for these two cases are (in 10 mM phosphate buffer, pH 7.0): 3.3×10^{-5} M substrate, 1.3×10^{-2} M donor and 10^{-9} enzyme for k_1; and 5.3×10^{-4} M substrate, 3.3×10^{-4} M donor, and 10^{-9} M enzyme for k_4.

The reduction of substrate produces cyclic tetraguaiacol with an E_{436nm} of 25.6 cm^{-1} mM^{-1} ($=a$, i.e. for 4 molecules of guaiacol). Therefore, the quantity of H_2O_2 to cause an absorption increase (A) of 0.05 at 436 nm is (Section 9.2.3.4):

$$\frac{dP}{dt} = \frac{A}{dt} = \frac{4 \times A}{a \times dt} \text{ mM} = \frac{4 \times 0.05}{25.6 \times dt} \text{ mM} = \frac{7.8}{dt} \mu M$$

In combination with eqs. 3 and 4, $k_1 = 2.36 \times 10^8$ M/dt and $k_4 = 2.36 \times 10^7$ M/dt is obtained. If the time required to obtain an A of 0.05 in these two determinations was, e.g., 25 and 68 sec, respectively, then $k_1 = 9.5 \times 10^6$ M^{-1} sec^{-1} and $k_4 = 3.5 \times 10^5$ M^{-1} sec^{-1}. Thus the requirements for $k_1[H_2O_2] \ll k_4[DH]$ and $k_1[H_2O_2] \gg k_4[DH]$ are fulfilled.

A disadvantage of the use of guaiacol is the fading of the color of tetraguaiacol a few minutes after its formation. Pyrogallol which forms purpurogallin is also frequently used to assess the POase activity (e.g., by Sigma). The activity is then expressed by the purpurogallin number (Purpurogallinzahl, PZ; Wilstätter and Stoll, 1917). However, in their test $k_1[H_2O_2] \approx k_4[DH]$ and the method is, therefore, not suitable: the PZ varies considerably. Maehly (1954) and Chance (1949) found that purpurogallin was still formed after all of compound II had disappeared. This reaction thus, does not reflect real activity, but a complex mechanism. Moreover, this H-donor is highly sensitive to trace metals.

Diaminobenzidine yields insoluble oxidation products and is, therefore, very well suited for EIH but not for EIA. However, this product, as some other H-donors, may be carcinogenic. A popular H-donor in EIA is 5-aminosalicylic acid (5-AS). Unfortunately, it is not offered in a pure form, while much can be gained by purification. After purification, it is readily soluble and very stable, in contrast to the original product, and background staining is significantly reduced. It is convenient to purify large quantities of 5-AS and to store (without H_2O_2) at $-20°C$ as ready-to-use solution.

Purification of 5-AS, according to Ellens and Gielkens (1980), is easy: 5 g of 5-AS and 5 g of sodium bisulfite are dissolved in 550 ml deionized water at 80°C. This temperature is maintained, while stirring, for 10 min. Activated charcoal is then added (2 g) and the suspension is mixed for 5 min. The hot solution is filtered and then cooled to 4°C. The precipitate is washed twice with 5 ml water at 4°C, and dried in the dark. The purified 5-AS is redissolved (very soluble) at a concentration of 1 g/l in 10 mM sodium phosphate buffer, pH 6.0, containing 0.1 mM EDTA, and stored at (20°C. Upon thawing a precipitate is usually present which readily redissolves by bringing the container in hot water to room temperature. Peroxide is added just before use.

o-Dianisidine (ODA) is occasionally employed as H-donor, but is not recommended since its solubility is low and it is sensitive to ammonium salts (Fridrovich, 1963).

Another popular donor is the diammonium salt of 2,2'-azino-di-(3-ethyl-benzthiazoline sulfonate-6) (ABTS; Boehringer Mannheim). ABTS is colorless with a maximum absorbance at 340 nm, whereas the oxidized product has an optimum at 414 nm.

A sensitive and versatile chromogenic assay for POase is based on the oxidative coupling of 3-methyl-2-benzothiazolinone hydrazone (MBTH) and 3-(dimethylamino)benzoic acid (DMAB) (Ngo and Lenhoff, 1980) in the presence of substrate. MBTH is the donor which, after oxidation, reacts with DMAB to form a cationic indamine dye, a purple compound with a maximum absorption at 590 nm. The coupled reaction has some advantages over other donors in solid-phase assays, such as high detectability and the lack of carcinogenicity, but background levels are somewhat higher (Tijssen et al., 1982).

o-Tolidine (OT), a frequently used H-donor, gives a blue color. It has a high detectability but is potentially carcinogenic.

o-Phenylenediamine (OPD) or 1,2-benzenediamine is a very suitable H-donor of which the oxidized form (orange) can be measured at low concentrations at 445 nm or 492 nm, depending on the pH. OPD should be white and stored in the cold. Tan-colored crystals should be recrystallized. Although background staining can be significant, OPD might be the most sensitive activity indicator (there is some controversy on this point; Section 14.4.1.1), but is photosensitive and possibly mutagenic.

The preparation of these substrates is presented in Section 14.4.1.1. for EIA and in Section 17.3.3 for EIH.

10.1.1.5. Activity determination of horseradish peroxidase   A method designed to obey $k_1[H_2O_2] \gg k_4[DH]$, in which, consequently, the activity corresponds to $k_4[DH][E]$, is given in Table 10.7.

The concentration of H_2O_2 in a '30% solution' is not very stable, even when stored at 4°C real concentration can be measured at 240 nm where its molar extinction coefficient is 43.6 M^{-1} cm^{-1} (Hilde-

TABLE 10.7
Determination of peroxidase activity

	ml	Final concentration (mM)
100 mM potassium phosphate buffer, pH 7.0	3.00	96.5
245 mg guaiacol/100 ml	0.05	0.3
Sample	0.02	
8 mM hydrogen peroxide (see text)	0.04	0.1

Total volume is 3.11 ml; $A_{436\,nm}$ is measured; extinction coefficient of guaiacol (tetra-guaiacol is formed) is 25.6/4 $cm^2/\mu mole$.

brandt and Roots, 1975), i.e. 8 mM H_2O_2 (0.025%) has an optical density of 0.35 (optical pathway of 1 cm). Peroxide should be added under stirring after the sample has been mixed with the rest of the assay mixture.

The volume activity (Section 9.2.3.4; using the a value of guaiacol from Section 10.1.1.4):

$$\frac{V}{v} \times \frac{1}{a \cdot b} \times \frac{A}{\min} = \frac{3.11}{0.02 \times 1 \times 6.4} \times \frac{A}{\min} = \frac{24.3 \times A}{\min} \, U/ml$$

Dividing the volume activity by the enzyme concentration yields the specific activity which is 250–300 U/mg. Convenient alternative methods using MBTH–DMAB (Ngo and Lenhoff, 1980) are: (i) rate method, in which the absorbance change at 590 nm is continuously measured. The enzyme is added to 100 mM sodium phosphate buffer, pH 6.5, containing 10 mM H_2O_2, 3.3 mM DMAB and 0.07 mM MBTH; or, (ii) fixed time method, in which the absorbance is measured at various time intervals against a blank (without enzyme) at 590 nm. The assay is carried out in the same buffer, containing 1 mM H_2O_2, 30 mM DMAB and 0.6 mM MBTH, before the enzyme is added (10 μl/3 ml). The operational molar extinction coefficient at 590 nm is 47600 $M^{-1}cm^{-1}$ (i.e., $a = 47.6$ cm²/μmole).

10.1.2. β-Galactosidase (BGase)

β-D-Galactoside galactohydrolase (EC 3.2.1.23), or β-Galactosidase (BGase), has been detected in numerous microorganisms, animals and plants. The most extensively investigated enzyme, from *Escherichia coli* (*E. coli*), is most popular for EIA, and will be discussed here. Its large size makes it less suitable for EIH.

10.1.2.1. Physicochemical properties of β-galactosidase   Native BGase, a tetramer, has a molecular weight of 465000 (from its complete amino acid sequence) and a p*I* of 4.6 (Fowler and Zabin, 1977). The tetramer dissociates into inactive monomers at pH < 3.5 or > 11.5 or with mercurials (Loontiens et al., 1970). Aggregated

forms of BGase, i.e. multiples of the tetramers (16 S) with $s^0_{20,w}$ values of 23, 27, 32, 36, and 41–45 S, are readily formed in purified preparations (Wallenfels et al., 1959; Marchesi et al., 1969), in particular in the absence of SH compounds (Sund and Weber, 1963). With 100 mM 2-mercaptoethanol (2-ME) and 10 mM $MgCl_2$ (2-ME alone inactivates the enzyme) the enzyme is also much more heat stable (Craven et al., 1965).

The enzyme is stable for at least 30 min at 40°C within pH 6–8 (Wallenfels and Weil, 1972), but its stability at 40°C falls sharply below pH 6.0 and slowly above pH 8.0. Heat stability is considerably lowered by various intermediates in the glucose metabolic cycle (Brewer and Moses, 1967).

It is of interest for EIA that BGase is an excellent immunogen, that anti-BGase antibodies do not inhibit enzymic activity (Cohn and Torriani, 1952) and that some inactive BGase mutants can be activated through the reaction with specific antibodies (Rotman and Celada, 1968).

10.1.2.2. Purification of β-galactosidase   In some *E. coli* strains about 5% of the total protein content is BGase if lactose is the sole source of carbon. The large size and stability of BGase render its isolation easy. The classical method of Craven et al. (1965) as well as a simple affinity chromatography procedure, are described here.

E. coli K 12 cells (1 kg wet weight), grown in lactose medium, are suspended in 2 l standard buffer (10 mM Tris–acetate, pH 7.5, containing 10 mM $MgCl_2$, 10 mM 2-ME, and 10 mM NaCl) and sonicated. The disrupted cell suspension is clarified by centrifugation at $2500 \times g$ overnight. $(NH_4)_2SO_4$ is added to 650 mM and the precipitate is removed by centrifugation. The $(NH_4)_2SO_4$ concentration in the supernatant is then raised to 1.3 M. The precipitate, collected by centrifugation, is resuspended in and dialyzed extensively against the standard buffer without NaCl. An eventual precipitate is removed by centrifugation. This sample (in 10 ml aliquots) is passed through a Sephadex G-200 column (5×100 cm); the enzyme elutes just after the void volume. The pooled fractions are applied to a DEAE–Sephadex A-50 (not DEAE–cellulose!) column (4 × 25 cm) equilibrated with standard buffer (without NaCl). The enzyme is then eluted with a standard buffer–NaCl gradient, using a 500 ml closed mixing chamber containing the standard buffer, and adding dropwise by gravity a 2% NaCl solution. The yield of practically pure enzyme is about 400 mg. The enzyme may be crystallized by the method of Wallenfels and Malhotra (1960).

Alternatively, the enzyme can be purified after precipitation with $(NH_4)_2SO_4$ by 2 cycles of affinity chromatography on p-aminophenyl-β-D-thiogalactopyranoside-agarose (Sigma; Villarejo and Zabin, 1974). Using this method, Steers et al. (1971) obtained the enzyme from a crude extract from 25 g bacteria in 95% yield. The TN (Section 9.2.3.4) of the purified enzyme is about 3×10^5 moles of o-nitrophenyl-β-D-galactoside (o-NPG) at 25°C in 50 mM potassium phosphate buffer, pH 6.8, containing 1 mM $MgCl_2$ and 2.6 mM substrate. This corresponds to a specific activity of about 500 U/mg (Section 9.2.3.4).

10.1.2.3. Catalytic properties of β-galactosidase   BGase follows Michaelis–Menten kinetics (Wallenfels and Weil, 1972) and $k_{cat} \ll k_{-1}$ so that $K_m = K_S$. However, additional enzyme complexes may be distinguished:

$$E + S \xrightleftharpoons{K_S} ES \xrightarrow[\substack{\downarrow P_1}]{k_2'} ES' \xrightleftharpoons{k_2} E + P_2$$

where P_2 is the free galactose and P_1 is either glucose or an aglyconic group. The enzyme displays a wide tolerance to the structure of P_1; the K_m value for its natural substrate, lactose, $(3.85 \times 10^{-3}$ M) is higher than for o-NPG and p-NPG $(9.5 \times 10^{-4}$ M and 4.45×10^{-4} M, respectively; Bergmeyer et al., 1974). The D-pyranoside is essential and the pH optimum of activity is 7.2–7.7 (Wallenfels et al., 1959).

Acceptor alcohols (methanol, glycerol, 2-ME, Tris) stimulate the cleavage of o-NPG, but not of other substrates. Heavy metals, organo-mercuric compounds, chelating agents (EDTA, citrate), prevent the inhibitory effect of 2-ME which in that case is an excellent activator of the enzyme. Studies on these parameters in solid-phase EIA are altogether lacking.

10.1.2.4. Assay of β-galactosidase   The standard assay of BGase is a coupled assay (Section 9.2.3.2) with the following sequence:

$$\text{lactose} + H_2O \xrightarrow{\text{BGase}} \beta\text{-D galactose} + \text{D-glucose}$$

$$\beta\text{-D-galactose} + NAD^+ \xrightarrow{\frac{\beta\text{-galactose}}{\text{dehydrogenase}}} \text{D-galactono-}\delta\text{-lactone} + NADH + H^+$$

For EIA, *o*-NPG, which is converted to *o*-nitrophenol (*o*-NP), is preferred since the relative catalytic rate is considerably higher and less solid-phase interference is expected. Composition of the assay mixture is given in Table 10.8. The coupled reaction is measured by the absorbance of NADH ($a = 6.22$ cm^2/μmole at 340 nm), whereas in the alternative assay *o*-NP is measured ($a = 18.5$ cm^2/μmole at 405 nm). The change of optical density, which is measured per minute, is used for the calculation of the volume activity in

TABLE 10.8
Assays for *β*-galactosidase

	Substrate	
	Lactose (ml)	*p*-nitrophenyl-*β*-D-galac-toside (p-NPG) (ml)
25 mM potassium phosphate buffer, pH 6.8	1.00	1.00
50 mM lactose	1.93	
14 mM *p*-NPG		1.95
100 mM MgSO$_4$	0.03	0.03
14 mM NAD$^+$	0.01	
β-Galactose dehydrogenase (5 mg/ml)	0.01	
Sample	0.02	0.02
Total volume (ml)	3.00	3.00

the sample (Section 9.2.3.4):

$$\text{volume activity} = \frac{3.00}{a \cdot b \cdot 0.02} \times \frac{A}{\min} \text{ U/ml sample}$$

The specific activity and the TN can be established after determining the enzyme concentration (Section 9.2.3.4).

10.1.3. Alkaline phosphatase (APase)

APases (orthophosphoric monoester phosphohydrolase, alkaline optimum, EC 3.1.3.1) are found primarily in animal tissues and microorganisms. APases used in EIA are isolated from bovine intestinal mucosa or from *E. coli*. These enzymes have considerable differences in their properties and should not, as often done, be assayed under identical conditions.

APases hydrolyze numerous phosphate esters, such as those of primary and secondary alcohols, phenols and amines (Levine, 1974). One unit of activity of APase corresponds to the hydrolysis of 1.0 μmole of *p*-nitrophenyl phosphate (*p*-NPP) per min (in 100 mM glycine, 1 mM $ZnCl_2$, 1 mM $MgCl_2$ and 6 mM *p*-NPP, pH 10.4; or in 1 M diethanolamine, 0.5 mM $MgCl_2$ and 15 mM *p*-NPP, pH 9.8). The bovine enzyme generally has a specific activity of 1000 and 2000 U/mg in these two buffers, respectively, at 37°C. At 25°C, activity is reduced to about half. This demonstrates that buffers may have a marked influence on the enzymatic activity of APases which explains the great differences in activity given for commercial preparations. Assays with *p*-NPP above 30°C suffer from the spontaneous hydrolysis of this substrate, with serious consequences for the enzyme kinetics (see below). The bacterial enzyme has lower activity than the bovine intestinal enzyme.

A major reason for the popularity of APase for EIA is its absence from higher plants. However, this enzyme is particularly abundant in animal and human tissues involved in nutrient transport (hence its isolation from intestinal mucosa), and in developing tissues and secretory organs, but it is not found in significant amounts in muscle, connective tissue or cartilage. Some pathological conditions increase APase activities in sera. For the same reason POase, which is abundant in plant but not in animal tissues, is popular for EIA with samples from human or animal origin.

10.1.3.1. Physicochemical properties of alkaline phosphatase

APases are dimeric proteins, the properties of which vary according to the origin of the enzyme (Table 10.9). They all seem to be zinc metalloenzymes with at least 2 atoms of Zn^{2+} per enzyme molecule. Three classes of metal-binding sites are distinguished (at least for the bacterial enzyme), the so-called catalytic (A), structural (B), and regulatory (C) sites (Otvos and Armitage, 1980). Binding at the two A sites only results in the phosphorylation of only one subunit, i.e. negative cooperative subunit interaction (Otvos et al., 1979). When metal ions, e.g. Mg^{2+}, are added to fill the B and the C sites, the negative cooperative regulation is abrogated and both subunits can be phosphorylated. Zn^{2+} binds to three essential histidyl residues per subunit (McCracken and Meighen, 1981), of which at least one seems to be in the A site. The intestinal and bacterial APase are 20 and 60 times more active in the dimeric form, respectively (Neumann and Lustig, 1980).

TABLE 10.9
Physicochemical properties of alkaline phosphatase

Property	Enzyme from bovine intestinal mucosa	Enzyme from E. coli
Mass (daltons)	84500[a]	80000[b]
pH optimum for activity	10.3[c]	8.0[d,e]
Sedimentation coefficient (S; pH 6)	6.0[a]	5.2[d]
Partial specific volume (ml/g)	0.73	0.73[e,f]
Isoelectric point	5.7[h]	4.5[d]
Structure		globular[i]
Extinction coefficient (1%; 278 nm; 1 cm)	7.8	7.2

References: a, Neumann and Lustig, 1980; b, Rothman and Byrne, 1963; c, Fernley, 1971; d, Reid and Wilson, 1971; e, Garen and Levinthal, 1960; f, Ullmann et al., 1968; g, Simpson et al., 1968; h, Lazdunski et al., 1965; i, Torriani, 1968.

10.1.3.2. Purification of alkaline phosphatase from E. coli   *E. coli* K10 is cultured in the medium of Echols et al. (1961) by the method of Torriani (1968). Under limiting phosphate conditions cultures may contain as much as 6% enzyme (Garen and Levinthal, 1960). APase is primarily localized in the periplasmic space and released by a 'shock' medium (Torriani, 1968).

The bacterial pellet obtained from the culture is suspended in 10 mM Tris–HCl buffer, pH 7.7, carefully washed three times with the same buffer and the final pellet resuspended in a solution (1 g/20 ml) of 500 mM sucrose in 30 mM Tris–HCl buffer, pH 8.0, containing 0.5 mM EDTA. The suspension is gently mixed in a 2 l flask for 10 min at room temperature. The pellet, obtained by centrifugation (10 min, $13000 \times g$), is resuspended in an equal volume of cold (3°C), distilled water. The cells are mixed for 10 min and again pelleted. About 80% of the enzyme is recovered in the supernatant.

$(NH_4)_2SO_4$ is added to 3.6 M (volume increase!). The precipitate, collected by centrifugation, is dissolved in Tris–HCl buffer, pH 7.4, containing 1 mM $MgSO_4$ in 1/50 of the original volume and dialyzed extensively against this buffer, if further purified on DEAE–cellulose, or against 10 mM Tris–HCl, pH 8.0, if further purified by affinity chromatography (see below). The sample is applied on a DEAE–cellulose column (80 ml), equilibrated with the buffer. The enzyme is eluted by gradually increasing the NaCl concentration in the buffer to about 125 mM, just before the nucleases. The final yield is about 60%.

10.1.3.3. Purification of alkaline phosphatase from bovine intestinal mucosa   Crude APase (Boehringer, grade II) can be purified 20-fold and completely recovered by the simple method of Landt et al. (1978) and Mössner et al. (1980). The enzyme is dialyzed against several changes of 10 mM Tris–HCl buffer, pH 8.0, over a 24 h period. The sample is applied to a column of L-histidyldiazo-benzylphosphonic acid–agarose (Sigma; capacity about 100 U/ml), washed with Tris buffer and the enzyme is eluted with 10 mM

Na_2HPO_4. The enzyme is then dialyzed against the Tris buffer containing 0.1 mM $ZnCl_2$ and 1 mM $MgCl_2$. The column is regenerated with Tris–HCl buffer.

10.1.3.4. Catalytic properties of alkaline phosphatases   The enzyme transfers the phosphoryl residue via a phosphoryl–enzyme intermediate, which can be repressed by inorganic phosphate (P_i; Fig. 10.3).

Under certain conditions the steady state has the form of the Michaelis–Menten equation (Section 9.1.2). Nevertheless, the equation for APase contains more factors than that of the simple reaction given in Section 9.1.2. For detailed kinetic considerations, Fernley (1971) and Reid and Wilson (1971) should be consulted. The simplified representation of Fig. 10.3 is also often complicated by other parameters; e.g. only one active site per dimer seems to be active for the bacterial enzyme at low substrate concentrations ($< 10^{-4}$ M), whereas at higher concentrations both sites are active. Substrate activation, at high substrate concentrations ($> 10^{-2}$ M), was noted by Heppel et al. (1962) but not at high ionic strength (Simpson and Vallee, 1970).

Fernley (1971) discussed the influence of different buffers on bovine

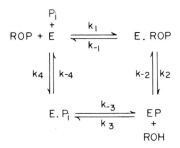

Fig. 10.3. Schematic representation of hydrolysis of a phosphate ester (ROP) by APase. P_i represents inorganic phosphate, ROP is substrate and EP is phosphoryl enzyme. Typical values for the various rate constants for the bacterial enzyme in 50 mM Tris–HCl buffer, pH 8.3, at 10°C with *p*-nitrophenyl phosphate as substrate (Bale et al., 1980) are $k_1/k_{-1} = K_s \geq 1.5 \times 10^{-4}$ M; $k_2/K_s = 1.6 \times 10^7$ M^{-1} sec^{-1}; $k_2 \geq 2.4 \, 10^3$ sec^{-1}; $k_3 = 78$ sec^{-1} and $k_{-4} = 7.6$ sec^{-1}.

APase activity. The pH optimum of the enzyme is shifted to higher values with increasing substrate concentrations, whereas with increasing pK values of the substrate, the pH optimum tends to shift to neutrality. Addition of ions, such as Mg^{2+}, may significantly enhance enzyme activity in some buffers, (glycine buffers, which have insufficient buffering capacity for APase) but not in others (diethanolamine, Bergmeyer, 1974). Tris buffers produce a sharp increase in enzyme activity (Neumann et al., 1975).

Many inhibitors may be present in biological samples or in buffers currently used for EIA. P_i is a competitive inhibitor of the enzyme and forms an intermediate with the enzyme which is indistinguishable from the intermediate formed during catalysis of the hydrolysis of phosphate esters (Caswell and Caplow, 1980). The K_i (i.e. the K_m for P_i) is lower than the K_m for the substrate, typically $K_i/K_m = 0.3$, i.e. a lower concentration of P_i than of the substrate is required to half-saturate the enzyme. Arsenate is a stronger competitive inhibitor than P_i, whereas phosphonates are weaker. Metal chelating products (EDTA, cysteine, thioglycolic acid) are also important inhibitors. Many amino acids show a mixed competitive or uncompetitive inhibition (Fernley, 1971).

10.1.3.5. A major flaw in the current methodology of EIA using alkaline phosphatase   In most solid-phase EIA methods, incubations and washings are performed in phosphate-buffered saline (PBS). PBS contains a relatively high amount of P_i (15 mM), and behaves as a highly concentrated solution of inhibitor for APase. Though the substrate is presented in another buffer, 5–10% of the PBS buffer (e.g. 10–20 µl) remains in the wells after washing, particularly in the unstirred layer where the enzyme is situated. The practice of 'shaking-dry' produces only the evaporation of water, not the removal of P_i.

The use of *p*-NPP as a substrate for this enzyme is popular, since: (i) its spontaneous hydrolysis is low below 30°C; (ii) it is soluble to a concentration 100 times higher than the K_m value, enabling zero-order kinetics; and, (iii) its hydrolysis product, *p*-nitrophenol (*p*-NP), absorbs strongly at 405 nm.

The production of p-NP ([P]) follows eq. 6 from Section 9.1.2:

$$v = \frac{d[P]}{dt} = \frac{k_{cat}[E][S]}{[S] + K_m} \tag{5}$$

which can be simplified if $[S] \gg K_m$, as is the case in the present assay, to $v = k_{cat} \cdot [E]$. In this ideal case, product formation is linear with the enzyme concentration, and thus with the immunoreactant. Moreover, small variations in $[S]$ do not affect the rate of product formation and $d[P]/dt$ remains fairly constant.

For the inhibited reaction, eq. 5 may be rewritten as (Section 9.1.6):

$$\frac{d[P]}{dt} = \frac{k_{cat} \cdot [E]}{1 + K_m/[S] + (K_m/K_i) \cdot ([P_i]/[S])} \tag{6}$$

This simplifies to eq. 5 if $[P_i] = 0$. In the experimental conditions described above, however, about 10% of the original P_i, i.e. 1.5 mM, may remain in the wells, whereas it is customary to use 4.6 mM substrate (Voller et al., 1979). A typical value of the K_i/K_m ratio for this enzyme–substrate–inhibitor combination is 0.3 (Section 9.2.3.4). Therefore:

$$\frac{d[P]}{dt} = \frac{k_{cat} \cdot [E]}{1 + 1/100 + (1/0.3) \cdot (1.5/4.6)} = 1/2 \, k_{cat} \cdot [E] \tag{7}$$

Thus, at the start of the reaction, only half the maximum catalytic activity is obtained. This effect may be more or less serious for different solid phases (Section 9.2.2).

Despite these obvious objections, virtually all EIA using APase continue to be performed in PBS. The type of reaction kinetics changes then from zero-order to mixed (first- and zero-) order, in which: (i) $d[P]/dt$ decreases much faster than in zero-order kinetics as can be shown by integration (Section 9.1.5); (ii) the lowered activity caused by the presence of P_i is due to random factors and depends on the amount of PBS remaining in the well; and, (iii) the presence of P_i invalidates the error structure of the assay. Though the amounts of P_i remaining in the wells can be expected to follow a skewed distribution, the effect of P_i on enzyme activity is more complex since the degree of inhibition is not linearly proportional to the P_i concentration.

For the same reasons, spontaneous substrate hydrolysis, producing P_i, should be prevented. The presence of only 1% P_i in the substrate (p-NPP) produces a significant inhibition of the enzyme (Jung and Pergande, 1980). Commercially supplied substrates may contain up to 6% P_i. The performance of the substrate should be tested, if necessary purified, and be stored at low temperature.

10.1.3.6. Assays of alkaline phosphatases   APases hydrolyze numerous phosphate esters, but not phosphodiesters. For activity measurements, p-NPP is now generally used. Enzyme activity is measured as indicated in Table 10.10, with a 50 mM solution of p-NP for calibration (696 mg p-NP in 100 mM NaOH to 1 l, and diluted 100 times with the same solution).

The concentration of P_i in the assay mixture should be lower than 0.05 mM. Tris buffers are preferred for the bacterial APase and diethanolamine (DEA) for the bovine enzyme, which gives, with excess substrate, about 15% higher activity in a 2 M DEA–HCl buffer than at 1 M. However, the background is also stronger (Walter and Schütt, 1974).

TABLE 10.10
Assay of alkaline phosphatase

	Origin of enzyme	
	E. coli	Bovine intestinal mucosa
3 M Tris–HCl buffer, pH 8.0	1.0 ml	
3 M diethanolamine–HCl buffer, pH 9.8		1.0 ml
20 mM p-nitrophenyl phosphate	1.9 ml	1.9 ml
Enzyme sample	0.1 ml	0.1 ml
Total volume	3.0 ml	3.0 ml

Mix and measure 30 sec later for 2 min (stopwatch) at 405 nm. If the increase in absorbance is significantly more than 0.2/min, dilute the sample with physiological NaCl solution (150 mM).

Jung and Köhler (1980) reported that the molar extinction coefficient (18.6×103 M^{-1} cm^{-1}) of p-NP depends on the assay temperature, concentration of the buffer, and the presence of proteins. Small, apparent differences reported in activities may, therefore, be due in part to a changing extinction coefficient.

The volume activity (Section 9.2.3.4) is:

$$\frac{3.00}{18.6 \times 1.0 \times 0.1} \times \frac{A}{\min} = \frac{1.61 \times A}{\min} \text{ U/ml sample}$$

and the specific activity (U/mg protein) is calculated from the volume activity by dividing with the enzyme concentration (mg/ml).

10.1.4. Glucose oxidase (GOase)

GOase (β-D-glucose:oxygen-1-oxidoreductase, EC 1.1.3.4) is frequently used in AA-type EIA. This enzyme can be obtained from fungal sources, in particular from *Aspergillus niger* and *Penicillium* species, of which virtually only that of *A. niger* is used for EIA. Some caution is warranted for the comparison of enzyme activity indicated by commercial suppliers: some express the unit activity based on the uptake of 1 or 22.4 µl oxygen per min (Sigma), whereas others (Boehringer) use an indicator reaction (POase) to express activity. It is important to realize that although the purest commercial GOase preparations contain less than 0.01% catalase, the latter, due to its high TN, competes for H_2O_2 with POase in the indicator reaction. It is, therefore, advisable to determine the catalase activity of the GOase preparation prior to use in EIA (Section 10.1.4.4). Other frequent contaminants (amylase, maltase, galactose oxidase, glycogenase and invertase) do not interfere significantly in the EIA. H_2O_2 may inactivate the enzyme (Kleppe, 1966).

10.1.4.1. Physicochemical properties of glucose oxidase   The

A. niger enzyme is a dimer with two very tightly bound coenzyme (FAD) molecules per dimer (Swoboda and Massey, 1965). The most salient properties of GOase are listed in Table 10.11. Only a small

TABLE 10.11
Physicochemical properties of glucose oxidase

Mass (daltons)	186000[a], 153000[b]
Number of subunits	2[a]
Coenzyme	FAD (2 molecules)[a]
Overall structure	globular[b]
Frictional ratio	1.21[b]
Stokes radius (nm)	4.3[b]
Carbohydrate content (mostly mannose)	12%[b]
Isoelectric point	4.35[c]
Sedimentation coefficient (S)	8.0[c]
Extinction coefficient (278 nm; 1 cm; 1 mg/ml)	1.8

References: a, Swoboda and Massey, 1965; b, Nakamura et al., 1976; c, Bentley, 1963.
FAD = flavine adenine dinucleotide.

portion of the enzyme has an ordered structure (helix or β-pleated sheat conformation; Nakamura and Hayashi, 1974) . Oxidation with periodate hardly affects the enzyme activity, immunological properties (antigenicity) and heat-stability. The oxidized enzyme, however, is somewhat less resistant to detergents than the native enzyme (Nakamura et al., 1976). The concentration of $NaIO_4$ used in these studies was about 25 times higher than needed for conjugation by the $NaIO_4$ method.

Crystalline GOase retains its activity for at least two years at $0°C$ and 8 years at $-15°C$ (Bentley, 1963) and it is stable for at least a year in an $(NH_4)_2SO_4$ solution at $4°C$. An aqueous solution of the enzyme is stable for a week at $5°C$. Moreover, the activity of GOase is not affected at $39°C$ for 1 h at pH 5.6 or by incubation with 0.2% sodium deoxycholate or SDS, or with 1% pepsin or papain. The enzyme is unstable above $40°C$ or at pH values above 8, though the presence of glucose may exert a protective action.

10.1.4.2. Purification and catalytic reaction of glucose oxidase
A. niger GOase may be obtained commercially at low prices. However, if desired, crude preparations of this enzyme may be purified as described by Nakamura and Fujiki (1968).

Early work by Keilin and Hartree (1948) demonstrated a bell-shaped profile for the pH-dependence of the initial velocity with a peak at pH 5.6. The enzyme is specific for β-D-glucose:

$$\beta\text{-D-glucose} + H_2O + O_2 \xrightarrow{\text{GOase}} \text{D-glucono-}\delta\text{-lactone} + H_2O_2$$

The solubility of oxygen in pure water after equilibration at 25°C with air or pure oxygen is about 0.24 mM and 1.2 mM, respectively, but corrections have to be made if other solutes are present (Robinson and Cooper, 1970). Since the K_m value for oxygen (Table 10.12) is usually not exceeded by much, oxygen is almost always the limiting substrate for the enzyme. The formation of H_2O_2 can be monitored at 235 nm ($a_{235} = 0.058$ mM^{-1} cm^{-1} (controversial, cf. Section 10.1.1.5; Bright and Appleby, 1969) if the enzyme concentration is less than 0.5 μM. Otherwise caution is warranted since FAD and FADH$_2$ absorb differently at this wavelength. If contaminating enzymes are absent, it is easier to detect the presence of H_2O_2 with an excess of POase and a suitable redox dye (DH; Section 10.2.1.5).

The complex kinetics of GOase have been described by Bright and Porter (1975). Some of the characteristics of the catalytic reaction of GOase are given in Table 10.12.

TABLE 10.12
Some characteristics of catalysis by glucose oxidase

Optimum pH	5.6 (broad range 4–7)[a]
Inhibitors (% inhibition at 10 mM)	2-deoxy-D-glucose (?)[a];
	p-chloromercuribenzoate (100%)[b];
	sodium nitrate (13%)[b];
	D-arabinose[c];
	8-hydroxyquinoline (11%)[a]
K_m (glucose)	28 mM[d]
(oxygen)	0.18 mM[d]

References: a, Keilin and Hartree, 1948; b, Bentley, 1963; c, Adams et al., 1960; d, Nakamura et al., 1976.

10.1.4.3. Assay of glucose oxidase and catalase   GOase activity can be determined by fluorimetric, manometric, electrochemical or spectrophotometric methods.

On oxidation, homovanillic acid, HVA (4-hydroxy-3-methoxy-phenyl-acetic acid), is converted to a highly fluorescent, stable compound with an excitation wavelength of 315 nm and an emission wavelength of 425 nm. Oxidized HVA is produced in an amount proportional to that of GOase between 0.001 and 0.25 U/ml (Guilbault, 1968). Guilbault (1976) showed that *p*-hydroxyphenylacetic acid has some advantages over HVA with respect to cost and fluorescence coefficient (fluorescence/concentration) and 0.01 U of enzyme could be assayed.

GOase activity is conventionally assayed in a Warburg apparatus to measure the uptake of oxygen (Guilbault, 1976). Electrochemical methods (potentiometric or amperometric) are less sensitive than the fluorimetric methods, but are well-suited for automation (Pardue et al., 1964; Blaedel and Olson, 1964).

The spectrophotometric assay is based on a POase indicator reaction to measure the amount of H_2O_2 liberated. For this reason an excess of POase and H-donor (Section 10.2.1.4.2) has to be used. One unit (U) is then expressed as the amount of enzyme liberating 1 μmole of H_2O_2 per min at 25°C.

In the spectrophotometric assay system (Bergmeyer et al., 1974; Table 10.17), the total reaction mixture (3 ml) should contain about 0.5 U GOase (about 2 μg active enzyme) per ml (at 25°C), added

TABLE 10.13
Assay mixture for glucose oxidase

Volume (ml)	Reagent	Final concentration
2.17	100 mM potassium phosphate buffer, containing 0.066 mg *o*-dianisidine/ml	82 mM
0.50	D-glucose (100 mg/ml)	0.17 mM
0.01	peroxidase (2 mg/ml)	1.2 U/ml
0.02	sample (added after mixing of reagents)	

in a volume of 20 μl. The optical density at 436 nm (1 cm light path) is measured after 1, 2, 3, 4, and 5 min and the mean A/min is calculated. The volume activity (Section 9.2.3.4.; a of o-dianisidine being 8.3 cm^2/μmole) is:

$$\frac{3}{8.3 \times 1.0 \times 0.02} \times \frac{A}{\text{min}} = \frac{18.07 \times A}{\text{min}} \text{ U/ml}$$

The specific activity in U/mg enzyme is obtained by dividing the volume activity by the enzyme concentration (mg/ml).

Contaminating catalase, which catalyzes the reaction $2H_2O_2 \rightarrow 2H_2O + O_2$, and interferes in the above assay, can be determined by the method of Bergmeyer (1955). Since little H_2O_2 is present, catalase follows a first-order reaction and the amount of H_2O_2 consumed is directly proportional to the concentrations of both H_2O_2 and catalase. Two solutions are prepared just before use: (i) about 1 μg pure catalase per ml in 50 mM phosphate buffer, pH 7.0; and, (ii) a solution containing 0.1 ml of 30% H_2O_2 in 50 ml of the same buffer (0.52–0.55 A in 1 cm cuvet at 240 nm; molar extinction coefficient: 0.040 cm^2/μmole). For the assay, 0.1 ml of the enzyme solution is added to 2.9 ml of the substrate solution, mixed, and the time needed for decreasing the optical density from 0.45 to 0.40 is noted. The amount of enzyme solution added should be adjusted so that the time needed for the desired decrease in absorbance is about 20 sec. The general formula for the determination of the volume activity (Section 9.2.3.4) has to be multiplied by 60 to obtain A/min:

$$\frac{3}{0.04 \times 1.0 \times 0.1} \times \frac{0.05}{\text{seconds}} \times 60 = \frac{2250}{\text{seconds}} \text{ U/ml}$$

and the specific activity is obtained by dividing this activity by the enzyme concentration (mg/ml).

10.1.5. Urease: a convenient enzyme for the visual determination of titration endpoints

Urease (urea amidohydrolase, EC 3.5.1.5) has the advantage that in the presence of the pH indicator bromocresol purple it produces a sharp unequivocal endpoint with its substrate, urea (Chandler et al., 1982). Moreover, it is absent from mammalian cells. Though urease can also be used for potentiometric EIA (Section 14.6.5), other deaminating enzymes, in particular asparaginase (Gebauer and Rechnitz, 1982), are more promising. The major drawback of urease is the possibility of rapid loss of enzyme activity. Type VII or C-3 urease (Sigma) from jack beans (*Canavalia ensiformis*) are the most frequently used enzyme preparations. The physicochemical properties of urease are compiled in Table 10.14.

The reaction catalyzed by urease is:

$$urea + H_2O \rightarrow CO_2 + 2NH_3$$

The substrate-indicator solution is prepared by dissolving 8 mg bromocresol purple powder (Gurr) in 1.48 ml 10 mM sodium hydroxide and made up to 100 ml with deionized water. Urea (100 mg) and EDTA (to 0.2 mM) are then added and the pH is adjusted to 4.8.

TABLE 10.14
Physicochemical properties of urease

Mass (daltons)	480000[a,b]
K_m (in phosphate buffer, pH 7.0, 25° C; mM)	10.3[c]
Inhibition by	Na^+, K^+, NH_4^+ [d]
Activation by	inorganic phosphate[d]
Specific activity of pure enzyme[g]	≈ 1000
Stability (lyophilized)	several months[d] at 4° C
Absorbance ratio (280/260 nm)	1.8–1.9[e]
Absorbance coefficient (278.5 nm; 1 cm; 0.1%)	0.6–0.8[f]

References: a, Reithel et al., 1964; b, Gorin et al., 1962; c, Peterson et al., 1948; d, Bergmeyer et al., 1974; e, Blakely et al., 1969; f, Reithel, 1971.
[g] Activity is expressed as: μmoles of NH_3 liberated from urea per min at pH 7.0 at 25° C. (1 μmole unit is 0.054 Sumner units).

The production of ammonia by urease is readily detected by a rise in pH, which is indicated by a vivid color change of the indicator from yellow to purple. The reaction may be stopped by the addition of thiomersal.

10.2. Enzymes used in activity modulation assays

The previously discussed enzymes may all be used for solid-phase AM assays. For homogeneous AM-type EIA, lysozyme, malate dehydrogenase (MDase), glucose-6-phosphate dehydrogenase (GPDase), and ribonuclease A (RNase A), are used in addition to BGase.

10.2.1. Lysozyme

Lysozyme (*N*-acetylmuramide glycano-hydrolase, EC 3.2.1.17) from hen-egg white was the first enzyme used in homogeneous EIA (Rubenstein et al., 1972) and is employed for a number of assays (Table 10.15).

TABLE 10.15
Activity-modulation assays using lysozyme

Substance	Detection limit (μg/ml)	Reference
Amphetamine	2.0	a,b
Barbiturate	2.0	a,c
Benzodiazapine	0.7	d
Benzoyl ecgonine (cocaine metabolite)	1.6	e
Methadone	0.5	a
Morphine	0.5	e,f
Propoxyphene	2.0	b

Lysozyme is used in rapid urine assays (total assay time < 60 sec), but has some important limitations. Sometimes urine samples are positive for lysozyme and blanks should be run for all positive samples. These assays may also be affected by the pH, salt concentrations, and lysozyme inhibitors in urine. Blood and serum have high lysozyme levels. Detection limits are given at 95% confidence levels of semiquantitative tests (Kabakoff and Greenwood, 1982).
References: a, Schneider et al., 1974; b, Ullman and Maggio, 1980; c, Walberg, 1974; d, Haden et al., 1976; e, Bastiani et al., 1973; f, Schneider et al., 1973.

Lysozyme has bacteriolytic properties. A small round bacterium, *Micrococcus lysodeikticus*, is particularly susceptible to this enzyme (Fleming, 1922) and is widely used as a substrate. The activity of the enzyme is determined by the decrease of light scattering ('absorbance') of a bacterial suspension at 450 nm. The polysaccharide polymers of the cell wall of *M. lysodeikticus* are made up of two alternating sugars, *N*-acetylglucosamine (NAG) and *N*-acetylmuramic acid (NAM; a derivative of glucosamine). Lysozyme, which possesses β(1→4)-glucosaminidase activity, hydrolyzes the bond between the C-1 of NAM and the C-4 of NAG, resulting in cell lysis, due to the high osmotic pressure inside, and consequently in a decrease of light scattering.

One of the 6 lysyl residues (residue 97) of lysozyme is near the active site. Conjugation of a hapten to this group does not affect the activity of the enzyme, but incubation of the enzyme–hapten conjugate with the specific anti-hapten antibody prior to the addition of the bulky substrate, produces serious inhibition. The smaller Fab is not as effective for inhibition as complete IgG.

10.2.1.1. Physicochemical properties of lysozyme   The amino acid sequence of lysozyme (Jollès et al., 1963; Canfield, 1963; Canfield and Liu, 1965) and its unusually stable three-dimensional structure (Phillips, 1966) provide a model for the detailed description of its interaction with inhibitors and substrate analogs (Johnson and Phillips, 1965; Blake et al., 1967). The enzyme has a deep cleft on one side, lined mostly with hydrophilic amino acid residues, to which the substrate (6 sugar residues) is bound.

Lysozyme has a tendency to form polymers. Between pH 5 and 9 it occurs predominantly as a dimer (Sophianopoulos and Van Holde, 1964), forming higher polymers above pH 9.0. The enzyme is stable between pH 1.2 and 11.3 (Jirgensons, 1952). Its physicochemical properties are listed in Table 10.16.

Modification of its lysyl residues with *O*-methylisourea has no effect (Geschwind and Li, 1957), but acetylation which removes positive charges from the enzyme, affects strongly the enzymic activi-

TABLE 10.16
Molecular properties of lysozyme

Mass (daltons)	14600	Jollès et al., 1963; Canfield, 1963
Number of amino acid residues	129	Jollès et al., 1963, Canfield, 1963
Radius of gyration	1.4	Krigbaum and Kügler, 1970
Volume (nm³)	17.5	Imoto et al., 1972
Sedimentation coefficient (S)	1.6–1.9	Imoto et al., 1972
Extinction coefficient (1%, 280 nm, 1 cm)	25.5	Canfield et al., 1974
Isoelectric point	11.1	Tanford and Wagner, 1954

ty, probably reflecting an alteration in the electrostatic interaction between the positively charged enzyme and the negatively charged cell wall (Imoto et al., 1972). Modification of the 11 arginines, located on the surface of the molecule, generally has no effect on the lytic activity (Imoto et al., 1972). In contrast, the modification of the carboxyl groups of glutamyl and aspartyl residues, which are involved in substrate binding, has a profound influence on the activity of lysozyme. Selective esterification of the carboxyl groups not involved may be possible by adsorbing lysozyme on chitin (Skujins et al., 1973). Alkylation of the single histidyl residue (His 15; not far from the catalytic site) does not abolish lytic activity. Under mild conditions, the 4 disulfide bonds are not exposed to the solvent and will not react with reducing agents.

10.2.1.2. Purification and catalytic properties of lysozyme   A simple, albeit crude, method for bulk preparation is the direct crystallization from hen-egg white solution by the addition of 5% NaCl at pH 9.5 (Alderton and Fevold, 1946). This heterogeneous preparation can be further purified (Green and Toms, 1971), though the very low cost of this enzyme is hardly an incentive.

Two side-chains, Asp 32 and Glu 35 are directly involved in the hydrolysis (Phillips, 1966). The carboxyl group of Glu 35, which is non-ionized and is located about 0.3 nm from the glucosidic oxygen atom between C-1 of NAM and C-4 of NAG, donates a proton to this oxygen and produces a C-1-OH in NAM and a

C-4$^+$–H carbonium ion intermediate in NAG. This enzymatic reaction is promoted by the presence of a negatively charged group (Asp 32) 0.3 nm away from the carbonium ion intermediate and by the distortion of the NAG ring into a half-chair form. During binding, the substrate is forced to assume the geometry of the transition state which is similar to that of the carbonium ion geometry. This mechanism explains the strong pH- and ionic strength-dependence of lysozyme action (Chang and Carr, 1971). Derivation of these groups abolishes enzyme activity.

Michaelis–Menten equations often do not apply for enzymatic reactions at surfaces, such as bacterial walls (McLaren and Packer, 1970). Precise kinetic parameters, which can only be obtained with well-characterized low molecular weight substrates, are complicated by non-productive binding of small substrates, i.e. binding outside of the catalytic site.

10.2.1.3. Assay of lysozyme   Selsted and Martinez (1980) reported a simple method with high detectability for lysozyme. The lytic activity against *M. lysodeikticus* is measured photometrically after an 18 h incubation period with a detectability as low as 5 pg/ml and is applicable for assays of enzyme in complex biological mixtures. *M. lysodeikticus* (Difco) is suspended in 50 mM phosphate buffer, pH 7.4, as a stock solution at such a concentration that a 10-fold dilution gives an optical density of about 0.6 at 450 nm. The reaction mixture contains 0.1 ml of this cell suspension, 0.1% NaN$_3$, 1 mg of BSA/ml and 0.1 ml of the lysozyme sample in 1 ml buffer. Duplicates are incubated (in snap-cap plastic tubes) at 37°C with mild agitation. After 18 h, the absorbance is measured at 450 nm. Plotting the optical density against the logarithm of the known lysozyme concentrations yields the standard curve.

Other methods have considerably less detectability. The photometric rate-of-lysis assays (Shugar, 1952; Selsted and Martinez, 1978; Carroll and Martinez, 1979) detect 20 ng of lysozyme in a matter of minutes, but suffers from a limited range of linearity. The so-called lysoplate assay (Osserman and Lawlor, 1966) is about 10^5 times less powerful (0.5 μg of lysozyme/ml) and is as long as the method of Selsted and Martinez (1980).

10.2.2. Malate dehydrogenase (MDase)

MDase (L-malate:NAD$^+$ oxidoreductase; EC 1.1.1.37), used in homogeneous EIA, is prepared from pig heart (mitochondria). The oxidation of L-malate is generally catalyzed by two distinct pyridine nucleotide-dependent enzymes: those of the malate–oxaloacetate class, which use NAD$^+$, and those of the malate–pyruvate class (commonly known as malic enzymes), which use NADP$^+$ (Banaszak and Bradshaw, 1975).

MDase catalyzes the general reaction:

$$\text{L-malate} + NAD^+ \rightarrow \text{oxaloacetate} + NADH + H^+$$

Enzyme activity can, therefore, be conveniently followed by measuring the formation of NADH at 340 nm. This enzyme is popular in AM-type EIA (Table 10.17). The reaction of anti-hapten antibodies with the hapten attached to the enzyme either inhibits or potentiates the enzyme activity, probably through changes in the conformation of the enzyme. MDase is detectable at 10^{-11} M during a 1-min measurement. (Lysozyme is detectable at 10^{-8} M during the same time interval).

TABLE 10.17
Applications of malate dehydrogenase in homogeneous EIA and detection range

Substance	Detectability	Reference
Thyroxine	20 ng/ml	Ullman et al., 1979
Morphine	2×10^{-12} moles/ml	Rowley et al., 1975
Codeine	2×10^{-13} moles/ml	Rowley et al., 1975
Triiodothyronine	20 ng/ml	Ullman and Maggio, 1980
Tetrahydrocannabinol	15 ng/ml	Rodgers et al., 1978

10.2.2.1. Physicochemical properties and purification of malate dehydrogenase MDase, as an enzyme of the citric cycle, is ubiquitous. The physicochemical and the kinetic properties of the mitochondrial enzyme (Table 10.18) differ considerably from the cytoplasmic enzymes (Banaszak and Bradshaw, 1975).

MDase is composed of 2 identical subunits of about 35000 daltons which are held together by secondary interactions. The 2 subunits have equivalent binding sites for NAD^+ (Holbrook and Wolfe, 1972) and each subunit binds a coenzyme. These subunits can dissociate without losing catalytic activity and reassemble in the presence of substrate (Shore and Chakrabarti, 1976; Bleile et al., 1977). The enzyme contains 14 SH groups, two of which are required to bind substrate (Sequin and Kosicki, 1967).

Commercial preparations are supplied as $(NH_4)_2SO_4$ precipitates with a specific activity of about 1000 U/mg with oxaloacetate as substrate and are stable for at least a year at 4°C. Once dialyzed against phosphate buffer, it should be stored at -20°C.

The earliest purification procedures used fractionation with

TABLE 10.18
Molecular properties of malate dehydrogenase

Mass (daltons)	70000[a,b]
Subunits	2[c]
Isoelectric point	6.2[d]
Dissociation constant,	
NADH (Tris buffer, pH 8.0)	2.16 μM[e]
NAD^+	480 μM[e]
Apparent K_m,	
oxaloacetic acid	4.5×10^{-5} M[f]
NADH	3.2×10^{-5} M[f]
pH optimum	7.4[d]
Activators	phosphate[g], arsenate[g], Zn^{2+} [g], malate[h]
Inhibitors	oxaloacetate[i], 8-hydroxyquinoline[j], adenine (AMP, ADP, ATP)[k], sulphite[l], thyroxine[a], phenols and substituted phenols[m]

References: a, Thorne and Kaplan, 1963; b, Banaszak and Bradshaw, 1975; c, Dévényi et al., 1966; d, Wolfe and Neilands, 1956; e, Holbrook and Wolfe, 1972; f, Rowley et al., 1975; g, Blonde et al., 1967; h, Telegdi et al., 1973; i, Kun et al., 1967; j, Vallee et al., 1956; k, Kuramitsu, 1966; l, Pfleiderer et al., 1956; m, Wedding et al., 1967.

$(NH_4)_2SO_4$ from ethanol or acetone powders (Ochoa, 1955). An additional zinc–ethanol precipitation step yielded apparently pure preparations (Wolfe and Neiland, 1956). More recently, large-scale purification of pig-heart MDase was achieved by fractionation on CM–cellulose, followed by further purification on Sephadex G-100 (Glatthaar et al., 1974). Mitochondrial MDase from acetone powders was also obtained by precipitation with $(NH_4)_2SO_4$, followed by chromatography on Bio-Rex 70 and DEAE–cellulose (Gregory et al., 1971).

10.2.2.2. Catalytic properties and assay of malate dehydrogenase
Dehydrogenases probably operate according to an, at least partially, ordered pathway (Banaszak and Bradshaw, 1975):

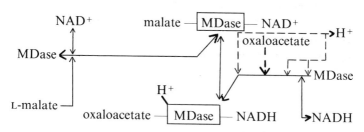

Substrate inhibition by oxaloacetate has been reported (Raval and Wolfe, 1963). Rate-limiting of both catalytic steps appears to be the dissociation of the coenzyme. Activation of MDase by malate is seen as a binding of malate to some effector site (other than the active site), resulting in a tighter binding of NAD^+ (Telegdi et al., 1973).

   MDase activity is monitored by the change in optical density at 340 nm per min due to the disappearance of NADH according to the reaction:

$$\text{oxaloacetate} + NADH + H^+ \rightarrow \text{L-malate} + NAD^+$$

The reaction is performed at 25°C in a 100 mM potassium phosphate buffer, pH 7.4, which also contains 0.5 mM oxaloacetate and 0.2

mM NADH. The enzyme stock solution is diluted with ice-cold phosphate buffer to a concentration of 1 μg/ml immediately before use and 6 μl of this solution are added for each ml of the assay mixture. The optical density change per min is recorded for 5 min and the mean is calculated (A/min).

If the final volume of the assay mixture is 3 ml and the optical pathway (b) 1 cm, the volume activity (Section 9.2.3.4) is:

$$\frac{3}{a \times b \times 0.018} \times \frac{A}{\min} = \frac{26.8 \times A}{\min} \; U/ml$$

The specific activity of the enzyme (U/mg protein) is obtained by dividing the volume activity by the enzyme concentration (mg/ml).

10.2.3. Glucose-6-phosphate dehydrogenase (GPDase)

GPDase (D-glucose-6-phosphate:NADP$^+$ oxidoreductase; EC 1.1.1.49) is frequently used for AM-type EIA, particularly for substances in sera (Table 10.19). This enzyme is widely distributed (Keller, 1971; Löhr and Waller, 1974). However, unlike its mammalian

TABLE 10.19

Applications of glucose-6-phosphate dehydrogenase and detection range (μg/ml) in homogeneous EIA

Lidocaine	(1–12)[a,b]	Carbamazepine	(2–20)[g]
Phencyclidine	(>0.025)[b,c]	Ethoxuximide	(10–150)[g]
Theophylline	(2.5–40)[d]	Gentamicin	(1–16)[j]
Digoxin	(0.5–6 ng/ml)[e]	Quinidine	(1–8)[k]
Cortisol	(0.02–0.5)[f]	Procainamide	(1–16)[l]
Phenytoin	(2.5–30)[g]	N-acetylprocainamide	(1–16)[m]
Phenobarbital	(5–80)[h]	Methotrexate	(0.09–0.9)[g]
Primidone	(2.5–20)[g]	Tobramycin	(1–16)[h,n]
Benzodiazepam	(2.5–30)[i]	Valproic acid	(10–150)[o,p]

References: a, Pape et al., 1978; b, Walberg and Gupta, 1979; c, Brunk et al., 1976; d, Oellerich et al., 1979; e, Chang et al., 1975; f, Finley et al., 1976; g, Ullman and Maggio, 1980; h, Oellerich et al., 1977; i, Tom et al., 1979; j, Kabakoff et al., 1978; k, Collins et al., 1979; l, Fanciullo et al., 1978; m, Izutsu et al., 1978; n, Leung et al., 1979; o, Schottelius, 1978; Isutzu et al., 1979.

counterpart, the bacterial enzyme (from *Leuconostoc mesenteroides*) may use NAD^+, and $NADP^+$ (DeMoss et al., 1953), avoiding interference by mammalian enzymes. GPDase activity, like that of MDase, seems to be affected through a conformational change of the enzymes, resulting in a change of their kinetic parameters (K_m and V_{max}).

GPDase consists of 2 subunits which have a combined molecular weight of 104000 (Olive and Levy, 1971). Each subunit contains a reactive lysyl residue near the active site (Milhausen and Levy, 1975). GPDase from *L. mesenteroides* contains no cysteine (Ishaque et al., 1974) and is very stable (1 year at 4°C).

10.2.3.1. Catalytic properties and assay of glucose-6-phosphate dehydrogenase   The reaction catalyzed by the bacterial GPDase is:

$$\text{glucose-6-phosphate} + NAD^+ \rightarrow$$
$$\text{6-phospho-D-gluconate} + NADH + H^+$$

The unit activity is defined as the amount of enzyme which oxidizes 1 μmole of glucose-6-phosphate to 6-phospho-D-gluconate per min in the presence of $NADP^+$ at pH 7.8 and 30°C (specific activity up to about 400 U/mg). If NAD^+ is used as coenzyme, activity increases by a factor of 1.8.

Mg^{2+} stimulates the enzyme up to 10 mM but inhibits its activity at higher concentrations. Other bivalent cations are often inhibitory. Another important inhibitor is phosphate, though $NADP^+$ may reverse to a certain extent this inhibition (Glaser and Brown, 1955). There is a rather pronounced pH dependence of the *L. mesenteroides* GPDase activity (Löhr and Waller, 1974), namely 7.8.

GPDase activity may be determined by several methods (Löhr and Waller, 1974), among which the spectrophotometrical determination of NADH at 340 nm is the most convenient.

In the assay, the use of phosphate buffer should be avoided, but magnesium (< 10 mM) should be included. Table 10.20 gives the composition of the assay mixture. For the assay, 10 μl containing

TABLE 10.20

Composition of assay mixture for glucose-6-phosphate dehydrogenase

Volume (ml)	Reagent	Concentration (mM)
2.59	100 mM triethanolamine buffer, pH 7.8	86.3
0.20	100 mM MgCl$_2$	6.7
0.10	35 mM glucose-6-phosphate	1.2
0.10	11 mM NAD$^+$	0.37
0.01	enzyme sample (see text)	

about 40 µg enzyme/ml is added and mixed. The volume activity and the specific activity are calculated as in Section 9.2.3.4 (extinction coefficient is 6.22 cm^2/µmole).

10.2.4. Ribonuclease A (RNase)

RNase (ribonucleate 3′-pyrimidino-oligonucleotidohydrolase; EC 3.1.27.5; Richards and Wyckoff, 1971) is a rather small enzyme (13683 daltons), which hydrolyzes a large substrate (RNA). It might, therefore, be expected that this enzyme is sensitive to steric exclusion of the substrate after the interaction of a RNase–protein conjugate with the relatively large antibody. The reaction of anti-hapten antibodies with the haptens attached to the enzyme directly affects the conformation of the enzyme and thus its activity, but antibodies may combine with large enzyme–protein conjugates, without affecting enzyme activity. The exclusion of a very large substrate by steric hindrance could, however, be achieved by large ligands.

A prototype assay for human IgG has been developed by Ullman and Maggio (1980), with a detectability of 10^{-10} M IgG (15 ng/ml). A serious problem with RNase is its ubiquitous nature, causing frequent interference and limiting its practical utility.

10.3. Enzymes used in enzyme immunohistochemistry

The most popular enzymes used in EIH are POase (Section 10.1.1), APase (Section 10.1.3), GOase (Section 10.1.4) and microperoxidase.

10.3.1. Microperoxidase (MPOase)

MPOases are used only in EIH and only when penetration of bulky antibody–enzyme conjugates into tissues poses problems (Section 17.2). MPOase is a proteolytic fragment of cytochrome c from horse heart containing the active site, with a molecular weight of only 1500–2000 (Fig. 10.4).

Three types of MPOases are used: 11-MPOase, a heme-undeca-peptide, containing beside the porphyrin, 11 amino acids from residue 11 through 21 (Harbury and Loach, 1959; Feder, 1971); 8-MPOase,

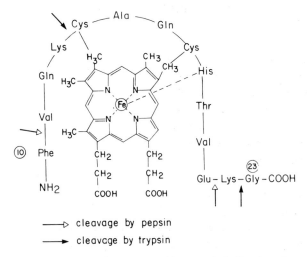

Fig. 10.4. Microperoxidase (MPOase) obtained by proteolytic digestion of cytochrome c. Cleavage by pepsin yields a fragment of the active site of the enzyme containing 11 amino acids (11-MPOase), whereas trypsin yields a fragment of 9 amino acids (9-MPOase). Combination of these digestions yields 8-MPOase. These MPOases have a peroxidatic activity several hundred times greater than the intact cytochrome c.

a heme–octapeptide from residue 14 through 21 (Kraehenbuhl et al., 1974; Tijssen and Kurstak, 1974); and 9-MPOase, a heme-nona-peptide from residue 14 to 22 (Plattner et al., 1977). All have much higher peroxidatic activity than the original enzyme, but somewhat lower than POase. Only 8-MPOase has a single amino group. MPO-ases are very expensive, but can be prepared at low cost by simple methods (Section 10.3.1.1).

10.3.1.1. Physicochemical properties and preparation of microperoxidases MPOases are readily soluble in water or buffer solutions. They can be repeatedly frozen and thawed or stored in solution at 4°C for one year, without change in activity.

Table 10.21 lists some of the physicochemical properties of these MPOases. The pI of these probes seems to lie slightly below 5.0

TABLE 10.21
Physicochemical properties of microperoxidases

	Microperoxidase[a]			References
	8	9	11	
Mass (daltons)	1502	1630	1857	from amino acid sequence[c]
pI	4.85	4.95	4.85	[d, e]
Wavelength (nm) of maximum absorbance[b]	396	397.5	400.5	[d, e]
Extinction coefficient $\times 10^{-5} (M^{-1} cm^{-1})$ at maximum absorbance[b]	1.05	1.11	1.23	[d, e]
pH of optimum activity with DAB	12–13	12.5	13.5	[d, e, f]

[a] 8, 9, 11 denotes length of peptide.
[b] At pH 7.0 and 22° C.
References: c, Margiolash et al., 1961; d, Plattner et al., 1977; e, Tiggeman et al., 1981; f, Simionescu, 1979.

(Gerber et al., 1975; Plattner et al., 1977), significantly lower than for cytochrome c (10.0, Theorell and Akesson, 1941).

A simple method to prepare 9-MPOase was reported by Plattner et al. (1977). Cytochrome c is digested on a column containing trypsin covalently linked to Sepharose or agarose, prepared by the method given in Section 7.1.8.2 (coupling 300 mg trypsin per g of CNBr-activated Sepharose) or purchased (Sigma). Cytochrome c at a concentration of 10 mg/ml 100 mM ammonium carbonate buffer, pH 8.5, is applied to a long, narrow column (50 × 0.25 cm) of trypsin–Sepharose at room temperature in the same buffer and is pumped slowly through the column (flow rate 0.5 ml/h). The red-colored effluent is collected and freeze-dried.

The purification strategy is based on the interaction of the 'unburied' heme group of 9-MPOase with Sephadex resulting in a considerable retardation of the 9-MPOase fragments (elution at almost twice the exclusion volume of the smallest molecules; > 99% pure). In detail, the freeze-dried degradation products are dissolved in a small volume of the same buffer, loaded on a column of Sephadex G-50 (150 × 0.8 cm) and eluted at a flow rate of 5 ml/h. The 9-MPOase which can be readily recognized as a red band elutes after about 40 ml. The overall yield is usually about 50% of the theoretical value.

Preparation of 8-MPOase is similar, with the inclusion of a step of digestion with free pepsin in 0.1 N HCl for 24 h at room temperature and gives high yields of 8-MPOase (Tijssen and Kurstak, 1974; Tiggemann et al., 1981). Alternatively, 8-MPOase can be prepared from the 11-MPOase, which is about 10 times cheaper than 8-MPOase, simply by passing it over the trypsin–Sepharose and the Sephadex columns as described above.

10.3.1.2. Measurement of peroxidatic activity of microperoxidases   The POase-like activity of the MPOases has a pH optimum different from that of both POase and cytochrome c which depends on the H-donor used and the type of MPOase (Fig. 10.5).

Gelatine-stabilized diaminobenzidine (DAB)–H_2O_2 medium (Herzog and Fahimi, 1973) is convenient to measure the various peroxi-

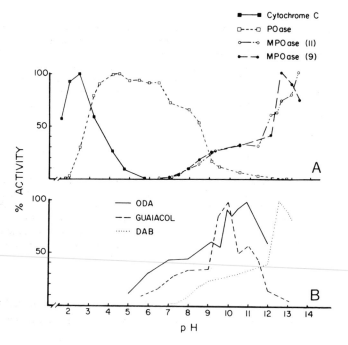

Fig. 10.5. pH-Dependence of POase activities. The maximum activity is fixed at 100%. A shows that large differences exist among cytochrome c, POase, 11-MPOase, and 9-MPOase in their activity in a gelatin-stabilized hydrogen peroxide-diaminobenzidine (DAB)-medium (Herzog and Fahimi, 1973). However, the activity also depends on the H-donor (ODA = o-dianisidine) as exemplified for 9-MPOase in B (courtesy Dr. H. Plattner and *Histochemistry*).

datic activities. A disadvantage of DAB is its 'auto-oxidation' at higher pH values, in particular above 12.5 (Fig. 10.5). The activities of the three MPOases, POase and cytochrome c at their pH optimum are compared in Table 10.22 which reveals that on a molar basis the isolated active site of cytochrome c is about 200 times more active than the complete enzyme but about 50 times less active than POase. Moreover, the number of these fragments which can be conjugated to an IgG or Fab molecule is much larger (20–50) than that of POase before diminishing the antigen-binding capacity.

TABLE 10.22

Comparative activities of microperoxidases, peroxidase (C) and cytochrome c at their optimum pH and with diaminobenzidine as hydrogen donor

Compound	pH	Activity relative to MPOase(9) per weight unit	Activity relative to MPOase(9) per mole unit
MPOase(8)	13	0.61	0.56
MPOase(9)	12.5	1.00	1.00
MPOase(11)	13.5	0.70	0.80
POase	4–6	1.82	44.37
Cyt c	2.5	0.00045	0.0035

Data compiled from Plattner et al. (1977) and Tiggeman et al. (1981) have been normalized to reflect relative activities. Both studies reported the activity for MPOase(9), which is, therefore, taken as a reference. However, the activity of MPOase(9) is probably somewhat too high since it is based on pure material (i.e., without residual water or salt) as calculated from amino acid analysis, whereas the other data were obtained for weighed samples. MPOase(8), (9), and (11) correspond to microperoxidase with 8, 9, and 11 amino acids, respectively; POase is horseradish peroxidase.

Thus, a highly substituted Fab molecule is only slightly less active than an IgG–POase conjugate but has only half the diameter of the latter.

The DAB-oxidation test medium (de-aerated before the addition of H_2O_2) contains per ml: 0.89 ml of 0.3% DAB (tetrahydrochloride form, filtered before use) in 0.1% gelatine in the appropriate buffer (50 mM citrate–NaOH for pH 2–7, 50 mM Tris–HCl between pH 7 and 9, and glycine–NaOH at higher pH values), 0.10 ml of 10 mM H_2O_2 (concentration determined as in Section 10.1.1.5), and 10 μl of the enzyme solution (about 50 μg/ml of MPOase or POase, or 10 mg/ml of cytochrome c). The change in optical density (A/min) is recorded at 465 nm.

Like POase, MPOase is also inhibited by high concentrations of substrate (H_2O_2). MPOases are also sensitive to cyanide (67% inhibition at 10^{-6} M) and, importantly, very sensitive to glutaraldehyde used in fixation or conjugation procedures. In contrast, MPOases are very heat-stable, e.g., resistant to boiling for 1 h.

CHAPTER 11

Preparation of enzyme–antibody or other enzyme–macromolecule conjugates

11.1 Conjugation procedures and their relative merits

An ideal conjugation procedure should yield 100% conjugate of well-defined composition without inactivation of the enzyme or the antibody, produce a stable link, and be practical (i.e., cost, simplicity). None of the present conjugation procedures responds fully to these requirements: large differences exist among the conjugation efficiencies, and in the relative detectabilities by the conjugates. It is, therefore, necessary to make a choice which depends on the given enzyme or the design of the assay. For EIH a 1:1 conjugate is more appropriate, since this probe penetrates more easily into tissue than more complex conjugates. On the other hand, for EIA the highest enzyme/antibody ratio without impairing either activity is desired.

Three fundamentally different conjugation methods exist. The original methods, in which chemical labeling was accomplished, are still the most popular. The development and application of new conjugation methods eliminated most of the problems of the original procedures. Direct conjugation by the periodate ($NaIO_4$) method is very convenient for glycoproteins. The second type of coupling reactions, frequently named 'unlabeled conjugation', is based on a reaction of anti-enzyme antibody with the corresponding enzyme without abrogating the enzyme activity. The enzyme–antibody conjugate is then linked to immune complexes by means of anti-Ig. This immunologic labeling method thus requires specific and more time-consuming designs, is only applicable in AA-type assays, but can increase detectability up to about 100-fold. In the third group of methods auxiliary molecules are used to introduce the enzyme. For example, both the enzyme and the immunoreactant can be biotinylated and linked by the bridging molecule, avidin. Table 11.1 lists the various methods and their relative merits for the different enzymes.

Lyophilized enzymes can be used directly, whereas those obtained as an $(NH_4)_2SO_4$ precipitate should be pretreated. For example, an excellent preparation of BGase is available from Boehringer Mannheim as a suspension (5 mg/ml) which can be centrifuged at $1000 \times g$ for about 15 min, the supernatant discarded and the enzyme dissolved in 100 mM phosphate buffer, pH 7.0, containing 10 mM $MgCl_2$ and 50 mM NaCl. Dialysis against this buffer removes the rest of the salt.

TABLE 11.1

Most popular and widely used procedures for the conjugation of enzymes to macromolecules[a,b]

Conjugation procedure	MPO-ase	POase	GAase	APase	BGase	Urease	GOase
Chemical							
NaIO$_4$[c]		+ +	+ +				*
GA[d]:							
1-step	+ / −		+	+ +	+	+ +	+
2-step		+					
PBQ[e]		+		+	+	+	+
OPDM[f]			+ +	+ +			
MBS[g]		+		+ +			+
NHS-FBA	+ +						
CHM-NHS		+ +		+ +	+		+ +
Immunological[h]							
Antibody		+		+			
Soluble complex		+ +		+ +			
Avidin bridge[i]							
biotinylation		+ +		+ / −	+		+ +
avidin-labeling				+ +			

[a] Legend: + + satisfactory method; + often used but not recommended method; + / −

11.2. Chemical conjugation

11.2.1. Strategy of chemical conjugation

Little systematic research has been done with respect to the factors governing the course of chemical conjugation and the yields. Table 11.2 lists some of these factors. There is a strong tendency in published procedures to aim at high conjugation rates (Section 11.2.2). However, this often results in excessive polymerization or immunologic inactivation. It can be shown with the law of mass action and the Poisson distribution that excellent conjugation can only be expected at definite (high) equimolar concentrations of activated enzyme and macromolecules.

---

method not very suitable due to rapid inactivation of enzyme; * should work well, since GOase has 12% carbohydrates and stability and activity seem not or hardly affected by $NaIO_4$ oxidation (Section 10.2.4.1). Preferred chemical methods: MPOase: NHS-FBA; POase: $NaIO_4$ or CHM-NHS; glucoamylase: $NaIO_4$; APase: none gives completely satisfactory results, least detrimental are GA (large degree of polymerization), ODPM or CHM-NHS; GOase: CHM-NHS; urease: GA.

[b] Enzyme abbreviations: MPOase, microperoxidase; POase, peroxidase; GAase, glucoamylase; APase, alkaline phosphatase; BGase, β-galactosidase; GOase, glucose oxidase. Other abbreviations: GA: glutaraldehyde; PBQ: p-benzoquinone; OPDM: N,N'-o-phenylenedimaleimide; MBS: m-maleimidobenzoic acid N-hydroxysuccinimide ester; NHS-FBA: N-hydroxysuccinimide ester of p-formylbenzoic acid; CHM-NHS: 4-(N-maleimidoethyl)-cyclohexane-1-carboxylic acid N-hydroxysuccinimide ester.

[c] $NaIO_4$ gives excellent yields in the labeling of glycoproteins, however, partial inactivation and polymerization are difficult to avoid.

[d] GA is widely used (also by commercial suppliers) but should be avoided. Generally, it yields inferior products, it is wasteful, but it is applicable to most proteins and is technically undemanding.

[e] PBQ resembles GA in its use and gives only slightly better results if PBQ of superior purity is used.

[f] OPDM gives superior results with BGase (100% conjugation of enzymes: stable for at least 1 year at 4° C and pH 6.5). However, with APase 20–40% of the enzyme activity is lost. OPDM can be used for conjugation of almost all proteins.

[g] MBS gives excellent results for BGase.

[h] Unlabeled antibody methods are very simple and give excellent results when monoclonal antibodies are used, otherwise soluble enzyme–anti-enzyme antibody complexes are far superior.

[i] Some enzymes (e.g., APase) are inactivated by biotinylation, thus making direct chemical coupling of avidin to enzyme preferable.

TABLE 11.2
Factors governing the course and yield in chemical conjugation

1. Concentration of the molecules to be conjugated (law of mass action).

2. The relative rate of intramolecular over intermolecular cross-linking increases at lower protein concentrations.

3. Molecular concentration ratio of the 2 molecules to be conjugated (formation of different conjugates follows Poisson distribution).

4. The relative reaction rates of the cross-linking agent with the two molecules (formation of homopolymers vs. heteropolymers).

5. Effective concentration of the cross-linking agent: the active fraction of the reagent depends on a large number of parameters, such as pH, medium, etc.

6. Purity of buffer solutions and reactivity of its components with the cross-linking agent.

7. Ionic strength and pH of the buffer solution to obtain the highest probability of the desired conjugation.

8. Protection of groups involved in the biological activity.

The law of mass action, which is widely ignored in conjugation methods, states that the forward rate of complex formation is proportional to the concentration of the reactants, i.e.,

$$\frac{[Ab\text{-}E]}{dt} = k_a[Ab][E]$$

in which [Ab] is the antibody concentration, [E] is the activated (not total!) enzyme concentration, and k_a is the association rate constant. For example, a lowering of the concentration of the proteins from 5 mg/ml to 1 mg/ml requires a prolongation of the incubation period by 25 times to obtain the same amount of conjugates. High concentrations of the proteins are, therefore, important to adequately shorten the incubation period.

A second problem which arises at low protein concentrations is the formation of relatively more intramolecular than intermolecular bonds. This, in turn, may lead to a higher degree of inactivation of the biological function of the proteins and to the necessity of prolonging the incubation periods more than dictated by the law of mass action.

The molar concentration ratio of the proteins is also important. If the activated enzyme has only one reactive group, which can serve as a bridge between the antibody and enzyme molecule, the enzyme molecules will not be evenly distributed over the antibody molecules, but according to the Poisson distribution. The restriction to be made is that the number of enzyme molecules coupled to an IgG molecule will also depend on the degree of saturation. However, as shown below, the molecular ratios of interest (at about 1) are small compared to the ratio at saturation, so that steric hindrance may be unimportant. In situations where higher attachment ratios are required, optimization may be achieved by an alternative binomial model originally derived for the kinetics of phage attachment to bacteria already carrying a number of phages (Yassky, 1962; Archer, 1976). The Poisson distribution (Section 5.4.3.2) can be expressed as:

$$P(r) = \frac{m^r \cdot e^{-m}}{r!}$$

in which $P(r)$ is the fraction of antibodies with r (0, 1, 2, etc.) enzyme molecules per molecule, whereas m is the molecular ratio (average) in the mixture. Table 11.3 and Fig. 11.1 demonstrate that irrespective of the molar concentration ratio of activated enzyme/antibody, not more than 36.8% of the IgG is conjugated with one enzyme molecule, with an optimum at a molar ratio of 1. Though increasing the molar concentration ratio of enzyme/IgG, as frequently advocated, will lower the fraction of unconjugated antibodies, the fraction of antibody molecules conjugated with 2 or more enzyme molecules increases even more, leading to larger conjugates (undesired for EIH).

It is often assumed that the two-step glutaraldehyde (GA) method is superior to the $NaIO_4$ method to obtain 1:1 conjugates of antibody–

TABLE 11.3

Fraction of antibody molecules with (1, 2, 3, etc.) enzyme molecules per antibody molecule according to the Poisson distribution[a]

Enzyme molecules attached per antibody	Input molecular ratio of activated enzyme/antibody					
	0.25	0.50	1.00	2.00	(2.00)	4.00
0	0.779	0.607	0.368	0.135	(0.090)	0.018
1	0.195	0.303	0.368	0.271	(0.263)	0.073
2	0.024	0.076	0.183	0.271	(0.329)	0.147
3	0.002	0.013	0.061	0.181	(0.219)	0.195
4	0.000	0.002	0.015	0.090	(0.082)	0.195
5	0.000	0.000	0.005	0.052	(0.017)	0.372

[a] These values have been calculated without considering hindrance of the attachment of additional enzyme molecules by the enzyme molecules already conjugated to the IgG molecule. For POase this influence will be significant at input ratios above 1–2, and can be calculated by rather complex mathematics (Archer, 1976). As an example the values obtained by these formulas for the fractions of antibodies with 0, 1, 2, etc. bound POase molecules are given between parentheses at the input molecular ratio of 2, where deviations become significant.

POase. The theoretical considerations above demonstrated that this reflects more the limited activation of POase by GA rather than the superiority of this method. A similar result can be obtained with the NaIO$_4$ method by a more limited activation of the enzyme. If POase, activated by GA, is added to the antibody preparation in higher excess than usual, additional higher polymers will be formed. Indeed, these considerations are supported by the results obtained by Nygren (1982) who observed that an 8-fold excess of GA-activated POase produced additional bands of polymers on SDS–PAGE gels, whereas a 4-fold excess produced primarily 1:1 conjugates; at both ratios the majority of antibodies remained unconjugated. Fig. 11.1 suggests that less than 1 out of every 10 enzyme molecules is activated by GA, whereas with the standard NaIO$_4$ method at least 80–90% of enzyme is activated (Section 11.2.2.1). On the other hand, a high degree of activation of the protein, i.e., the introduction of several cross-linking groups per molecule, enhances its action as a bridge between other proteins. Exceedingly large aggregates can then be formed.

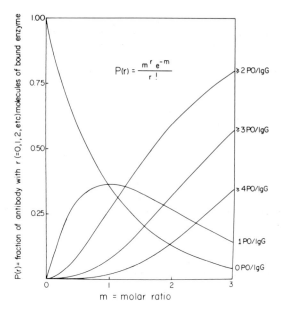

Fig. 11.1. Fractions of antibody with 0, 1, 2, 3, or more POase molecules (PO) bound as dictated by the Poisson distribution at different molar ratios (POase/IgG) of admixture. The steric interference for successive binding of enzyme molecules to the same antibody molecule is not considered.

It is also important to take into account the reactivity of the proteins towards the cross-linker. POase is poorly activated with GA, even at a large excess, whereas APase or IgG easily yields cross-links and polymers; 4,4′-difluoro-3,3′-dinitrophenyl sulfone (FNPS) reacts 66 times faster with IgG than with POase (Modesto and Pesce, 1971). An IgG molecule activated with FNPS has, therefore, a 66-fold greater chance to cross-link with another IgG molecule than with a POase molecule at equimolar concentrations of the two proteins. Consequently, the predominant conjugates are IgG polymers, only to some of which POase may be attached. In EIA, enzymatically non-active polymers compete in the immunological reaction with the relatively few enzyme–antibody conjugates. Although larger polymers have a greater probability to contain both antibody and enzymic activities, loss of activity due to steric factors or chemical modification is substantial with increasing polymerization (Clyne et al., 1973). The formation of large polymers can be limited by decreasing the relative concentration of the more reactive protein. Though it is mostly impossible to separate enzymatically active from non-active large polymers, free IgG can and should be removed prior to use in EIA.

The effective concentration of the cross-linking agent is of paramount importance, not only due to the law of mass action (using the concentration of reactive groups, not the protein concentration), but also to other characteristics as solubility and stability. For example, GA is very soluble in water, in contrast to hydrophobic reagents such as FNPS, cyanuric chloride, and tolylene diisocyanate, which is one of the reasons for the higher reactivity of GA. Another reason may be the higher rate of hydrolysis of the active groups of hydrophobic reagents. Background staining may increase due to the introduction of hydrophobic cross-linking agents.

Unsuccessful conjugation can often be traced to the presence of contaminants or of buffer constituents which may react with the cross-linking agent.

The nature of the buffer used may affect considerably the conjugation yield. For example, if amino groups of the protein are involved, conditions should be chosen in which these groups are least protonated. In addition, for linkage of unlike proteins, such as enzyme to antibody, buffer conditions should be maintained so as to provide maximum opposite charges to favor the interaction between unlike proteins and repellent action between the like proteins, i.e.: (i) a pH not to close to the pI of the proteins to decrease homopolymer formation; (ii) a pH between the pI values of the two proteins to increase heteropolymer formation; and, (iii) an ionic strength of an appropriate buffer to optimize attraction between unlike charged proteins. The one-step conjugation of POase to IgG, which have quite similar pI values (close to 8), is a practical example. An intermediate pH between their pI values (pH 8.0–8.2) would hardly induce repellent action among like proteins. However, POase has very few charges and a lower pH can be chosen to increase repellent action among the IgG while hardly affecting the IgG–POase interaction. The optimum buffer composition is, therefore, quite important and highly dependent on the nature of the proteins. The procedures for the conjugation of different enzymes rarely reflect these considerations, e.g., for coupling APase, GOase, or BGase to IgG by GA, the same buffer is often used as for POase.

Buffers are also important for the activity of the coupling agent. For example, to promote the reaction of FNPS with the free amino groups of proteins, a pH of 10.5 should be maintained. GA also reacts better at higher pH than generally chosen for conjugation (Molin et al., 1978). Activation of glycoproteins by $NaIO_4$ is highly pH dependent, with an optimum between pH 4–5.

Some effective cross-linking agents are less suitable for the conjugation of enzyme to antibody. Diazonium salts of aromatic compounds react preferentially with histidine and tyrosine which are very often located in or near the active site of the enzyme. Protecting the active sites with inhibitors (Jansen et al., 1971) is often cumbersome and, consequently, not very popular.

Similarly, paratopes of the antibody molecule may be protected by adsorption to an immunosorbent (Mannik and Downey, 1973); this approach, however, suffers from poor recovery of high-avidity antibodies (Section 7.1.9.2) and does not provide the advantages theoretically expected (Mannik and Downey, 1973; Kennedy et al., 1976b).

The best methods are not universally applicable and tend to be restricted to a few enzymes. Thus, the $NaIO_4$ method can only be used with glycoproteins while N,N'-o-phenylenedimaleimide (OPDM) is very well suited for BGase, but much less for other enzymes.

A low number of enzyme molecules per antibody generally does not affect the antigen-binding activity of the conjugated antibody, though the conjugate reacts slower than free antibodies (Tijssen et al., 1982). Several approaches to favor the yield of 1:1 conjugates have been investigated. Low-level conjugation with subsequent purification of conjugates is one approach. Another is the use of a two-step procedure in which one of the molecules is first treated with the cross-linking agent ('activated') and then conjugated to the second protein. Such two-step procedures can be based on three fundamentally different principles: (i) one of the macromolecules (e.g., enzyme), which is not highly reactive with the cross-linking agent, is treated with an excess of reagent and free cross-linker is removed before the addition of the activated enzyme to IgG to prevent polymerization of IgG; (ii) to activate the remaining free site of the cross-linker attached to the macromolecule by a change in the buffer conditions so that it reacts with a second protein (a possible complication may be that some groups of the macromolecule which did not react with the cross-linking agent under the first condition will become reactive in the second buffer, leading to the formation of homopolymers); (iii) the use of heterobifunctional reagents. Such reagents are first reacted with one of the macromolecules under conditions in which only one of the two groups is reactive; then, after removal of free cross-linking reagent, the conditions are changed so as to render the free group of the bifunctional reagent active with the other macromolecule.

11.2.2. Direct conjugation procedures after activation of one of the two macromolecules with periodate (NaIO$_4$)

11.2.2.1. Original NaIO$_4$ method and its principles   An elegant chemical conjugation procedure, which is applicable and very efficient for glycoproteins, is the method devised by Nakane and Kawaoi (1974). This method has been most significant for the development and application of EIA and immunoperoxidase procedures, due to its high efficiency compared to the GA methods. With the NaIO$_4$ method, yields are at least 3–4 times higher (e.g., Voller et al., 1979), and conjugates were reported to have 5 times higher detectabilities in spot-ELISA tests than the conjugates prepared with GA (Nygren, 1982), despite the significant inactivation (about 50%) of the enzyme by NaIO$_4$, noted, among others, by Nygren. The NaIO$_4$

method was originally used for the conjugation of horseradish POase to antibodies but may be applied to other glycoproteins, such as amyloglucosidase (Harper and Orengo, 1981), and GOase (Section 10.1.4.1).

In this procedure (Fig. 11.2) all the amino groups of POase are first irreversibly blocked with 1-fluoro-2,4-dinitrobenzene ('Sanger's reagent'). The carbohydrates of this enzyme (21% of total weight,

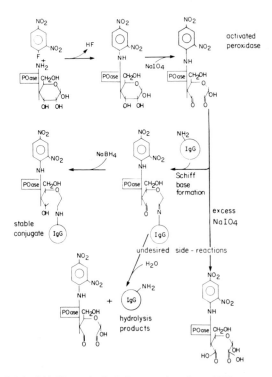

Fig. 11.2. Original NaIO₄ method of direct conjugation of POase to antibody (IgG). The amino groups are first blocked with Sanger's reagent, whereafter the carbohydrate groups of the enzyme are oxidized. (Overoxidation leads to acidic instead of aldehyde groups.) The aldehyde groups of the enzyme are allowed to react with amino groups of the IgG (Schiff's bases). The conjugates are stabilized with NaBH₄ to prevent hydrolysis. The exact nature of the linkage between the two macromolecules is not known.

Welinder, 1979) are then oxidized by *meta*-NaIO$_4$, producing alde-hyde and carboxyl groups. The aldehyde groups form Schiff's bases with the free, non-protonated amino groups of added protein (e.g., IgG or SpA) but not with its own blocked amino groups. These unstable amino–carbonyl adducts can be stabilized by reduction with NaBH$_4$. The details of this method (Nakane and Kawaoi, 1974) are in Table 11.4. They reported that about 70% of the POase and approximately 99% of the IgG was conjugated, with a maximum of 5–6 POase molecules per IgG molecule. The amount of activated POase to be added to antibody to achieve a definite ratio of bound

TABLE 11.4

Original method of Nakane and Kawaoi (1974) to couple peroxidase to IgG

---

1. Dissolve 5 mg POase (*RZ* 3.0) in 1.0 ml freshly made 300 mM NaHCO$_3$, pH 8.1.

2. Add 0.1 ml 1% DNFB (in absolute ethanol) and mix gently for 1 h at room temperature.

3. Add 1.0 ml of 40–80 mM NaIO$_4$ in distilled water and mix gently for 30 min at room temperature (brown solution will turn yellow-green).

4. Add 1.0 ml of 160 mM ethylene glycol (or 0.1 ml of 1.6 M ethylene glycol) in distilled water and mix for 1 h at room temperature.

5. Dialyze activated POase at 4° C against 3 changes of 1 l of 10 mM sodium carbonate buffer, pH 9.5.

6. Add 5 mg IgG to the solution of activated POase (molar ratio input ratio of POase/IgG of about 4). IgG may be added as a salt-free powder or dissolved in 1 ml of 10 mM sodium carbonate buffer, pH 9.5. Mix gently for 3 h at room temperature.

7. Add 5 mg NaBH$_4$ and incubate at 4° C for 3 to 18 h[a].

8. Dialyze against PBS. If a precipitate forms, remove by centrifugation.

9. Purify and store the conjugate as described in Section 11.2.2.3.

---

[a] The stabilization of Schiff bases by reduction with NaBH$_4$ may, in some cases, inactivate up to about 50% of the antibodies (Hevey et al., 1976; Saunders, 1979). Unreduced Schiff bases are quite stable provided the conjugate is stored in glass tubes at 4° C in the dark under sterile conditions.

enzyme molecules per IgG molecule can be predicted on theoretical grounds.

The experimental relation between the molecular ratio POase/IgG in the conjugate and the molar concentration ratio of input POase/IgG (Nakane and Kawaoi, 1974) can be expressed in a mathematical form (Fig. 11.3). At equilibrium:

$$K = \frac{[\text{IgG}'-\text{PO}]}{[\text{IgG}'] \cdot [\text{PO}]} \tag{1}$$

in which IgG' represents a coupling site on the antibody for the activated POase (PO). Eq. 1 may be rearranged (as shown in Section 8.5) to express the fraction of coupling sites which are occupied

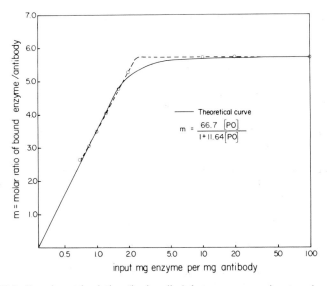

Fig. 11.3. Experimental relation (broken line) between enzyme input and enzyme bound per mg antibody as reported by Nakane and Kawaoi (1974). The theoretical curve follows the experimental curve very closely (Section 11.2.2.1). This theoretical curve is calculated from observations at 2 input values (1 mg POase and 50 mg POase per mg antibody) and yields the equation derived in the text.

(Langmuir adsorption isotherm):

$$\frac{[IgG'-PO]}{[IgG'-PO] + [IgG']} = \frac{K \cdot [PO]}{1 + K \cdot [PO]} \qquad (2)$$

The fraction of occupied coupling sites also equals m/N in which m represents the average number of bound POase molecules per IgG molecule ($= [IgG'-PO]/[IgG]_{total}$) and N the number of coupling sites per IgG molecule ($= [IgG']_{total}/[IgG]_{total}$):

$$\frac{m}{N} = \frac{[IgG'PO]/[IgG]_{total}}{[IgG']_{total}/[IgG]_{total}} = \frac{[IgG'-PO]}{[IgG'-PO] + [IgG']} \qquad (3)$$

combining eqs. 2 and 3 yields:

$$\frac{m}{N} = \frac{K \cdot [PO]}{1 + K \cdot [PO]} \quad \text{or} \quad m = \frac{N \cdot K \cdot [PO]}{1 + K \cdot [PO]} \qquad (4)$$

Numerical values are obtained from experimental curves. At high concentrations of free POase, $1 + K[PO]$ in the denominator is not significantly larger than $K[PO]$, yielding $m = N$. Therefore, $N = 5.73$ can be read directly from the experimental curve of Fig.11.3 and K can be calculated at sub-saturation conditions of conjugation. For example, at an input of 1 mg activated POase per mg IgG, which corresponds to 4 enzyme molecules per IgG molecule, a molecular ratio of bound POase/IgG of 3.47 was found by Nakane and Kawaoi (1974), which, according to the conservation law, leaves $0.1325 (= 1 - 3.47/4)$ mg POase free. Using eq. 4, K (in ml/mg) can be calculated, and the general form which relates the amount of excess of POase required to obtain the desired number of POase molecules bound per IgG molecule (m) can be expressed as:

$$m = \frac{66.7[PO]}{1 + 11.64[PO]} \qquad (5)$$

For example, to obtain a molecular ratio of 2, the excess PO per mg IgG should be 0.046 mg and the total input of the POase required per mg IgG would be 0.5 mg (2 molecules POase per molecule of IgG) + 0.046 mg, for a total of 0.546 mg POase, i.e. an input of about 2.2 molecules of POase per IgG molecule. The excess required at the various ratios, is represented in Fig.11.4. The estimation of the fraction of POase remaining free at each input ratio produces a theoretical curve (Fig. 11.3), which correlates very well with the experimental curve.

These theoretical considerations reflect only upon the activated enzyme molecules. In reality, after $NaIO_4$ treatment (Table 11.4) usually only about 85% of the enzyme molecules are activated (Archer, 1976). The efficiency of the conjugation can be optimized by

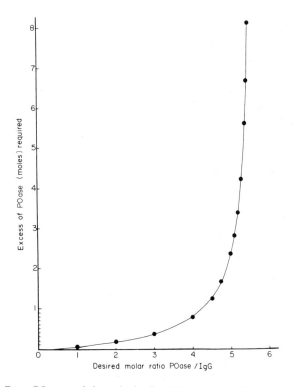

Fig. 11.4. Extra POase needed to obtain the desired molar ratio enzyme/antibody as calculated from the formula given in Fig. 11.3. It can be seen that the excess required of POase is low unless high conjugation rates are wanted.

taking into account: (i) the degree of activation of enzyme; (ii) the molecular ratio desired and the excess of activated enzyme required; and, (iii) the distribution of POase molecules among the various IgG–POase conjugates as discussed in Section 11.2.1. Figs. 11.1 and 11.4 reveal that at low molar concentration ratios (POase/IgG) relatively little POase but a high fraction of IgG remains free, whereas the contrary is observed at high molar ratios.

11.2.2.2. Optimized NaIO₄ methods for the conjugation of peroxidase   The original NaIO₄ method often produced large polymers since, (i) the input molar concentration ratio (POase/IgG) was 4; and, (ii) the strong oxidation of POase yielded many attachment sites so that POase acted as a bridge between several IgG molecules (Section 11.2.1).

Wilson and Nakane (1978) modified their initial method mainly: (i) by omitting the blocking of the amino groups since very few of these groups are accessible; and, (ii) by lowering the molecular concentration ratio of POase/IgG to 2. This method (Table 11.5) is simpler than the original method and results in less inactivation of POase.

TABLE 11.5

NaIO₄ method (II) for the conjugation of peroxidase (Wilson and Nakane, 1978)

1. Dissolve 4 mg POase in 1 ml distilled water.

2. Add 0.2 ml freshly made 100 mM NaIO₄ and stir for 20 min at room temperature.

3. Dialyze overnight at 4° C against 1 mM sodium acetate buffer, pH 4.4. Auto-conjugation at this pH is reduced about 7-fold.

4. Add 20 μl 200 mM carbonate buffer, pH 9.5, 8 mg IgG (dissolved in 1.0 ml of 10 mM carbonate buffer, pH 9.5) and stir for 2 h at room temperature.

5. Add 0.1 ml fresh NaBH₄ solution (4 mg/ml in water) and incubate for 2 h at 4° C. (See footnote to Table 11.4 for remarks on reduction of Schiff bases).

6. Purify and store the conjugate according to Section 11.2.2.3.

The central problem in the $NaIO_4$ method is the sensitivity of the carbohydrate moiety to oxidation. This varies from lot to lot of POase, but the enzyme is over-oxidized in all current methods. Too little oxidation will not activate sufficiently the enzyme, but an excessive oxidation may have harmful consequences. Firstly, stronger oxidation produces progressively more carboxyl groups, since the aldehyde groups are more sensitive to oxidation than the original glycol groups, resulting in less activation of the enzyme (Fig.11.5). Secondly, POase is gradually inactivated by increasing $NaIO_4$ concentrations and its three-dimensional structure is affected since some amino acid residues may also be oxidized (De la Llosa et al., 1980; Yamasaki et al., 1982). Thus, methionine is readily oxidized by $NaIO_4$ at concentrations used for conjugation into methionine sulfoxide, which is much more hydrophilic, altering the conformation of the protein. Thirdly, excessive oxidation favors the formation of polymers, as well as creates problems for the purification of conjugates by affinity chromatography on Con A–Sepharose.

The oxidation conditions were investigated in more detail (Tijssen and Kurstak, 1984). Beside the $NaIO_4$ concentration, several factors

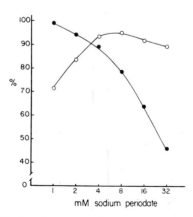

Fig. 11.5. Relationship between the concentration of $NaIO_4$ used for oxidation and the conjugation efficiency (○) and enzyme activity remaining (●). Results from Tijssen and Kurstak (1984).

are important: (i) the pH of the solutions has a profound effect on the degree of oxidation (strongest oxidation at pH 3–5; Dyer, 1956); (ii) the use of double-distilled water to avoid contamination by weakly oxidizing metals, as well as by other impurities, such as bacteria, bacteriostatic agents, polystyrene, etc., to which POase is sensitive; (iii) oxidation should be carried out in the dark; and, (iv) the use of closed containers in order to avoid pH fluctuations when carbonate buffers are used. For a constant 2 h incubation at 20°C and pH 8.1, the optimum concentration for m-NaIO$_4$ is 4 mM for many POase lots, though some lots required a slightly higher concentration (about 5–15 times lower than currently used). With this procedure (Table 11.6), about 90% of the POase is conjugated while about 90% of its activity is retained (Fig. 11.5). The subsequent step, in which dry Sephadex G-25 is added to the combined

TABLE 11.6

Simplified NaIO$_4$ method (III), with reduced inactivation of peroxidase and improved yield of conjugate

---

1. *Activation of peroxidase*
   a. Dissolve 5 mg POase (purified according to Section 10.1.1.2) in 0.5 ml freshly prepared 100 mM NaHCO$_3$ in a small tube.
   b. Add 0.5 ml of 8–16 mM NaIO$_4$ (depending on lot of POase), close tube and incubate at 20° C for 2 h in the dark.

2. *Conjugation*
   a. Dissolve 15 mg IgG in 1–2 ml of 100 mM sodium carbonate buffer, pH 9.2.
   b. Add the activated POase and IgG to the tube, or preferably to a glass-wool-plugged Pasteur pipet (tip closed with flame) and add rapidly dry Sephadex G-25 (1/6 of the combined weight of solutions).
   c. Incubate for 3 h at room temperature.

3. *Stabilization*
   a. Elute conjugate from Sephadex.
   b. Add, with mixing, 1/20 volume of freshly prepared NaBH$_4$ (5 mg/ml in 0.1 mM NaOH) and 30 min later another volume (1/10) of freshly prepared NaBH$_4$ solution.
   c. Incubate for 1 h at 4° C.

4. *Purification*
   Purify and store the preparation according to Section 11.2.2.3.

POase and IgG solutions (Fig. 11.6), serves several purposes. The Sephadex G-25 beads swell almost immediately, leading to a two-fold increase in the concentration of the proteins (and, consequently, accelerating the conjugation rate about four-fold, Section 11.2.1), and to an uptake of the $NaIO_4$ molecules, followed by the consumption of $NaIO_4$ by the vicinal glycols of the dextran. However, the raise of the pH to about 9.2, needed due to the pK_a of the amino groups, reduces also the oxidative power of $NaIO_4$. The conjugation is continued for 3 h if the concentration of the POase is higher than 2 mg/ml, otherwise the incubation is adjusted as discussed in Section 11.2.1.

The Schiff bases formed are stabilized by reduction with borohy-

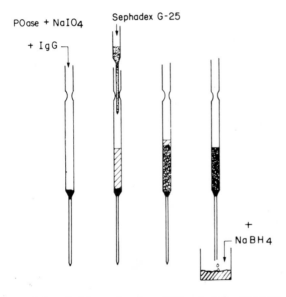

Fig. 11.6. Simplified method for conjugation of POase to IgG with $NaIO_4$. A Pasteur pipet is closed at the outlet by flaming and a glass-wool plug is inserted. Activated POase and IgG solutions are added, followed by dry Sephadex G-25 to an amount 1/6 of the weight of the 2 solutions. After incubation, the sealed tip of the pipet is broken and the conjugate is eluted. $NaBH_4$ can be added for stabilization of the conjugate.

dride (beware of health hazards, Chapter 18). Although its potassium salt is much more stable in solution than sodium salt, the latter is generally used. The current long incubation periods with sodium borohydride are useless since it is hydrolyzed almost instantaneously. The modified method is similar to that used for reductive methylation (Biocca et al., 1978; Table 11.6, step 3).

This method yields a maximum of close to 37% of the IgG conjugated with 1 POase molecule (Table 11.3), since the molar concentration ratio of activated enzyme/IgG is about 1. A similar fraction of the IgG remains free, whereas smaller fractions of the IgG are conjugated with 2 or more molecules of POase. Sometimes, though, it may be advantageous to increase the molar ratio of enzyme/IgG to about 1.5 to lower the fraction of unconjugated IgG to about 22%. On the other hand, free IgG can be recovered by simple methods and reused.

11.2.2.3. Purification and storage of peroxidase–IgG conjugates
Free POase is soluble in solutions of $(NH_4)_2SO_4$ up to 70–80% saturation (Section 10.2.1.2). Therefore, the addition of an equal volume of saturated $(NH_4)_2SO_4$ solution (Section 7.1.2) to the preparation precipitates free and conjugated IgG but not free POase. After an equilibration period of 1 h, the precipitate is collected by centrifugation (15 min, $6000 \times g$), washed with a half-saturated $(NH_4)_2SO_4$ solution and recentrifuged. [Sometimes, free POase can be separated from IgG and conjugates by a simple passage on SpA–Sepharose (Section 7.1.8.1)].

For the separation of free IgG from the IgG–POase conjugates, the pellet is equilibrated with a buffer containing 100 mM sodium phosphate, pH 7.2, and 100 mM NaCl (PBS–C) or with 'Con-A buffer' (100 mM acetate buffer, pH 6.0, supplemented with 1 M NaCl, 1 mM $CaCl_2$, 1 mM $MgCl_2$, and 1 mM $MnCl_2$) by dialysis or passage over Sephadex G-25. The separation is then achieved by affinity chromatography on Con A–Sepharose, which has an affinity for POase or POase-containing conjugates (if POase is not over-oxidized). Unfortunately, Con A also has an affinity to a small fraction (about 5%) of the IgG (Arends, 1981). This reactive IgG can be removed from the IgG pool by a passage over Con A–Sepharose prior to labeling.

Con A–Sepharose is commercially supplied as a suspension in Con A-buffer and 0.02% merthiolate. The bed volume of the Con A–Sepharose column should be 1 ml per 3 mg of POase. The column should be rinsed prior to use with about 5 volumes of PBS–C or Con A buffer. The passage of free IgG is monitored at 278 nm. After all IgG passed, POase complexes are desorbed with α-methyl-D-mannopyranoside, at 10–100 mM in PBS–C or Con A buffer. This sugar competes with POase at the binding sites, and needs not to be removed from the conjugate prior to EIA. The difference in detectabilities in EIA using conjugates with or without free IgG is considerably more than expected from relative concentrations of free IgG and conjugate (Tijssen et al., 1982).

The conjugates can be stored at $-70°C$ after the addition of stabilizing proteins. However, activity disappears rather fast when frozen in dilute solutions. The addition of NaN_3 is not recommended since it is a potent inhibitor (above 10^{-3} M) of the enzyme. The addition of an equal volume of glycerol and storage at $-20°C$ in convenient aliquots also proved satisfactory in our laboratory. The sample then remains liquid and the required small quantities can be retrieved without the harmful, repeated freezing–thawing or the wasteful dispensing in very small aliquots.

Spectrophotometric determination of POase and IgG content of the conjugates, according to the method used for the PAP complexes (Section 11.3.2), is not reliable for chemically linked conjugates since the RZ of the enzyme changes during conjugation. Usually, conjugates with an RZ of 0.30–0.45 are satisfactory.

11.2.3. Cross-linking agents for the conjugation of enzymes to antibodies or other proteins

All cross-linking agents have at least two reactive groups. In homobifunctional reagents the reactive groups are the same, whereas in heterobifunctional reagents the two reactive groups are different and each group may, therefore, react under different conditions. Theoretically, the latter group of reagents should lead to a better controlled conjugation. Some homobifunctional reagents can be used in two-step procedures if the activation of the second group requires a change in conditions (Sections 11.2.3.1.2, 11.2.3.1.3), or when one of the proteins is not very reactive with the cross-linker (Section 11.2.1). Otherwise, homobifunctional reagents are used in one-step procedures, in which the enzyme and the other protein (e.g., antibody, antigen, SpA, or avidin) are reacted with the cross-linker after their admixture. These one-step methods provide poor control on the size and composition of the conjugates.

11.2.3.1. Homobifunctional reagents

11.2.3.1.1. Glutaraldehyde (GA)   GA is an extensively used cross-linking agent, primarily because its use is simple and quite effective with some proteins. There are large variations with respect to the concentration of GA (0.01 to 8%), the incubation period (1–24 h) and temperature (4–25°C) used for conjugation (Morris and Saelinger, 1982) and the cross-linking ability of different lots of GA.

GA, a dialdehyde with the basic structure of pentanedial, exists mostly in a hydrated form at or below room temperature (Korn et al., 1972). Monsan et al. (1975) analyzed commercial preparations of aqueous 25% GA by NMR spectroscopy and found 79% water, 18% polymers and only 3% free GA. The polymers, which regenerate easily at higher temperatures to the free monomeric form (Korn et al., 1972), are formed particularly at higher pH, and will precipitate in alkaline conditions as poly(GA). GA should, therefore, be stored as a slightly acidic solution (pH 3–4). Purification of GA by vacuum distillation does not increase its cross-linking ability (Siess et al., 1971). The monomer absorbs at 280 nm (4.2 $M^{-1}cm^{-1}$), while its polymers absorb strongly at 235 nm ($1.53 \times 10^3 M^{-1}cm^{-1}$).

GA reacts irreversibly with the ε-amino group of lysine (Quiocho and Richards, 1966). Since this bond is stable to hydrolysis, formation of Schiff bases as well as Michael-type addition of a resonance-stabilized carbanion to a conjugated double bond can be ruled out (Monsan et al., 1975). Other studies (Hardy et al., 1976) on the reaction mechanism of GA with 6-aminohexanoic acid suggest that polymeric quaternary pyridinium structures are reactive. It is also noteworthy that an average of 4 GA molecules are bound per lysine residue (Korn et al., 1972).

The reaction of a protein with GA is favored by a rise of (i) the pH above 7.0 (stable rate below pH 7.0; Molin et al., 1978); (ii) of the temperature (Bowes and Cater, 1966); and, (iii) of the concentrations of GA (law of mass action). However, the enzymatic and antibody activity of the conjugates may decrease significantly when the formation of polymers is beyond control (Boorsma and Streefkerk, 1976; Molin et al., 1978).

The GA method is most suitable for APase (one-step procedure), and for the antibody-chimera method (Section 11.5), whereas for EIH the POase–Fab or POase–IgG conjugates are frequently prepared by the two-step GA procedure.

The technical details of the one-step procedures (Avrameas, 1969) for various enzymes are given in Tables 11.7 and 11.8. This method cannot be recommended for POase: only 1% of the POase and 5% of the immunoreactivity were recovered in the conjugates (Clyne

TABLE 11.7
One-step conjugation procedure using glutaraldehyde

1. Dialyze the enzyme and antibody solutions extensively against 100 mM phosphate buffer, pH 6.8, until complete elimination of interfering substances. Buffers should be prepared with double- or triple-distilled sterile water. The enzyme and antibody solutions may be mixed prior to dialysis, in the proportions given in Table 11.8.

2. Add dropwise the GA solution (EM grade; e.g., TAAB Lab., Reading U.K.), as indicated in Table 11.8.

3. Incubate at room temperature for 2–3 h and add an excess of L-lysine (1/20 volume, 1 M) to block reactive sites.

4. Dialyze extensively to remove reagents and store as described in Section 11.2.2.3.

TABLE 11.8
Amounts of proteins and glutaraldehyde used in the one-step conjugation procedure
(Avrameas et al., 1978)[a]

	Total volume (ml)	Enzyme (mg)	IgG or (mg)	Fab (mg)	1%GA (ml)
POase	1	10	5	2.5	0.05
APase	2	10	5	2.5	0.05
GOase	1	10	5	2.5	0.15
BGase	2	10	5	2.5	0.10

[a] The conjugation of POase with this method is not recommended. A wide variation in the recommended concentrations of both protein and GA is found in the literature.

et al., 1973; Boorsma and Kalsbeek, 1975; Adams and Wisdom, 1979). The efficiency with APase is significantly higher, whereas conjugation of GOase is intermediate between the two (Guesdon and Avrameas, 1977). On the other hand, lactoperoxidase is efficiently conjugated (to about 50%) with 0.3 μmol GA per mg protein and retains about 60–70% of the immunoreactivity.

Though the dominant isozyme in virtually all POase preparations is isoperoxidase C, its 6 lysine groups (Section 10.2.1.1) seem to be shielded from reacting with GA, possibly by the allylisothiocyanates or by the carbohydrates surrounding the molecule. Conjugation of POase with GA may be restricted to minor isozymes, to microheterogeneity of isoperoxidase C, such as the C-terminal variants noted by Welinder (1979), to single-base mutations from asparagine (21 residues) to lysine, as noted for turnip POase (Welinder and Mazza, 1977) or to biosynthetic or degradative differences in its carbohydrate composition.

A number of modifications have been introduced into the original coupling method, all aimed at finding a better compromise between labeling and inactivation. Avrameas and Ternynck (1971) introduced the two-step procedure which reduced polymerization of IgG and activated more POase. They observed that, even at high concentrations of GA, POase was not polymerized. Following treatment of POase with an excess of GA, free GA is removed and activated

POase added to the IgG in suitable proportions. This method gives mostly 1:1 conjugates if the molecular concentration ratio enzyme/ IgG is 4, but low yields (see Section 11.2.1). The one- and two-step GA reactions are illustrated in Fig. 11.7 and details of the two-step procedure, as described by Avrameas and Ternynck (1971), are given in Table 11.9. A feature this method shares with the single-step procedure is the extremely wasteful use of both enzyme and antibody.

A 4-molar excess of enzyme gives also best results for the two-step conjugation of SpA (Nygren and Hansson, 1981); conjugation of APase to SpA is given in Table 11.10.

11.2.3.1.2. p-Benzoquinone (PBQ).   This agent is primarily employed in two-step procedures, since at neutral pH it reacts only through one of its two reactive sites (Fig. 11.8). The excess of PBQ is then removed from the activated protein. A raise in the pH (to

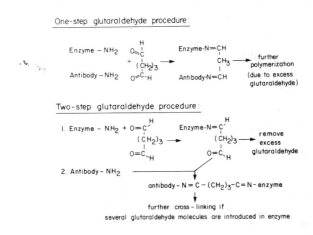

Fig. 11.7. One- and two-step conjugation procedures by glutaraldehyde. The one-step procedure, in which reagents and proteins are mixed, is poorly controlled and generally leads to excessive polymerization of antibody or of enzyme and antibody. In the two-step procedure, used primarily for POase which is relatively unreactive with GA, the enzyme is first treated with an excess of cross-linker, which is removed prior to admixture with the antibody so that no polymers of the latter are formed. However, if the enzyme has several activated groups, it can act as a bridge between antibodies and cause large polymers.

TABLE 11.9

Two-step procedure for the conjugation of peroxidase to proteins (IgG, SpA, etc.) with glutaraldehyde

---

1. Activate POase (10 mg enzyme in 0.2 ml 100 mM phosphate buffer, pH 6.8) with excess GA for 18 h at room temperature.

2. Remove excess of GA by exhaustive dialysis or by passage through a Sephadex G-25 column (40 ml) equilibrated with 0.9% NaCl. Concentrate recovered POase to 1 ml.

3. Add 5 mg antibody or 2.5 mg Fab (1 ml, equilibrated with 0.9% NaCl) and 0.2 ml of 500 mM sodium carbonate buffer, pH 9.5 (Note that the molar ratio of POase/IgG is about 7:1 or POase/Fab is about 4:1).

4. Incubate for 24 h at 4° C and block then remaining activated groups with 0.1 ml 1 M lysine (neutralized to pH 7.0) for 2 h.

5. Dialyse overnight against PBS, filter through sterile Millipore membrane (0.22 μm). Purify and store as described in Section 11.2.2.3[a].

---

[a] Though it has not been attempted in this laboratory, SpA–POase conjugates are most probably obtained in high purity by two affinity chromatography steps, namely Con A–Sepharose (Section 11.2.2.3) to eliminate free SpA, and rabbit IgG–Sepharose (normal IgG; prepared according to Section 7.1.8.2) to eliminate free POase (desorption conjugates from column according to Section 7.1.8.1.1).

TABLE 11.10

Conjugation of alkaline phosphatase to protein A by the two-step glutaraldehyde method (Engvall, 1978)

---

1. Dialyze 0.5 ml of an $(NH_4)_2SO_4$ suspension of APase (2.5 mg of type VII from Sigma) against several changes of PBS for 1 day.

2. Transfer dialysis bag to beaker containing 100 ml of 0.2% GA in PBS. Stir overnight at room temperature.

3. Dialyze against several changes of PBS to remove excess of GA.

4. Transfer contents of the bag (activated enzyme) to a tube containing 0.5 mg SpA in 0.1 ml PBS, mix and incubate overnight at room temperature.

5. Purify and store conjugate as described in Section 11.2.4.

6. Use conjugate in EIA at a dilution of about 1–1.5 μg of SpA per ml.

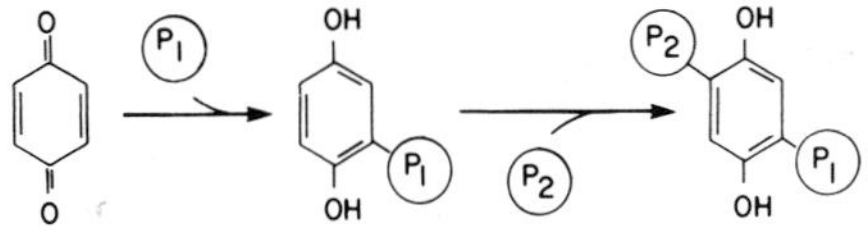

Fig. 11.8. Conjugation with *p*-benzoquinone. This cross-linker reacts at pH 6.0 at one of its 2 reactive sites. The other site reacts after raising the pH to 8.0. Removing excess reagent before raising the pH enables a better control of the reaction than is possible with glutaraldehyde.

8–9) activates the other reactive site of PBQ which might then link the activated protein to another protein (Table 11.11).

This conjugation method is almost as wasteful as the similar two-step procedure with GA, but PBQ seems to have a wider reaction spectrum, since it also reacts with carbohydrate and sulfhydryl groups (Brandt et al., 1975). This method is, therefore, an excellent choice to label polysaccharides.

The yield of POase–antibody conjugates with PBQ has been reported to be 15% with 90% of the 1:1 type with a recovery of about half the specific activities (per mg) of the enzyme and antibody (Ternynck and Avrameas, 1977). Conjugation with POase is best accomplished using a 3- to 4-fold molar excess of enzyme over IgG, Fab, or SpA (Nygren and Hansson, 1981).

PBQ can also be used in two-step procedures for enzymes other than POase (Table 11.11). In general, the protein, the activity of which is least affected by the free cross-linker, is activated in the first step.

11.2.3.1.3. N,N′-o-Phenylenedimaleimide (OPDM).   Proteins into which thiol groups can be introduced, or which contain thiol groups, may be conjugated by OPDM (Fig. 11.9). Though this procedure may share problems encountered with other homobifunctional reagents, it may, like PBQ, be used in selective two-stage coupling reactions. However, OPDM is superior to GA and PBQ and has a high reactivity under mild conditions.

This cross-linking agent is primarily used for BGase, which is one of the best enzymes for EIA, and does not affect enzymic activity

TABLE 11.11
Two-step conjugation procedure with p-benzoquinone (Avrameas et al., 1978)

A. *If enzyme is activated in the first step:*
   1. Add dropwise 0.1 ml of PBQ (30 mg/ml in ethanol) to 0.4 ml enzyme solution (10 mg/ml) in 100 mM phosphate buffer, pH 6.0. Only PBQ of highest purity (Fluka) gives satisfactory results and PBQ crystals should be stored in a cool, dark place, otherwise they turn brown. The PBQ solution is prepared just before use and should be bright yellow, but is discarded if brown.
   2. Incubate for 1 h in the dark at room temperature.
   3. Remove excess of free cross-linking agent as in step 2 of Table 11.9 and concentrate to 1 ml.
   4. Add the following amounts of IgG or Fab (for SpA see Section 11.2.3.1.2):

Enzyme (4 mg)	Fab (mg)	IgG (mg)
POase	1	4
APase	0.50	2
GOase	0.25	1
BGase	0.07	0.30

   5. Add 1/10 volume of freshly prepared 1 M $NaHCO_3$ and incubate for 48 h at 4° C.
   6. Stop reaction by adding 1/10 volume of 1 M lysine solution, pH 7.0 and proceed as in step 5 of Table 11.9.

B. *If IgG or Fab is activated in the first step:*
   1. Add 0.05 ml freshly prepared PBQ (30 mg/ml) in ethanol to 1 mg of Fab or 3 mg of IgG dissolved in 0.15 ml of 150 mM NaCl, containing 0.05 ml of 1 M phosphate buffer, pH 6.0.
   2. Proceed as in steps 2 and 3 of section A.
   3. Add either of the following amounts of enzyme: 4 mg POase, 8 mg APase, 16 mg GOase, 40 mg BGase.
   4. Add 1/10 volume of 1 M carbonate buffer, pH 9.0 and incubate for 48 h at 4° C.
   5. Proceed as in step 6 of Section A.

(Kato et al., 1975). Although BGase should contain about 40 cysteine residues, commercial enzyme preparations often contain far less free thiol groups, e.g. only 3 per molecule (O'Sullivan et al., 1978). The number of free thiol groups should, therefore, be determined (Section 11.2.3.1.3.1), irrespective of whether or not they are expected, intro-

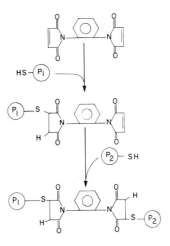

Fig. 11.9. Conjugation of antibody to enzyme (particularly BGase) by N,N'-o-phenyl-enedimaleimide. This method requires the presence of sulfhydryl groups on the macro-molecules to be conjugated.

duced by thiolation of the amino groups, or by reduction of the disulfide groups.

Conjugation with OPDM (Table 11.15) is still not very widely used, even if it gives better results than other homobifunctional reagents. With the use of Fab′–BGase conjugates in EIA, antigens can be detected in the femto- to attomole (10^{-15}–10^{-18}) range (Adachi et al., 1978).

11.2.3.1.3.1. Introduction of thiol groups and their quantitative determination. Introduction of thiol groups with *S*-acetylmercaptosuccinic anhydride (AMSA) under mild conditions (Klotz and Heiney, 1962), or with methyl-4-mercaptobutyrimidate (MMBI) (Traut et al., 1973), are both suitable (Kato et al., 1978; O'Sullivan et al., 1979).

The number of thiol groups introduced with AMSA may vary from limited to complete coverage of all amino groups, depending on the molar ratio of reagent to amino groups of the protein. The reaction is schematically represented in Fig. 11.10. A small fraction of the AMSA may be hydrolyzed but most will be coupled to the

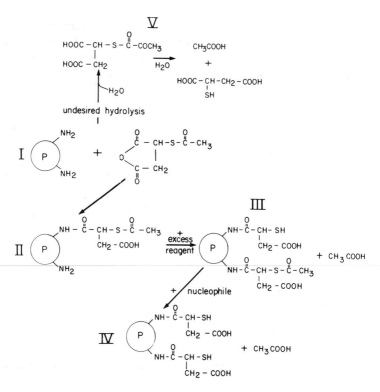

Fig. 11.10. Thiolation of proteins with S-acetylmercaptosuccinic anhydride (I → V). Most of the groups introduced will be acetylthio groups (III), although a few free thiol groups are also formed. The acetyl groups can easily be removed with appropriate nucleophilic reagents, yielding thiolated proteins IV. This reaction is accompanied by an undesired hydrolysis of the anhydride (V).

amino groups. This reagent can also form ester linkages with hydroxyl groups, so that thiolation in the absence of suitable amino groups is feasible.

The marked dependence on the pH is not surprising since protons are liberated in this reaction. Maximum thiolation, observed above pH 7.0, remains essentially constant in the pH range of 7 to 9, and is hardly affected by temperature changes in the 0–30°C range. Although the suitability of various buffers was not systematically studied, 125 mM phosphate buffer, pH 6.8, is satisfactory (Klotz and Heiney, 1962). Relatively high concentrations of proteins are used (10–80 mg/ml, depending on the protein) with a 5–10-fold molar excess of AMSA over the amino groups for complete thiolation, whereas at a molar ratio of 0.2 to 1.2, only about one-third of the amino groups are thiolated. The degree of thiolation also depends on the accessibility of the amino groups. Details are given in Table 11.12.

Though the name MMBI ('Traut's reagent') should be 2-iminothiolane (Jue et al., 1978), the original designation is still widely used. To minimize blocking the antigen-binding site, O'Sullivan et al. (1979) thiolated the amino groups of antibodies adsorbed onto an immunosorbent (Section 7.1.8.2), using MMBI (Table 11.13).

Thiol groups can sometimes be generated in proteins through

TABLE 11.12

Mercaptosuccinylation of proteins (according to Fig. 11.10; version adapted from Klotz and Heiney, 1962)

1. Dissolve 6 mg AMSA (MW = 174.2) in 0.1 ml DMF.

2. Dissolve or equilibrate 10 mg of IgG (or equivalent of other protein) in 1 ml of degassed 125 mM phosphate buffer, pH 7.0.

3. Add AMSA (50–100 molar excess over IgG) to IgG solution (under nitrogen gas) and close tube with Parafilm (resulting in 2–3 to 5–8 thiol groups/IgG).

4. Stir gently during 30 min at room temperature. The acetyl group of the AMSA keeps the thiol protected during coupling to the macromolecule until one wishes to expose the mercaptan for further reactions (following steps).

5. Add 0.2 ml of 100 mM Tris-HCl buffer, containing 500 mM hydroxylamine (nucleophile to expose mercaptan) and 10 mM EDTA (added to prevent oxidation of thiol), and adjust to pH 7.0.

6. Incubate mixture for 4 min at 30° C and separate by-products from macromolecule by passage over Sephadex G-25 column (1 × 30 cm), equilibrated with 100 mM sodium phosphate buffer, pH 6.0, containing 5 mM EDTA.

7. Concentrate the fractions containing macromolecules prior to conjugation.

TABLE 11.13
Thiolation of proteins with methyl-4-mercaptobutyrimidate (O'Sullivan et al., 1979)[a]

1. Mix 1 ml of immunosorbent (Section 7.1.8.2), to which about 5 mg antigen were coupled, with 3 ml of antiserum and incubate for 1 h at room temperature.

2. Remove non-specifically bound or non-adsorbed proteins by washing 10 times with 10 ml of 50 mM phosphate buffer, pH 7.0, containing 200 mM NaCl.

3. Suspend gel in 9 ml of 50 mM N-ethylmorpholine-HCl buffer, pH 7.5, to which 0.1 ml of a 10 mg/ml solution of methyl-4-mercaptobutyrimidate in ice-cold 100 mM sodium carbonate is added.

4. Mix for 1 h at room temperature and wash five times with 10 ml aliquots of distilled water.

5. Pack the gel into a 5 ml disposable syringe fitted with a glass-wool filter and wash the gel with 10 ml of dilute HCl, pH 3.5, supplemented with 100 mM NaCl.

6. Elute the antibodies with suitable buffer (Section 7.1.8.2). Keep thiolated proteins under nitrogen in degassed buffer.

[a] Correct name of reagent is 2-iminothiolane.

the reduction of their disulfide bonds. For example, IgG has no free thiol groups but it has numerous S–S bridges (Section 6.2.3). The intradomain S–S bonds are very stable (Sections 6.2.2; 6.2.3), in contrast to the interchain bridges. Although complete IgG also gives satisfactory results, best results are obtained with Fab' fragments (yield about twice of that with IgG). F(ab')$_2$ is prepared with pepsin as described in Section 7.5, followed by reduction with 10 mM 2-mercaptoethylamine at pH 5.0 (100 mM sodium acetate) at 37°C for 90 min, and by gel filtration on a Sephadex G-25 column (30 ml, in 100 mM phosphate buffer, pH 6.0). As discussed in Section 7.5, Fab' offers the advantage in EIA of producing less background staining in the presence of rheumatoid factors. IgG is reduced in exactly the same way (4–8 mg/ml). The addition of 5 mM EDTA generally stabilizes the thiol groups produced.

Thiol groups may be determined with 5,5′-dithiobis(2-nitrobenzoic) acid ('Ellman's reagent') (Anderson and Wetlaufer, 1975) or 4,4′-

dithiopyridine (Grassetti and Murray, 1967; Table 11.14). Stabilizing proteins in the preparations should be taken into account.

11.2.3.1.3.2.   Cross-linking   with   N,N′-o-phenylenedimaleimide (OPDM). One of two maleimide residues of OPDM, added in excess (10 μM) to the protein, reacts with the thiol group, whereas the other remains inactive. The number of maleimide-reacted thiol groups in the protein can be estimated by the determination of the number of unmodified sulfhydryl groups. Subsequently, the maleimide-derivatized protein is conjugated with BGase.

Since the introduction of this method by Kato et al. (1975), several improvements have been made. Hamaguchi et al. (1979) observed that maleimide decomposes from the derivatized protein at a significant rate at a pH above 6.5 or at 30°C instead of 4°C. Their observation that BGase from Worthington or from Boehringer Mannheim contains one or 11–13 thiol groups per molecule of enzyme, respectively, illustrates the necessity to determine the number of thiol groups prior to use. The addition of *N*-ethylmaleimide-treated bovine serum albumin as a stabilizing protein, and of $MgCl_2$ decreases the loss of enzyme activity. Conjugation of IgG to BGase is given in Table 11.15. This enzyme is coupled almost completely, virtually without loss of activity, whereas 15% of the IgG or 40% of the

TABLE 11.14
Determination of number of sulfhydryl groups in proteins

---

1. Incubate 20 μl aliquots of the sample(s), containing known amounts of (modified) proteins, with 0.2 ml 4,4′-dithiopyridine in 0.48 ml of 100 mM sodium phosphate buffer, pH 7.0 for 20 min at room temperature (0.15–0.60 mg protein per ml).

2. Determine absorbance at 324 nm for both treated and control samples.

3. Calculate number of sulfhydryl groups (molar extinction coefficient of 19800 for the modified, pyridine-4-thione, thiol groups).

4. The decrease of the number of thiol groups due to the maleimide derivatization (Section 11.2.3.1.3.2; Table 11.15) may also be determined with this method (the determination of the number of maleimide groups introduced into proteins without thiol groups is given in Table 11.18).

TABLE 11.15
Cross-linking of thiol-containing antibodies with β-galactosidase by N,N'-o-phenylenedimaleimide (slightly modified from Hamaguchi et al., 1979)[a]

---

1   Dialyze 4–8 mg of IgG or F(ab')$_2$, in 0.9 ml, against 100 mM sodium acetate buffer, pH 5.0.

2   Degas sample, add slowly 0.1 ml of 100 mM 2-mercaptoethylamine and incubate for 90 min at 37° C under nitrogen. (The lower pH and the nitrogen are more effective in the prevention of oxidation than the conditions of the published method.)

3. Remove reducing agent by filtration through a Sephadex G-25 column (30 ml), using the same acetate buffer, degassed and kept under nitrogen.

4. Monitor and collect the effluent (with stirring, under nitrogen) in a saturated solution (≈ 0.75 mM) of OPDM in 100 mM sodium acetate buffer, pH 5.0[b].

5. Incubate for 20 min at 30° C.

6. Remove excess reagent by filtration through a Sephadex G-25 column (30 ml) in 20 mM sodium acetate buffer, pH 5.0.

7. Pool the maleimide-derivatized antibodies and concentrate the solution in a dialysis bag (at about 20 torr) in the cold to about 0.3 ml[b].

8. Adjust the pH to 6.5 with 250 mM sodium phosphate buffer, pH 7.5.

9. Add successively 20 μl of N-ethylmaleimide–BSA, 1 μl of 1 M MgCl$_2$ and 0.1 ml of BGase (5 mg/ml). (N-ethylmaleimide–BSA is prepared by incubating a 10% BSA solution in 100 mM sodium acetate buffer, pH 5.0, with 100 mM N-ethylmaleimide at 30° C for 60 min and then at 4° C overnight, followed by gel filtration through a column, containing 30 ml Sephadex G-25 equilibrated with 10 mM sodium phosphate buffer, pH 7.0, and 100 mM NaCl.)[b]

10. Incubate for 16 h at 4° C.

11. Bring the volume of the sample to 1 ml with 10 mM sodium phosphate buffer, pH 7.0, containing 100 mM NaCl, 1 mM MgCl$_2$, 0.1% BSA and 0.1% NaN$_3$ (NaN$_3$ will destroy excess of maleimide groups).

12. Purify by chromatography on a Sepharose 6B column (80 ml) equilibrated with the buffer of step 11.

---

[a] Instead of the method presented here, it is possible to treat the enzyme with an excess of OPDM, which is then allowed to react with thiol groups in the antibody. This alter-

Fab′ is recovered in the conjugates (Hamaguchi et al., 1979).

Similar to the results with other homobifunctional reagents, conjugates are quite heterogeneous and about one-third is aggregated. Such aggregates may be harmful in EIA, particularly in the presence of rheumatoid factors. The selective two-stage conjugation procedure reduces, however, the degree of heterogeneity obtained with the GA methods.

After minor modifications, OPDM may be used for other enzymes though it may not be equally suitable. For example, β-glucosidase and APase lose their activity by thiolation and are only partially conjugated (Ishikawa et al., 1978).

Conjugates prepared with OPDM are stable over long periods (1–2 years) at 4°C. The cross-linker is, however, not sufficiently stable during the preparation of the conjugates, which prompted the synthesis of more stable maleimide derivatives (Section 11.2.3.2.1).

11.2.3.1.4. Bis-succinic acid N-hydroxysuccinimic ester (BSNHS)
The bifunctional ester BSNHS (Fig. 11.11) is useful for the conjugation of the heme–octapeptide, 8-MPOase (Section 10.4.1), to antibodies (Ryan et al., 1976). Since 8-MPOase has only one reactive amino group (Fig. 10.4) its treatment with a large excess of BSNHS results in a complete conversion of 8-MPOase to an intermediate monoactive ester without significant cross-linking, which is then added to the antibody or Fab′-fragment. The biological activity of the conjugate is retained to a high degree. Details are given in Table 11.16.

11.2.3.1.5. Carbodiimides (CDI)   The general formula of CDI, which can be regarded as *N,N′*-disubstituted anhydrides of

---

native approach is particularly useful for the labeling of Fab′ where small amounts are available. Similar amounts of proteins should then be used, but the concentration of OPDM (step 4; added in DMF) should be lowered 10–20 times.
[b] Step 4: alternatively, a 1/10 volume of 0.4 M OPDM in DMF can be added. Step 7: Do not use NaN_3 as a preservative, since it causes rapid decomposition of maleimide. Step 9: Determine if sufficient thiol groups are present in enzyme (Table 11.14). Lyophilized, commercial BGase preparations tend to contain more thiol groups than those in suspension.

TABLE 11.16
Conjugation of microperoxidase to antibodies by bis-succinic acid N-hydroxysuccinimic ester (Ryan et al., 1976)

---

1. Dissolve 16 μmol (5 mg) of BSNHS in 300 μl of DMSO.

2. Dissolve separately 5 mg (125 μmol) of 8-MPOase in 250 μl pyridine and add dropwise to the stirred solution of BSNHS over a period of 2.5 h.

3. Continue incubation under stirring for another 2.5 h at room temperature.

4. Add 4 volumes of diethylether and allow product to precipitate overnight at 4° C.

5. Remove carefully the supernatant and dissolve the precipitate in DMSO (400 μl).

6. Store at $-25°$ C (stable for at least 5 months).

7. Add activated MPOase in small aliquots (5 μl) to IgG solution (15 mg/ml) upto 12.5% of the original volume over a period of 90 min and stir subsequently for 4 h at room temperature.

8. Allow to stand overnight at 4° C.

9. Purify by gel filtration (Bio-Gel P300, 2.5 × 70 cm, in 100 mM Tris-HCl buffer, pH 7.4) to remove small by-products or reagent.

10. Purify on DEAE–cellulose, equilibrated with 10 mM sodium phosphate buffer, pH 7.4. Free antibody passes directly, while conjugate can be eluted subsequently with same buffer containing 300 mM KCl. Substitution rate will be about 1.6.

---

urea, is $R-N=C=N-R'$. The R and R' groups may be aliphatic or aromatic, like (homobifunctional) or unlike (heterobifunctional), and their nature determines the solubility of the CDI reagents.

The reaction of CDI with proteins is not completely understood, but links one molecule via its amino group directly to the carboxyl group of the other molecule (Section 7.1.8.2.3). The γ-amino group of the lysyl residue is mostly involved, as are the carboxyl groups from the acidic side-groups of aspartyl or glutamyl residues. Carboxyl groups can also be introduced after thiolation of proteins (Section 11.2.3.1.3.1), followed by a reaction with bromo- or iodoacetic acid (Gurd, 1967).

Various water-soluble CDI were effectively used for the conjugation of POase or APase to antibodies or protein antigens (Avrameas and Uriel, 1966; Nakane et al., 1966; Clyne et al., 1973). These conjugates, however, are quite unstable and deteriorate after a few days of storage (Avrameas et al., 1978). Therefore, this method is not recommended for the conjugation of proteins, although it may be well suited for haptens (Chapter 12).

11.2.3.1.6. Tolylene-2,4-diisocyanate (TDIC) TDIC (Fig. 11.11) is a homobifunctional reagent, the two isocyanate groups of which have different reactivities due to the presence of the methyl group. Thus, this reagent can be used both in one-step and two-step procedures (Modesto and Pesce, 1973).

The more reactive *p*-isocyanate group reacts with a protein, whereas heating to 37°C is usually necessary to activate the *o*-isocyanate group. This method is occasionally employed for the coupling of MPOase to IgG or Fab in a one-step method (Tiggemann et al., 1981), using 2 μl of TDIC for 1 mg MPOase and 1 mg Fab per ml (Schick and Singer, 1961). About 12–16 MPOase molecules per Fab or 60 molecules per IgG can be conjugated while retaining 70-80% of the enzyme activity.

11.2.3.1.7. Other homobifunctional reagents The reagent 4,4′-difluoro-3,3′-dinitrophenyl sulfone (FNPS), represented in Fig. 11.11,

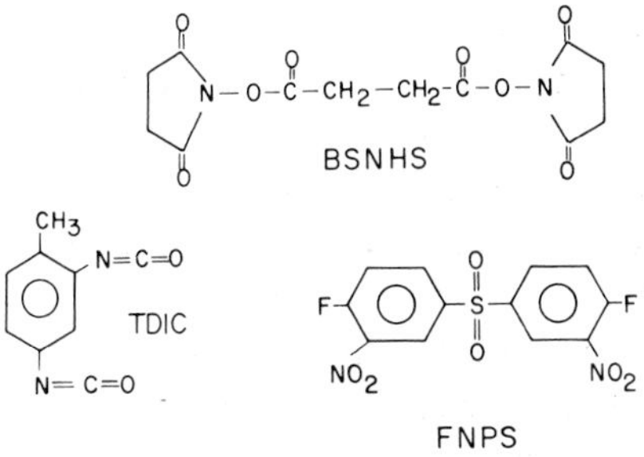

Fig. 11.11. Other reagents occasionally used for conjugation. BSNHS is bis-succinic acid *N*-hydroxysuccinimic ester, TDIC is tolylene 2,4-diisocyanate, and FNPS is 4,4′-difluoro-3,3′-dinitrophenyl sulfone.

has been widely used in the initial conjugation experiments (Nakane and Pierce, 1967). It has several disadvantages, such as low solubility, necessity of alkaline media (pH 10–11), low yields of conjugation and rapid hydrolysis of the fluorine groups to the detriment of the conjugation reaction. Cyanuric chloride, used for several enzymes (Avrameas and Lespinats, 1967) has similar disadvantages.

Diazonium compounds, which are formed from aromatic amines with nitrous acid, may react with proteins by electrophilic substitution of the aromatic amino acid residues. Among these, bis-diazotized benzidine (BDB), o-dianisidine, benzidine-(2,2′ or 3,3′)-disulphonic acid have been used extensively for protein conjugation (Kennedy et al., 1976a), but they may inactivate the enzyme or the antibody (coupling occurs mainly via the histidyl and tyrosyl residues).

Extensive lists of other reagents used for protein–protein coupling have been compiled by Kennedy et al. (1976a). Although for some of these reagents the potential for EIA remains to be established, most are of limited value.

11.2.3.2. Heterobifunctional reagents   The use of heterobifunctional reagents may result in better conjugation than with other chemical compounds. The different reactive groups of such reagents may make well-controlled, sequential reactions possible, thus avoiding undesired cross-linking (Kurstak et al., 1975).

A most promising group of such reagents contains maleimide derivatives (Ishikawa et al., 1978). They produce results far superior to GA (Deelder and De Water, 1981).

The heterobifunctional reagent N-succinimidyl-3-(2-pyridyldithio) propionate (SPDP) did not give, in our hands, satisfactory results, despite the strong recommendation in the literature. Although the conjugation efficiency with this reagent is quite high, the stability of the conjugate leaves much to be desired.

N-Hydroxysuccinimide ester of p-formylbenzoic acid, on the other hand, is satisfactory for the labeling of MPOase to antibody (Kraehenbuhl et al., 1974; Tijssen and Kurstak, 1974).

11.2.3.2.1. N-Hydroxysuccinimide (NHS) esters of maleimide deriv-atives   Maleimide groups react rapidly under mild conditions with thiol groups and, thence, may yield a high degree of conjugation, explaining the success of OPDM, but cannot be used with proteins in which thiol groups are essential for activity. Its instability is, however, a major drawback and expedited the search for more stable derivatives. One such compound, the 4-(*N*-maleimidomethyl)-cyclo-hexane-1-carboxylic acid *N*-hydroxysuccinimide ester (CHM–NHS), yielded largely monoconjugates of POase and Fab′ with an efficiency of close to 75% for both proteins (Yoshitake et al., 1982). Another derivative, now often used for BGase, is the *m*-maleimidobenzoyl-*N*-hydroxysuccinimide (MBS) ester (Kitagawa and Aikawa, 1976; Kita-gawa et al., 1978).

11.2.3.2.1.1. Conjugation with m-maleimidobenzoyl-N-hydroxysucci-nimide ester (MBS). Though MBS is not as stable as CHM–NHS, it has the advantage over OPDM that only one of the two proteins needs to contain free thiol groups. It is very suitable for BGase–antibody conjugation.

MBS contains a reactive NHS ester and a reactive maleimide residue (Fig. 11.12) both of which react under mild conditions. Acyla-tion of the free amino groups of one protein (e.g., IgG) occurs

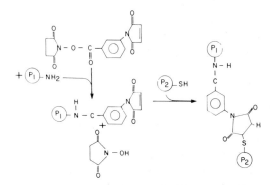

Fig. 11.12. Conjugation of enzyme to antibodies with *m*-maleimidobenzoyl-*N*-hydrox-ysuccinimide ester (MBS) as described in Section 11.2.3.2.1.1.

via the active NHS ester, whereas in the second step the thio-ethers are formed through the reaction of the free thiol groups of the other protein (e.g., BGase) with the double bond of the maleimide. Since the antibody does not contain free sulfhydryl groups, no cross-linking occurs in the first step. Excess reagent is removed prior to the addition of the enzyme which contains the free thiol groups. Several versions of the MBS technique have been described (Kitagawa and Aikawa, 1976; Shechter et al., 1978; O'Sullivan et al., 1979); the latter, with minor modifications, is given in Table 11.17. Yoshitake et al. (1982) removed excess reagent from POase with Sephadex using 50 mM sodium acetate buffer, pH 5.0, instead of the buffer of Table 11.17. It is advisable to determine the number of free thiol groups in the enzyme (Table 11.14) prior to the conjugation.

The conjugates are purified by chromatography on a Sephadex G-200 column (70 ml; sample < 1.5 ml), equilibrated with 10 mM Tris–HCl buffer, pH 7.0, containing 10 mM $MgCl_2$ and 50 mM NaCl. The conjugate elutes with the void volume and can be stored in the presence of 0.1% BSA and 0.02% NaN_3 for at least a year at 4°C. This method will separate free IgG from free enzyme and the conjugates. SpA–Sepharose may, in some cases, be used to separate enzyme from conjugate (Section 11.2.4).

This method gives high yields, both for the enzyme (80%) and for the antibody (60%), although 25% may be present in the form of aggregates, some of which may have pre-existed. Conjugation with MBS, however, is somewhat less efficient than with CHM–NHS for POase, APase, or GOase. For proteins which lack sulfhydryl groups, thiolation or reduction of disulfide bonds is required (Yoshitake et al., 1982).

11.2.3.2.1.2. 4-(N-Maleimidomethyl)-cyclohexane-1-carboxylic acid N-hydroxysuccinimide ester (CHM–NHS): a stable maleimide cross-linker. Ishikawa et al. (1978) synthesized alternative maleimide compounds of which CHM–NHS was particularly stable (decomposition rate less than 4% in 2 h at 30°C at pH 7.0, compared to 53% for OPDM and MBS. This cross-linker has been adopted successfully for the conjugation of GOase, APase, and POase (Yoshitake et

TABLE 11.17
Conjugation of β-galactosidase and peroxidase to antibody using m-maleimidobenzoyl-
N-hydroxysuccinimide ester (MBS)[a]

A. *BGase*

1. Dialyze purified IgG (1 mg/ml) against 100 mM phosphate buffer, pH 7.0, containing 50 mM NaCl.
2. Add dioxane, containing 20 mg MBS/ml, in the proportion of 1 μl for each ml of antibody solution, mix and incubate at 25°C for 1 h (degradation of MBS in the original method at 30°C can be extensive).
3. Remove excess of reagent by passing the sample through a Sephadex G-25 column equilibrated with 100 mM phosphate buffer, pH 7.0, containing 10 mM MgCl$_2$ and 50 mM NaCl (15 ml gel for each ml serum) and elute with the same buffer.
4. Pool the antibody-containing fractions, mix immediately with BGase (weight equal to weight of IgG) and incubate for 1 h at 30°C.
5. Terminate reaction by the addition of 1 M 2-ME to a concentration of 10 mM. Purify and store as described in Section 11.2.4.

B. *POase*

This method differs from BGase conjugation in that POase is treated with an excess of MBS, followed by conjugation to thiolated antibody. This method is less efficient than the CHM-NHS method (Table 11.19).

1. Dissolve 8 mg POase in 1 ml of 100 mM sodium phosphate buffer, pH 7.0 and 8 mg MBS in 0.1 ml of DMF.
2. Add reagent to POase and incubate the mixture for 1 h at 25°C.
3. Centrifuge the mixture to remove precipitate, remove by-product by gel-filtration on Sephadex G-25 (40 ml), equilibrated with 50 mM sodium acetate buffer, pH 5.0. (No NaN$_3$!.) Concentrate to 1 ml.
4. Add 10 mg Fab′ or 20 mg thiolated (Table 11.12 and 11.13) IgG in 1 ml of 100 mM sodium phosphate buffer, pH 6.0, containing 5 mM EDTA.
5. Incubate for 1 h at 30°C or 20 h at 4°C.
6. If thimerosal is used as preservative, it is recommended to treat the conjugate first with 1 mM N-ethylmaleimide (to block remaining thiol groups) for 10 min at 37°C.
7. Purify the conjugate according to Section 11.2.2.3.

[a] For pretreatment of BGase see Section 11.2.3.2.1.1.

al., 1982; Ishikawa et al., 1983), but it is not suited for BGase. POase conjugates are largely monomeric, in contrast to GOase, but the yields are high in both cases. Chemical reactions are shown in Fig. 11.13. The number of maleimide groups introduced per molecule is determined by the method given in Table 11.18.

TABLE 11.18
Determination of number of maleimide groups introduced into peroxidase

Principle: POase-maleimide is reacted with a known amount of 2-mercaptoethylamine and the fraction of thiol groups remaining free is determined with the method presented in Table 11.14.

1. Prepare a 0.15 ml sample of a known amount of derivated POase in 100 mM sodium phosphate buffer, pH 6.0. The concentration should be about 0.4 mg/ml.
2. Prepare a 500 mM solution of 2-mercaptoethylamine in a solution containing 50 mM EDTA (adjusted to pH 6.0 by adding 1 M NaOH).
3. Add 50 μl of the 2-mercaptoethylamine solution to the POase sample and incubate for 15 min at 30° C.
4. Determine the number of sulfhydryl groups present in the protein and the control samples according to steps 1–3 of Table 11.14.

The use of CHM–NHS is essentially similar to that of MBS. The incubation temperature for the introduction of the maleimide groups may, however, be raised to 30°C since CHM–NHS is more stable. The methods of Yoshitake et al. (1982), Imagawa et al. (1982b), and Ishikawa et al. (1983) for the conjugation of POase, GOase, and APase are given in Table 11.19. The principles of the reaction are given in Fig. 11.13. Treatment of POase with CHM–NHS at pH 7.0 is more effective than at pH 6.5, introducing 1–1.2 groups

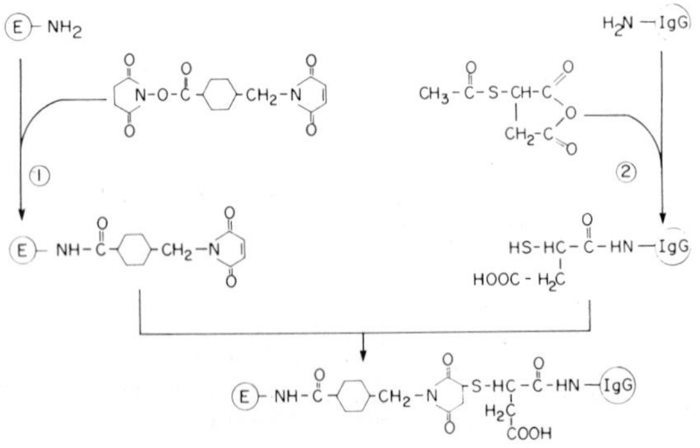

Fig. 11.13. Conjugation of enzyme (1) to thiolated antibody (2) by 4-(N-maleimidomethyl)-cyclohexane-1-carboxylic acid N-hydroxysuccinimide ester.

TABLE 11.19
Conjugation of enzymes to Fab or IgG using the N-hydroxysuccinimide ester of 4-(N-maleimidomethyl)cyclohexane-1-carboxylic acid (CHM-NHS)

A. Peroxidase

1. Dissolve 2 mg POase in 0.3 ml of 100 mM sodium phosphate buffer, pH 7.0, and add 1.6 mg CHM-NHS in 20 μl DMF. (Warm DMF to 30° C for a few min before the addition of CHM to prevent precipitation of the reagent.) Stir and incubate at 30° C for 1 h.

2. Remove precipitate that may have formed by centrifugation and pass POase through a column containing 30 ml Sephadex G-25 equilibrated with 100 mM phosphate buffer, pH 6.0, and elute with the same buffer.

3. Concentrate the pooled POase fractions in the cold.

4. Add the Fab′ (in the same buffer supplemented with 5 mM EDTA) so that the final concentration of both POase and Fab′ is between 0.05 and 0.15 mM (2–6 mg/ml). Thiolated IgG (Table 11.12 or 11.13) can be used at the same concentration.

5. Incubate for 20 h at 4° C (or 1 h at 30° C). Add, after incubation, 1 ml 2-mercaptoethylamine to block remaining maleimide groups.

6. Purify conjugates by gel filtration (e.g., on Ultrogel AcA 44, from LKB) or by the methods given in Sections 11.2.2.3 or 11.2.4. Do not use NaN₃ as preservative since it decomposes maleimide (Table 11.12).

B. β-Galactosidase

The conjugation of BGase to IgG by CHM-NHS is not as suitable as the OPDM method since the number of maleimide groups introduced is not easily controlled, particularly when Fab fragments are used. Large polymers are formed with increasing concentrations of IgG and BGase.

1. Dissolve 3 mg IgG in 1 ml of 100 mM sodium phosphate buffer, pH 7.0, and add 0.1 ml of 0.1% CHM-NHS in DMF.

2. Incubate for 30 min at 30° C.

3. Apply sample to a Sephadex G-25 column (40 ml) equilibrated with 100 mM sodium phosphate buffer, pH 6.5, and concentrate the pooled fractions containing IgG to 1 ml.

4. Dissolve 3 mg BGase (pretreated as described in Section 11.2.3.2.1.1) in 1 ml of

the buffer of step 3 and add to IgG sample (molar ratio IgG/enzyme is 3:1) and proceed as in steps 5 and 6 for the POase conjugation.

C. *Glucose oxidase*

The method is essentially similar to POase conjugation (protocol A), the most notable difference being the larger number of amino groups available on GOase. Therefore, the CHM-NHS concentration in step 1 of protocol A is lowered 5-fold for the GOase conjugation. Another modification necessary (due to the difference in MW for GOase and POase) for the conjugate of GOase using protocol A is the relative amount of enzyme and antibody used in step 4, namely per mg GOase, 1.3 mg Fab or 2 mg thiolated or reduced IgG.

D. *Alkaline phosphatase*

The CHM-NHS method adapted for APase conjugation (Ishikawa et al., 1983) differs in several respects from the above methods. To maintain an active enzyme, 50 mM sodium borate buffer, pH 7.6, containing 1 mM $MgCl_2$ and 0.1 mM $ZnCl_2$ (BMZ buffer) is used.

1. Enzyme obtained in suspension (in 3.2 M $(NH_4)_2SO_4$) is pelleted by centrifugation and taken up in BMZ buffer or dialyzed against this buffer (4 mg enzyme in 0.5 ml).

2. Dissolve 0.7 mg CHM-NHS in 30 μl N,N'-DMF and add to enzyme solution.

3. Incubate for 1 h at 30° C.

4. Remove by-products by passage over Sephadex G-25 column (40 ml) equilibrated with 100 mM Tris–HCl buffer, pH 7.0, containing 1.0 mM $MgCl_2$ and 0.1 mM $ZnCl_2$. Concentrate enzyme-containing fractions to 2 mg/ml. About 4 maleimide residues will be introduced per molecule and 30% of the enzyme activity will be lost.

5. Add 4-fold excess of Fab′ or thiolated IgG (10 mg/ml in 50 mM sodium acetate buffer, pH 5.0).

6. Incubate for 20 h at 4° C.

7. Block remaining maleimide groups by adding 100 mM 2-mercaptoethylamine.

8. Purify according to Section 11.2.4 using the buffer of step 4.

per POase molecule. (In contrast, MBS produces only 0.63 maleimide residues per POase molecule and it is less effective at 30°C than at 25°C). Recovery of POase and Fab′ in the conjugate is close to 75% with no loss of enzyme activity (Yoshitake et al., 1982). Compared to the $NaIO_4$ method, the recovery rate of conjugates is about equal for both, and while the $NaIO_4$ method is simpler, it decreases POase activity slightly, and yields significantly more polymers. The CHM–NHS method, on the other hand, produces mainly monoconjugates, resulting in lower levels of background staining (Imagawa et al., 1982b).

11.2.3.2.2. Conjugation of microperoxidase to antibody using the N-hydroxysuccinimide ester of p-formylbenzoic acid (NHS–FBA)

The two-step procedure for the conjugation of MPOase to Fab or IgG using NHS–FBA (Kraehenbuhl et al., 1974; Tijssen and Kurstak, 1974) is given in Table 11.20 and the two steps of the reaction (activation of MPOase; coupling to IgG) are shown in Fig. 11.14. About 50% of the MPOase is conjugated, while 70% of the immunological activity is retained.

Considerable differences exist with respect to the Michaelis–Menten parameters reported for MPOase (Kraehenbuhl et al., 1974; Plattner et al., 1977; Tiggemann et al., 1981).

11.2.3.2.3. N-Succinimidyl-3-(2-pyridyl-dithio)propionate (SPDP)

SPDP conjugates proteins under mild conditions, without producing homopolymers. The method (Table 11.21), as adapted from Nilsson et al. (1981) and Pain and Surolia (1981), consists of three steps: (i) the separate derivation of both proteins to be conjugated; (ii) the reduction of the SPDP group on one of the two proteins; and, (iii) the reaction of the SPDP group on one protein with the reduced SPDP group on the other when the derivatized proteins are brought into contact (Fig. 11.15). The titers obtained in EIA with conjugates prepared by this theoretically attractive method are disappointing despite the high conjugation efficiency.

11.2.4. Purification, assessment of quality and storage of conjugates obtained by chemical linkage

There is no single, general method for the purification of conjugates,

TABLE 11.20
Conjugation of the heme-octapeptide (8-MPOase) to Fab using the N-hydroxysuccin-
imide ester of p-formylbenzoic acid

A. *Derivatization of 8-MPOase*

1. Dissolve 4.5 g of p-formylbenzoic acid and 3.5 g of N-hydroxysuccinimide in 15 ml DMF and dilute with 40 ml of dichloromethane.

2. Cool the solution to $0°$ C and add 6.18 g N,N'-dicyclohexylcarbodiimide in 6 ml dichloromethane.

3. After 5 h, remove the precipitate (dicyclohexyl urea) by filtration and bring the filtrate to dryness under high vacuum (in a rotary evaporator).

4. Dissolve the residue in 200 ml of boiling propanol, filter the hot solution and cool the filtrate. The yield of the N-hydroxysuccinimide ester of p-formylbenzoic acid is about 3.7 g (m.p. about $165°$ C).

5. Dissolve 10 mg of the ester in 0.5 ml pyridine and add to 10 mg of 8-MPOase in 0.5 ml pyridine.

6. Incubate at room temperature for about 12 h.

7. Purify the derivatized 8-MPOase on a Sephadex G-25 column (about 70 ml gel). Lyophilize and store at $-20°$ C. About 80% of the 8-MPOase will be derivatized.

B. *Conjugation of the derivatized 8-MPOase to Fab*

1. Add 5 mg of the derivatized 8-MPOase to 10 mg of Fab in 1 ml borate buffer (100 mM; pH 9.5) and incubate for 5 h at $37°$ C.

2. Reduce the Schiff bases formed with 100 μl of freshly prepared $NaBH_4$ (5 mg in 0.1 mM NaOH) for 15 min at room temperature.

3. Purify conjugate on DEAE–cellulose (≈ 4 ml) equilibrated with 10 mM phosphate buffer, pH 7.4. The conjugate is retained and can be eluted with 1.5 M KCl.

---

since the numerous enzymes, as well as the different proteins to which they may be coupled, have quite different physicochemical properties. Moreover, a large variety of homo- and heteropolymers is usually present after conjugation.

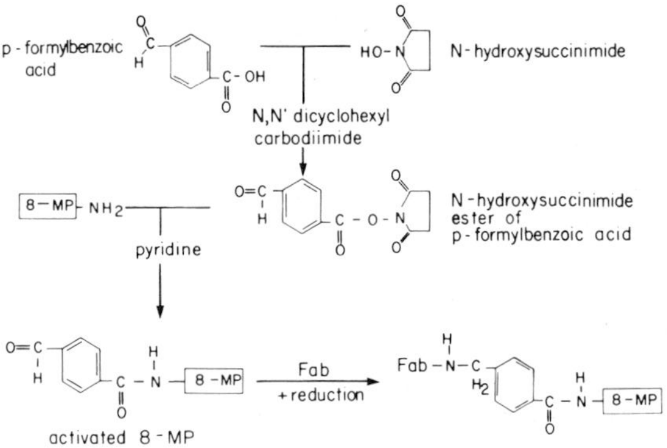

Fig. 11.14. Conjugation of MPOase to Fab by N-hydroxysuccinimide ester of p-formylbenzoic acid prepared from N-hydroxysuccinimide and p-formylbenzoic acid by N,N'-dicyclohexylcarbodiimide.

TABLE 11.21

Conjugation of enzyme to protein A or IgG using N-succinimidyl-3-(2-pyridyldithio)-propionate (SPDP)[a]

---

1. Dissolve each protein separately at a concentration of 10 mg/ml in 100 mM sodium phosphate buffer, pH 7.4, containing 100 mM NaCl.
2. Dissolve as much SPDP as possible in absolute ethanol (up to about 30–40 mM).
3. Add SPDP solution to each protein solution to obtain a suitable degree of substitution, i.e., about 6 μg SPDP per mg of protein for most proteins, such as antibodies, but about 15 times as much for POase.
4. React for 30 min at room temperature with occasional stirring.
5. Remove excess reagent and by-products by filtration through Sephadex G-25 equilibrated with the buffer used in step 1.
6. Concentrate proteins to about 6 mg/ml.
7. Reduce the SPDP-derivative of one of the two proteins (the least sensitive to reduction, e.g. POase) with dithiothreitol (DTT) at a final concentration of 50 mM (but not less than 2.5 mM DTT per mg protein).
8. Pass the reduced derivatized protein through Sephadex G-25 equilibrated with 100 mM sodium acetate buffer, pH 4.5, containing 100 mM NaCl to remove excess reagent, oxidized reagent and pyridine-2-thionine.
9. Concentrate pooled fractions to 4–5 mg/ml.
10. Mix the reduced and the non-reduced activated proteins and incubate for 20–24 h at room temperature.
11. Purify and store the conjugate as described in Section 11.2.4.

---

[a] If one of the two proteins has already SH-groups (e.g. Fab') it is not necessary to treat that protein with SPDP and steps 7–9 can then be omitted.

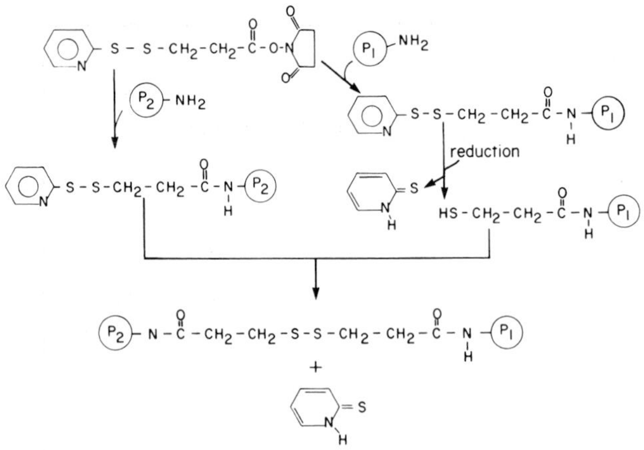

Fig. 11.15. Activation of both enzyme and antibody with N-succinimidyl-3-(2-pyridyl-dithio)propionate and subsequent conjugation.

In the AA-type EIA, competing free antibody reduces the detectability of the assays (Fig. 11.16), whereas free enzyme, and particularly polymers (Imagawa et al., 1982b), may increase background staining. Most of the purification methods are, therefore, primarily designed to remove free antibody. This is generally carried out by gel filtration under conditions where free IgG is not eluted with the void volume (e.g., 200 ml of Sephadex G-200 or Ultrogel AcA-44, with a maximum sample size of about 4 ml). Such gel filtration should be performed with buffers of a relatively high ionic strength, in order to avoid non-specific interactions between the matrix and the proteins (Section 7.1.4). However, it is virtually impossible with this approach to separate large enzymes from monoconjugates due to the relatively small differences in the molecular weights.

In some cases it is possible to purify conjugates by density gradient centrifugation, provided that the buoyant densities or sedimentation coefficients are sufficiently different (Mannik and Downey, 1973; Ford et al., 1978).

Ion-exchange chromatography may also be successful in some cases, although the method of Yamashita et al. (1976) recommended

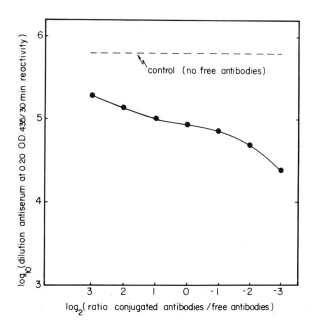

Fig. 11.16. Influence of free IgG on the detectability of antigen with peroxidase-conjugated antibodies in solid-phase EIA. An equal concentration of free and conjugated IgG causes an almost 10-fold reduction of the detectability. Courtesy *Archives of Virology*.

by Kabakoff (1980) for the purification of POase conjugates was quite unsatisfactory in our hands.

Affinity chromatography is increasingly used for the purification of conjugates (Section 11.2.2.3), and is well-suited for POase-containing conjugates (Tijssen et al., 1982).

Free enzyme may, in some cases, be removed by salt fractionation (Section 11.2.2.3) whereas SpA columns (e.g., SpA–Sepharose) may prove useful for the elimination of free enzyme in systems where IgG and IgG–enzyme complexes are adsorbed to such columns (Table 7.1). This might also be a simple method to separate IgG–BGase complexes from free BGase which is virtually impossible by gel filtration.

Purity of the conjugates may be assessed by common techniques, such as: (i) SDS–PAGE (Section 16.1), which is, however, not applicable for complexes larger than 5×10^5 Da; (ii) immunodiffusion (volume I, part III in this series); and, (iii) immunoelectrophoresis, using the microtechnique of Scheidegger (1955). After separation of the conjugates, they are revealed by adding the substrate to the central trough (Tijssen and Kurstak, 1974); for POase: 22 mM guaiacol and 0.03% hydrogen peroxide. The enzyme can be localized in a few minutes and the position of IgG can be revealed with an anti-IgG reagent. In general, enzymes and IgG move in opposite directions upon electrophoresis and the conjugates are mostly found close to the point of application.

Storage of the conjugates should be adapted to that of the enzyme including the buffer and ion requirements for optimal activity (Chapter 10). The addition of BSA (0.1–0.5%) to the conjugate is usually beneficial, particularly if the conjugate is stored frozen. It is often preferable to add an equal volume of glycerol to the solution of the conjugate, to prevent freezing, and to store at $-20°C$.

11.3. Immunological conjugation of enzyme to antibody

The enzyme activity is often not abrogated by a reaction with antibodies. Thus, an enzyme–anti-enzyme complex can be introduced by an anti-Ig into the complex and eliminates the inactivation of the enzyme or of the antibody by the chemical linkage, reduces background staining caused by the introduction of chemically reactive groups and, at the same time, enhances detectability.

Two approaches are possible in such techniques: (i) the sequential addition of the antibodies and enzyme (unlabeled antibody method); and, (ii) the preparation of enzyme–anti-enzyme complexes, prior to their application, followed by their linking to the primary antibodies (Section 11.3.2); the latter approach has become very convenient with the advent of monoclonal antibodies.

11.3.1. Unlabeled antibody method

The sequential application of the primary antibody, the excess of the linking antibody and the anti-enzyme antiserum has the problem that the linking antibody will also adsorb non-specific Ig and that only a fraction of the complexes will be able to react with the enzyme in the last step (low detectability).

Specific antibodies to the enzyme may be purified with immunosorbents (Section 7.1.8.2) and should, theoretically, give better results (Sternberger, 1969). However, this is not the case with POase. Only antibodies with low affinity will be obtained which will not retain efficiently the enzyme in the EIA. It has been estimated (Sternberger, 1979) that about 75% of the POase is lost from low-affinity antibodies during washing. Consequently, this method cannot be strongly recommended for POase.

In contrast, this method is suitable for APase (Mason and Sammons, 1978). Antibodies to bovine intestinal APase (type VII from Sigma, or type I purified according to Section 10.2.3.3) were produced in the rabbit (Sections 5.3.3.1 and 5.3.4). The enzyme (2.5 mg) was coupled to CNBr-activated Sepharose (0.25 ml; Section 7.1.8.2.2) and the specific anti-APase antibodies from 0.5 ml aliquots of rabbit antiserum (or Ig preparation) were retained on such minicolumns which were eluted subsequently with 100 mM glycine–HCl buffer, pH 2.5. The total yield over 7 adsorption/elution cycles is about 1–1.5 mg of antibody per ml of antiserum. In the test, APase and the specific anti-enzyme antibody could then be added simultaneously with the linking antibody (Mason and Sammons, 1978). The specificity of the purified antibody made it also possible to use a crude preparation of the enzyme without any decrease in detectability. Nevertheless, this method is quite involved for routine applications of EIA and is primarily used in EIH, such as in the simultaneous immunoenzymatic detection of two different antigens or epitopes (Section 17.3.2.3).

Most of these problems can be circumvented with monoclonal antibodies. This very promising approach provides the means for:

(i) the selection of antibodies which do not interfere with the activity of the enzyme; (ii) the elimination of the purification of specific anti-enzyme antibodies; and, (iii) the production of virtually unlimited quantities of identical antibodies. A possible drawback of this technique may be that primary antiserum must be produced in the same species as the monoclonal anti-enzyme antibodies. This restriction would limit the application of this technique to cases where the primary antiserum is from mice. Fortunately, this requirement is not absolute (Section 17.3.4.1) and Ig of many different species interreact with a given anti-Ig serum (linking antibody). It is also possible to haptenate both the primary and the anti-enzyme antibody and to use antihapten antibody for linking, instead of the anti-Ig antibody. With these simple methods (Section 12.5), about 15 hapten groups may be attached to each IgG molecule, producing a considerable amplification of the detectabilities. The use of anti-hapten antibodies renders the reaction very specific and makes it universally applicable. A variant of this method is the use of the avidin/biotin system (Hsu et al., 1981). Biotinylation of IgG is simple and does not adversely affect its activity (Section 3.2.2.3). Alternatively, SpA is used as the linking molecule between the primary antibody and the anti-enzyme antibody (Notani et al., 1979), if SpA is reactive with both IgG (Table 7.1).

11.3.2. Preformed, soluble complexes of enzyme with polyclonal or monoclonal antibodies

An elegant method for the preparation of PAP from polyclonal antisera was developed by Sternberger et al. (1970; for review, see Sternberger, 1979). Soluble PAP complexes are useful as tracers in EIA, but particularly in EIH. In general, their activity is superior, sometimes by several orders of magnitude, to that of chemically linked conjugates.

This procedure is based on the observation that the immune precipitate, obtained after the addition of POase to an anti-POase antiserum, can be solubilized, after the removal of non-specific proteins by washings, by the simultaneous acidification and addition of a 4-fold excess of POase (Fig. 11.17). The solubilized complexes contain 3 POase and 2 antibody molecules and remain stable and soluble for very long periods (for years at $-20°C$ in 50% glycerol/PBS).

It is necessary to determine the equivalence zone of the anti-POase antiserum to obtain optimum results (Table 11.22). If antiserum is used in excess, the yield of POase is higher, if POase is used in excess the yield of antibody is higher. At equivalence, the yield of PAP is 30%, both for the antibody and the antigen. PAP in good yields is obtained if anti-POase is precipitated with POase at 1.5 times the amount of equivalence (Table 11.23). In all cases PAP will be of the same composition (3:2 molecular ratio).

The composition of PAP can be determined spectrophotometrically by measuring the absorbance (A) at 401 nm (Soret band of POase; $a = 2.25$ cm²/mg; Table 10.4) and at 278 nm [protein absorbance by both POase ($a = 0.75$ cm²/mg) and IgG ($a = 1.4$ cm²/mg)] of a sample diluted with a neutral buffer. The POase content of the PAP (in mg per ml) is calculated according to Section 9.2.3.4: $A_{401 \text{ nm}} \times$ dilution factor $\times 2.25^{-1}$. Using this value, the contribution of POase (P) to the absorbance of the PAP at 278 nm (mg POase $\times 0.75$) can be calculated and, thence, the contribution of the anti-POase

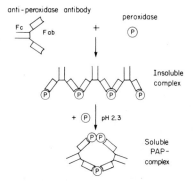

Fig. 11.17. Preparation of soluble POase-anti-POase (PAP) complex. Anti-POase antibody is mixed with POase (P) in appropriate ratios to obtain an insoluble complex. This is solubilized by simultaneously lowering the pH and adding an excess of POase.

TABLE 11.22
Determination of the equivalence zone of the antiperoxidase antiserum (Sternberger, 1979)

---

1. Place in a series of 10 small test tubes 0.2 ml aliquots of a serial dilution of POase in 0.15 NaCl, e.g., 0.05, 0.10, 0.15, ..., 0.50 mg POase per ml, respectively.

2. Add to each tube 0.2 ml antiserum and incubate overnight at 4° C.

3. Centrifuge tubes and transfer supernatants to a second series of 10 test tubes. Transfer from each tube 0.15 ml of solution to another series of 10 test tubes (third series).

4. Add to each tube of the second series 0.1 ml of the antiserum and to each tube of the third series 0.1 ml of the POase solution containing 0.1 mg/ml POase.

5. Incubate for 1 h at room temperature.

6. Observe excess antigen in second series and excess antibody in third series by quali-tatively reading precipitation after 1 h.

7. Three zones are observed: excess antigen, excess antibody and equivalence or near equivalence. Record the concentration of POase (in mg/ml) in the tube of the equiv-alence zone nearest to the antigen excess zone. This is the 'equivalence' concentra-tion used for the procedure in Table 11.23.

---

antibody (AP): $A_{278\,nm}$ of PAP $-$ mg POase $\times$ 0.75. The antibody content of the PAP complexes (in mg per ml) is, consequently, $A_{278\,nm;\,AP} \times$ dilution factor $\times 1.4^{-1}$, and the molecular ratio of POase to anti-POase:

$$\frac{mg\,P}{MW_P} : \frac{mg\,AP}{MW_{AP}} = \frac{mg\,P \times 150\,000}{mg\,AP \times 44\,000}$$

These PAP complexes have a sedimentation coefficient of 11.5 S, corresponding to a molecular weight of about 410 000–430 000 and a cyclic structure (Sternberger et al., 1970).

PAP complexes have been prepared with antibodies from rabbits (Sternberger et al., 1970), baboons (Marucci and Dougherty, 1975), goats (Rojas-Espinosa et al., 1974), mice (Marucci et al., 1977) and hamsters (Dougherty et al., 1974). The preparation of PAP with

TABLE 11.23

Preparation of PAP complex[a] (Sternberger et al., 1970; Sternberger, 1979)

1. Add and mix with 40 ml antiserum in a 250 ml centrifuge bottle the volume of POase solution (4 mg/ml; in 150 mM NaCl, referred to hereafter as saline) which contains 1.5 times the amount of 'equivalence' for 40 ml of serum.

2. Incubate for 1 h at room temperature and collect the precipitate by centrifugation at $6000 \times g$ for 20 min at $4°$ C. Remove the supernatant by gentle suction.

3. Resuspend the precipitate with 6 ml of cold saline by repeated pipetting and wash with about 200 ml of cold saline.

4. Centrifuge as in step 2 and repeat washing two more times.

5. Resuspend pellet in a solution of POase (4 mg/ml), using a volume 4 times that used in step 1, by repeated pipetting with 1 10 ml pipet.

6. Bring the pH of the solution to 2.3 by adding first about 2 drops of 1 N HCl (or about 30 μl 0.1 N HCl) and subsequently 0.1 and 0.01 N HCl for fine adjustment. The precipitate will dissolve almost instantaneously.

7. Neutralize with NaOH; proceed as for the acidification.

8. Add 1/10 volume of a solution containing 80 mM sodium acetate and 150 mM ammonium acetate. Chill on ice.

9. Centrifuge for 10 min at $40000 \times g$. Perform this and following steps at $1°$ C.

10. [b]Collect supernatant, add slowly an equal volume of saturated $(NH_4)_2SO_4$ (prepared according to Section 7.1.2.2) and stir for 25 min.

11. Collect precipitate by centrifugation (as in step 9) and wash once with a half-saturated $(NH_4)_2SO_4$ solution.

12. Dissolve precipitate in bidistilled water (volume equal to that of step 5).

13. Dialyze against several changes of a solution containing 135 mM NaCl, 7.5 mM sodium acetate and 15 mM ammonium acetate.

14. Remove precipitate by centrifugation as in step 9, collect supernatant and determine concentration.[c]

[a] Horseradish POase should be purified by the simple method given in Section 10.2.1.2 which yields a more active enzyme (by elimination of less active isozymes) and at a considerably lower cost than the commercial preparations.

[b] Bosman et al. (1980) replaced the purification steps by a step of chromatography on Sephacryl S-200 (1.5×90 cm) equilibrated with PBS. This simple method is practical with small samples (less than 5 ml).

[c] Measurement of the A_{401} nm/A_{275} nm absorbance ratio of the preparation facilitates the analysis of the PAP complex by the method given in Section 11.3.2.

chicken antibodies may pose some problems since the admixture of POase at the amount of equivalence to chicken sera produces a gelatinous precipitate which has to be resuspended, after the various centrifugation steps, with a needle-probe oscillator for about 10 sec. The final dialysis step may lead to the formation of a large precipitate which apparently is due to a non-specific protein co-precipitating with chicken immune precipitates (Dougherty et al., 1972).

PAP complexes with antibodies from different species are commercially available. Though they are expensive, only small amounts of PAP are required due to the high detectability of the assays using PAP; moreover, quantities needed in EIH are generally small.

In the case of monoclonal antibodies, the PAP or APase–anti-APase (APAAP) complexes can be readily obtained by adding crude enzyme to the supernatant of the hybridoma cell culture, or to ascitic fluid (Mason et al., 1983). This method is very simple, once such a producing hybridoma is obtained (Table 11.24). However, no cyclic structures are obtained with such monoclonal antibodies, since they are directed against a single epitope. The molecular weights of such complexes are, consequently, considerably lower. Table 11.25 gives some of their advantages.

TABLE 11.24

A simple method for the production of PAP with monoclonal anti-peroxidase antibodies

---

1. Antibody-producing cells are induced in mice by a series of i.p. injections of POase (20 μg) emulsified with an equal volume of Freund's complete adjuvant (Section 5.3.3.1). The final injection (3 days before removal of spleen) is given i.v. (200 μg POase in saline). The preparation of hybridomas and the selection and propagation of cells producing monoclonal anti-POase antibodies are by the methods given in Section 5.5.

2. Mouse PAP is prepared by adding 0.005 to 0.05 mg of POase/ml to undiluted culture supernatants of the anti-POase-secreting hybridoma line. This material can be stored and used at a dilution of more than 1:1000 without prior purification. If monoclonal antibodies are used from ascitic fluid, antibodies are first precipitated with 50% $(NH_4)_2SO_4$ and the enzyme is added (0.04–0.2 mg/ml) to the isolated antibodies.

TABLE 11.25
Characteristics of monoclonal PAP complexes.

— Gives a more satisfactory staining than polyclonal PAP.

— May be used for a wide range of monoclonal antibodies, e.g., for screening of monoclonal antibodies.

— Composition of PAP is two enzyme molecules and antibody (smaller than conventional polyclonal PAP complexes).

— Anti-POase antibodies may be selected with high affinities.

— A possible theoretical objection to this method is the fact that the monoclonal antibody is of a single class. However, there are a number of epitopes common to all mouse IgG.

11.4. Avidin–biotin–peroxidase complexes

In current procedures using the avidin–biotin method, an excess of the quite expensive avidin is needed, i.e., either in the incubation step with avidin or in the production of preformed avidin–biotin–POase complexes (Hsu et al., 1981; Section 17.3.2.2.3).

A simple and economical way to obtain complexes of optimum activity consists of the use of small column of iminobiotin saturated with avidin according to Section 3.2.1.3 (crude extract from egg whites can be used directly). One of the binding sites of avidin is occupied by the iminobiotin while the other remains free for reaction with the subsequently added biotinylated POase. Avidin is then added to saturate additional free biotin groups on POase. Complexes are then eluted from the column with 50 mM ammonium acetate (pH 4.0).

11.5. Combined procedures for conjugation

From the procedures discussed, it is evident that large differences exist in the ease and success with which macromolecules may be conjugated.

In some cases it may be possible to bind the enzyme to the immune complex by conjugating an enzyme-binding molecule (e.g., lectin or antibody) to the primary or anti-Ig antibodies. Conjugation of Con A, which has an affinity for POase, to antibody (Guesdon and Avrameas, 1980) may not be suitable for all situations since a small fraction of IgG has an affinity for Con A (Arends, 1981). In the antibody-chimera technique (Porstmann et al., 1984), monoclonal anti-POase antibodies are conjugated to the primary antibodies by a cross-linker which is much more efficient with IgG than with POase. In this method, 0.1 mg primary antiserum IgG is mixed with 0.8 mg monoclonal anti-POase IgG in 1 ml of 100 mM phosphate buffer, pH 6.8, containing 0.1% GA, for 2 h at room temperature. Then, 0.05 ml of 2 M glycine is added, incubated for a further 2 h, and dialyzed overnight against PBS. Precipitates are removed by centrifugation. POase (crude preparation) is then added at a 10-fold molar excess. This method, however, is much less suitable for polyclonal anti-POase antisera.

Conjugation of haptens

Macromolecules are haptenated for the preparation of: (i) immuno-genic hapten–carrier complexes for the production of anti-hapten antibodies; (ii) reagents for the detection of haptens by EIA; and, (iii) reagents which, in conjunction with anti-hapten antibodies, re-strict the specificity or increase the applicability of solid-phase EIA or EIH. The properties required of the hapten-conjugates are quite different for the three different situations. The haptenation proce-dures will be described according to the functional group of the hapten.

12.1. Basic concepts

Haptens are substances with a great diversity of reactive groups. These groups may be used for conjugation but are also frequently their specific immunodeterminants which distinguishes the hapten from related molecules. The use of these groups for linkage decreases the specifity of the anti-hapten antibodies (Murphy, 1980). Assays for morphine and theophylline are illustrative of this aspect. For the original morphine assay (Rubenstein et al., 1972), antibodies were raised against 3-O-carboxymethyl morphine coupled to BSA, which, however, recognized better the closely related codein than morphine. Substitution at the 6- or 3-oxygen sites of morphine do not provide selectivity, whereas substitution on the nitrogen produces minimal cross-reactivity with codein (Morris et al., 1974; Findlay et al., 1977). Similar problems exist for theophylline and the closely related caffeine. Although in some situations (e.g., in opiate abuse), the recognition of a wider range of haptens is desirable, specificity is often required. Choosing the group common to related molecules as the site of linkage provides superior specificity (Cook et al., 1976). The use of a spacer between the hapten and the protein may also improve specificity (Exley et al., 1971; Lindner et al., 1972) and recognition of the hapten (Mould et al., 1977).

Different factors governing the reactions and yields of conjugation (Table 11.2) apply equally to haptenation. The stability and solubility of the hapten, and the nature of the groups available for conjugation also influence the yield.

Many of the basic rules for haptenation were established by Landsteiner (1945). For immunization, a certain number of hapten groups per protein molecule is optimal (e.g., 8–25 for BSA) which may be quite different for EIA. Landsteiner observed that the antibody is directed primarily to the portion of the hapten farthest removed from the linkage. Nevertheless, immunogens prepared by haptenation of proteins often generate antibodies against the linkage (Eisen and Siskind, 1964). Van Weemen and Schuurs (1975), who noted similar effects, defined three types of heterologies any of which improved detectability: (i) different cross-linkers for the haptens used in immunization and EIA (bridge heterology); (ii) linkage at different positions of the hapten (site heterology); and, (iii) different but related haptens attached through the same site by the same linkage. However, the sequential saturation assay generally gives a lower specificity (Section 8.8.1.2).

The choice of the carrier is important. The most common carriers are serum albumin of various species (generally quite soluble; Erlanger et al., 1959), keyhole limpet hemocyanin, thyroglobulin, ovalbumin, or fibrinogen. Different carriers can be used for immunization and assays or, alternatively, antibodies to the carrier can be removed by absorption.

The linkage of haptens to proteins generally occurs at the most reactive groups of the proteins: ε- and α-amino (pK_a 10 and 8, respectively), phenolic, sulfhydryl (pK_a 9), imidazol (pK_a 7), carboxyl (pK_a 2–4). The pK_a, i.e., the pH at which half of the groups is protonated, determines the change of their reactivity with the pH; the unprotonated forms of the nucleophilic groups are reactive. The reactivities of these groups also depend on the micro-environment of the residue.

Many of the techniques are borrowed from the fields of protein chemistry (Glazer et al., 1975, vol. 4 of this series). The protein-modifying reagents have been classified into 4 broad groups (Kaba-koff, 1980): (i) acylating; (ii) alkylating; (iii) oxidizing and reducing; and, (iv) electrophilic reagents.

12.2. Choice of reagent used for conjugation

Acylating reagents form stable derivatives primarily with amino groups (deprotonated lysine) and tyrosyl residues, and unstable derivatives with cysteyl or histidyl residues under alkaline conditions, due to the pK_a of the groups involved (Section 12.1). Modified tyrosine can be regenerated by treatment with hydroxylamine (Riordan and Vallee, 1963).

The general formula of acylating reagents is $R-C(=O)-X$, obtained by activation of carboxyl groups. Examples are acetic or mixed anhydride, N-hydroxysuccinimide esters (NHS; Fig. 11.11 and 11.14) and S-acetylmercaptosuccinic anhydride (Fig. 11.10). In general, anhydrides are rapidly hydrolyzed and acylation is, therefore, in competition with the hydrolysis of the reagent.

Important alkylating reagents, used under mildly alkaline conditions (pH 7–8.5), are the maleimides (Section 11.2.3.1.3), the prototype of which is N-ethylmaleimide, and the aryl halides, such as DNFB or TDIC. Here again, hydrolysis competes with the alkylation reaction.

Redox reactions, which take advantage of the ease of reduction and oxidation of disulfides, are rarely used for the conjugation.

The best known among the electrophilic reagents are the diazonium salts.

Cross-linking reagents can also be classified (Table 12.1) according to the nature of the bridge formed between the hapten and the carrier: (i) those activating carboxyl groups (mostly on haptens) to render them reactive towards amino groups; (ii) those forming a bridge between two amino groups; and, (iii) those producing azo linkages with tyrosyl or histidyl residues. Among these, the carboxyl-activating reagents are the most widely used; their high versatility was illustrated in Fig. 3.1.

Like for conjugation of proteins, reagents should be used at high concentrations in order to increase the probability of the formation of the appropriate conjugates. Relatively insoluble reagents may be added in 5–25% organic solvent (dioxane for alkyl chloroformates,

TABLE 12.1

Some reagents for the conjugation of haptens to proteins
(modified after Parker, 1976)

Bond formed	Reagent[a]	Reaction steps	Water solubility	Optimal pH
	Carbodiimides			
	1. EDC	1 or 2	high	5.5–6
	2. DCC	1 or 2	low	–
	3. CMC	1 or 2	high	5.5–6
–CO–NH–	alkyl chloroformates	2	low (first step)	9.0 (second step)
	isoxazolium salts	1 or 2	high	5.5
	diisocyanates	2	low	7.5 (first step)
–NH–R–NH–	GA	1 or 2	high	9.0
	dihalonitrobenzene	1 or 2	medium-low	8–10
–X–R–X–	diazonium salts	1	high	7.5

[a] Abbreviations: EDC, 1-ethyl-3-(3-dimethylaminopropyl)carbodiimide; DCC, N,N'-dicyclohexylcarbodiimide; CMC, 1-cyclohexyl-3(2-morpholinylethyl)carbodiimide metho-p-toluenesulfonate

acetone for dihalonitrobenzenes). Regardless of the procedure used, cross-linking of the carrier (proteins) should be avoided as much as possible, e.g., by a two-step procedure (Table 12.1).

Haptens with carboxylic or amino groups can be directly used for conjugation if these groups are not essential for the specificity. Other haptens may require the introduction of such groups. Some haptens, nevertheless, may be difficult to conjugate with common reagents and hapten derivatives should be synthesized or very reactive reagents, such as arylnitrenes (Knowles, 1972), employed. Nitrenes become extremely reactive when exposed to light and may break C–H bonds which normally are not reactive. The same effect can be achieved by irradiation (radical formation), but such reactions have a low specificity and purification of the desired derivative is required.

The enormous variety of haptens excludes a comprehensive treatment of their conjugation. The methods described here are only representative of a given approach and may have to be modified for particular haptens.

12.3. Conjugation of haptens to proteins

12.3.1. Haptens containing carboxyl groups or which can be carboxylated

If a hapten does not contain free carboxyl, such group(s) may often be introduced. Alkylation of oxygen or nitrogen substituents with halo-esters, followed by hydrolysis of the ester, is frequently used for this purpose (Kabakoff, 1980). For steroids, carboxyl groups may be introduced to the hydroxyl or keton groups, through the formation of hemisuccinate esters or (carboxymethyl)oximes, respectively.

Widely used methods to conjugate carboxyl group-containing molecules to proteins are : (i) the mixed anhydride method; (ii) the CDI method; and, (iii) the NHS ester method.

The popular mixed anhydride method is a simple, direct procedure. The carboxyl group of the hapten can be converted to an acid anhydride which reacts with the amino groups of the protein (Table 12.2). Usually 10–20 mol of hapten per mol of enzyme are added (Rowley et al., 1975; Rajowski et al., 1977). This method was applied for the preparation of the estradiol-POase (Numazawa et al., 1977); cortisol-BGase (Comoglio and Celeda, 1976); morphine-lysozyme (Schneider et al., 1973); morphine-MDase (Rowley et al., 1975); progesterone-POase (Joyce et al., 1977); Yields are often around 25%, though values as high as 90% (Marks et al., 1978) have been reported.

The CDI method (Section 11.2.3.1.5) yields about 20% conjugate and is frequently used (Erlanger, 1980). It has been used to conjugate haptens to glucoamylase (Tateishi et al., 1977), BGase (Exley and Abuknesha, 1978) and APase (Ogihara et al., 1977), as well as for the conjugation of nucleic acids to proteins through the formation of a P–N bond (Khan and Jacob, 1977). The conditions of conjugation are simple: the carrier, an excess of hapten and the reagent are stirred for at least 30 min in a buffer at pH 6.0.

A variant of the CDI method is the NHS ester procedure, in

TABLE 12.2

Mixed anhydride method

Coupling of methotrexate (MTX) to BGase (Marks et al., 1978)

1. Dissolve 5.8 mg MTX in 0.1 ml DMF, cool to 10 °C, add 2 µl isobutyl chloroformate and stir for 30 min at 10 °C.

2. Add 1.5 mg BGase in 2 ml 50 mM Na_2CO_3.

3. Incubate for 4 h at 10 °C (maintain the pH of the solution at 9.0 by adding NaOH as required) and then overnight at 4 °C.

4. Separate conjugates from unreacted compounds by gel filtration on Sephadex G-25, equilibrated with 50 mM Tris–acetic acid buffer, pH 7.5, containing 100 mM NaCl, 10 mM $MgCl_2$, and 10 mM 2-ME. Pool enzyme fractions, purify by methods discussed in Section 12.4, and add 0.1% (w/v) BSA and 0.02% (w/v) NaN_3.

which dicyclohexylcarbodiimide (DCC), or another CDI (Section 7.1.8.2.3), is esterified with NHS. This superior method is applicable where water-soluble CDI fail (Erlanger, 1980), e.g. DL-10,11-epoxy-farnesoic acid (insect juvenile hormone) was first coupled to NHS with DCC and allowed to form amide bonds with the added proteins (Lauer et al., 1974). The isolation of the NHS ester prior to its mixing with the protein permits control of the hapten/protein ratio and the elimination of the interference by free CDI. Furthermore NHS esters are stable if stored dry. Examples of this procedure are given in Section 11.2.3.1.4 and in Tables 11.16 and 12.3 (Gross et al., 1974; Ullman et al., 1979).

12.3.2. Haptens with amino groups or reducible nitro groups

Haptens with amino groups can be divided into two classes: (i) aromatic amines; and, (ii) aliphatic amines. Nitro groups can also be reduced to amino groups (e.g., Section 13.3.3).

The classical work of Landsteiner (Section 12.1) was largely performed with aromatic amines. These are converted to diazonium salts by the slow addition of nitrous acid and reacted with proteins at a pH of about 9 (Table 12.4).

Haptens with aliphatic amines can be conjugated to proteins by

TABLE 12.3
N-Hydroxysuccinimide ester procedure

Coupling of progesterone to BGase (Gros et al., 1976)

1. Dissolve progesterone-11-hemisuccinate (from Steraloids; Wilton, NH, U.S.A.) in dioxane to a concentration of 100 mM.

2. Incubate with 100 mM N-hydroxysuccinimide in the presence of 200 mM DCC for 16 h at 14°C.

3. Purify the ester by thin layer chromatography (chloroform/ethanol; 9:1).

4. Add ester to BGase in a steroid/enzyme molar ratio of about 10 (in 50 mM phosphate buffer, pH 7.4).

TABLE 12.4
Diazotization of haptens
(modified from Pinckard, 1978; applicable to aromatic amines)

---

1. Dissolve 4 mmol hapten in 100 ml 0.1 N HCl.

2. Add dropwise 1% NaNO$_2$ with constant stirring at 4°C. Large excess of NaNO$_2$ should be avoided. This can be checked with starch–iodide paper or, alternatively, with 1% starch and 50 mM KI on a white tile. Free nitrous acid oxidizes iodide to iodine which reacts with starch to give a blue-black color.

3. Free nitrous acid should be present 15 min after the last addition of NaNO$_2$.

3. Dissolve protein in 200 mM borate or carbonate buffer, pH 9.0.

5. Add diazotized hapten slowly, with gentle agitation, to prevent local excess of acid. Monitor the pH and readjust to 9.5 each time it decreases to 7.0.

6. Mix for 2 h in the cold, check and adjust pH to 9.0.

7. Dialyze against PBS for about 2 days with frequent changings.

8. Store at −20°C at 20 mg/ml.

---

various methods adapted from the conjugation of proteins, such as CDI (Bartos et al., 1978; Kobayashi et al., 1978), TDIC (Section 11.2.3.1.6; Peskar et al., 1972), maleimide compounds (Section 11.2.3.2.1; Kitagawa and Kanamaru, 1978) or the NaIO$_4$ method (Section 11.2.2; Borrebaeck et al., 1978).

Another approach is to convert aliphatic amines to aromatic amines by reacting with *p*-nitrobenzoylchloride and subsequently reducing to a *p*-aminobenzoylamide (Anderer and Schlumberger, 1966). These amines can then be coupled to proteins after diazotation as in Table 12.4.

Bifunctional imidate esters react with amino groups to form amidines. Thus, desmethylnortriptyline was conjugated to BGase by dimethyladipimidate (Al-Bassam et al., 1978) and 75% immunoreactivity and 80% enzyme activity were recovered in the conjugate (Table 12.5).

TABLE 12.5

The use of bifunctional imidate esters: preparation of
desmethylnortriptyline-β-galactosidase (Al-Bassam et al., 1978)

1. Dissolve 570 μg desmethylnortriptyline and 488 μg dimethyladipimate in 0.4 ml dry methanol containing 5% (v/v) N-ethylmorpholine at room temperature.

2. After 30 min, add 0.1 ml of the ester for 100 μg BGase in 100 mM carbonate buffer, pH 9.9, containing 10 mM MgCl$_2$ and 10 mM 2-ME.

3. Incubate for 90 min at 20 °C and terminate the reaction by adding 1 ml 50 mM Tris–acetate buffer, pH 7.5, containing 100 mM NaCl, 10 mM MgCl$_2$ and 10 mM 2-ME.

4. Remove small molecules by dialysis or passage through Sephadex G-25. About 75% of the enzyme is conjugated to hapten (using nortryptyline instead of des-methylnortryptyline, only about 15% is conjugated).

12.3.3. Haptens with sulfhydryl groups

Maleimides (Section 11.2.3.2.1.2) are particularly useful for the conjugation of thiol-containing haptens. Other approaches are based on the activation of the protein with bromoacetamide groups (Singh et al., 1978) or on the formation of disulfide bonds between the carrier and hapten in acetate buffer, pH 4.0, in the presence of hydrogen peroxide, as used for the conjugation of penicillenic acid (De Weck and Eisen, 1960).

12.3.4. Haptens with hydroxyl groups

This group includes sugars, nucleosides, phenols and alcohols. Direct conjugation is generally not possible.

The conversion of alcohol to the half ester of succinic acid ('hemisuccinate') introduces a carboxyl group available for conjugation. This method (Table 12.6) has been used for a large number of haptens (Steiner et al., 1969; Den Hollander et al., 1974; Okabayashi et al., 1977). The bifunctional reagent, sebacoyldichloride, converts alcohol to acid chloride which, at pH 8.5, reacts readily with proteins (Bailey and Butler, 1967).

TABLE 12.6

Conversion of alcoholic hydroxyl group to carboxyl group through the formation of hemisuccinate (Okabayashi et al., 1977)

1.	Dissolve 15 g 2,2,2-trichloroethanol, 12 g succinic anhydride and 8.7 ml triethylamine in 100 ml ethylacetate.
2.	Heat and reflux for 1 h.
3.	Evaporate solvent and take up residue in 5% aqueous $NaHCO_3$.
4.	Wash twice with ether and acidify subsequently to pH 2.0 with H_2SO_4.
5.	Wash resulting solid (2,2,2-trichloroethylhemisuccinate) twice with water and recrystallize from chloroform–hexane (yield about 75%; mp 88–89 °C).
6.	Add 2.5 g of the hemisuccinate to 6.5 ml thionyl chloride and heat for 30 min at 65 °C.
7.	Evaporate to dryness in vacuum and keep residue under high vacuum for 1 h.
8.	Dissolve the solid (2,2,2-trichloroethylsuccinyl chloride) in 15 ml N,N-dimethylethylacetamide and react with the hydroxyl group of the hapten (i.e., the 5′-OH of 1-β-D-arabinofuranosylcytosine, 2.79 g), by stirring for 2 h at room temperature.
9.	Evaporate under high vacuum at 65 °C and recrystallize from isopropanol (yield: about 84% of crystalline 5′ ester in the hydrochloride form; mp 160 °C).
10.	Cleave the trichloroethylester with zinc and acetic acid in DMF in order to obtain the hapten-hemisuccinate (Woodward et al., 1966). The carboxyl group thus introduced can be coupled to protein, e.g., by the carbodiimide method.

Phenols can be activated with diazotized *p*-aminobenzoic acid (Section 12.3.2.2), which introduces a carboxyl group, and can then be reacted with the carrier or enzyme molecule by a mixed anhydride reaction (Levy et al., 1976; Table 12.2).

Sugars can be activated by Landsteiner's method (1945), forming a *p*-nitrophenyl glycoside, followed by the reduction of the nitro group and the conjugation after diazotization. A simpler method is based on the cleavage of vicinal glycols of sugars to aldehydes (Section 11.2.2) which are then coupled to amines by reductive alkylation. This method (Table 12.7) has been successfully applied for the conjugation of nucleosides and nucleotides (D'Alisa and Erlanger, 1976) and of digoxin (Butler and Chen, 1967).

Conjugation of haptens through the highly reactive chlorocarbonates, prepared with an equimolar amount of phosgene, is an alternative which has been used for testosterone (Erlanger et al., 1957).

12.3.5. Haptens with aldehyde or keton groups

Carboxyl groups can be readily introduced into ketones and aldehydes through the formation of O-(carboxymethyl)oximes (Table 12.8). Keton groups can also be derivatized with p-hydrazinobenzoic acid (Africa and Haber, 1971) to produce carboxyl groups which can be conjugated to the carrier by the method discussed in Section 12.3.1. Haptens containing aldehydes can be directly conjugated through the formation of Schiff bases which are stabilized by reduction with $NaBH_4$, as in Table 11.7, steps 4 and 5 (Còrdoba et al., 1966; Ungar-Waron and Sela, 1966).

TABLE 12.7

Oxidation of vicinal glycols of haptens with $NaIO_4$ and conjugation to protein

Coupling of adenosine to BGase (Lauer and Erlanger, 1971)

1. Dissolve 20 mg adenosine in 1 ml 100 mM $NaIO_4$ and incubate for 30 min at 4°C in the dark.

2. Add one drop of ethylene glycol.

3. Add the activated adenosine to the solution of BGase (20 mg/ml of 150 mM NaCl and 10 mM $MgCl_2$, adjusted to pH 9.0 with 3% K_2CO_3).

4. Incubate for 2 h at 4°C and maintain at pH 9.0.

5. Add 1/10 volume of fresh $NaBH_4$ (50 mg/ml) and incubate overnight at 4°C.

6. Dialyze against 50 mM phosphate buffer, pH 7.4, containing 10 mM $MgCl_2$, 10 mM 2-ME and 100 mM NaCl (several changes).

TABLE 12.8

O-(Carboxymethyl)oxime derivatives from keton-containing steroids (Erlanger et al., 1957)

---

1. Dissolve 10 mM O-(carboxymethyl)hydroxylamine (sold as (aminooxy)acetic acid or carboxymethoxyl amine) and 4 mM keto-hapten in a mixture of 200 ml ethanol and 20 ml 5% NaOH.

2. Heat and reflux for 90 min.

3. Reduce volume by rotary film evaporation, add water to 40 ml and extract with ether.

4. Wash ether extract with water and dry white powder over Na_2SO_4.

12.4. Purification of hapten conjugates

For EIA, it is important to establish the degree of substitution, the specific and the total activity of the enzyme recovered, as well as the extent of recovery of the immune reactivity. The number of amino groups substituted with haptens in carrier molecules is conveniently established by the determination of the number of free amino groups before and after substitution (Habeeb, 1966; Table 12.9). Another method is provided by the use of radioactive haptens (Abraham et al., 1971).

Small haptens can be removed from the conjugate by a variety of methods, the simplest being dialysis against a buffer to which 1–2% Norit A is added to increase efficiency. Exley and Abuknesha (1978) used a series of affinity chromatography steps. A simpler purification procedure, which is applicable to many conjugates, consists in dialysis to remove free hapten, followed by adsorption of the conjugate to affinity column (immunosorbent with anti-hapten antibodies), its elution by competition with the free hapten, and the final removal of free hapten by dialysis. Comparitive studies of EIA with purified and unpurified conjugates are scarce (van Weemen and Schuurs, 1972).

TABLE 12.9

Determination of amino groups in proteins by the color development due to the reaction of 2,4,6-trinitrobenzenesulfonic acid (TNBS) with ε-amino groups

This determination is performed under more gentle conditions than the ninhydrin method and is linear up to 1 mg/ml. SDS interferes, particularly when the pH of the sample is below pH 8.5 in the first step.

Method
1. Add 1 ml 4% NaHCO$_3$ and 1 ml 0.1% TNBS, respectively, to 1 ml of protein solution (0.6–1.0 mg/ml). The blank contains 1 ml water instead of protein solution.

2. Incubate for 2 h at 40°C.

3. Add 1 ml SDS (10%) to solubilize the protein and prevent its precipitation by addition of 0.5 ml 1 N HCl.

4. Read at 335 nm (molar extinction coefficient of TNBS modified amino group of different proteins are all close to $10^4\,M^{-1}\,cm^{-1}$).

12.5. Haptenated antibodies for improved specificity or generalized application

Haptenation of antibodies and the use of anti-hapten antibodies may increase the specificity and applicability of EIA. An enzyme-labeled anti-hapten antibody may amplify the reaction with haptenated first layer antibody, may be applied to antibodies of any origin since after haptenation they are specifically recognized by the same anti-hapten conjugate, may eliminate the quite common cross-reactivity among primary antibodies of different origin for the same anti-Ig antibodies, and can be used for the study of alloantigens for which conventional methods are often difficult due to cross- or shared-reactivity. These methods are generally named 'hapten-sandwich labeling'. The increased detectability of EIA may reveal extremely weak shared reactivity between antibodies to two haptens (e.g., *p*-azobenzoate and *p*-azobenzenearsonate). Therefore, the choice of haptens is crucial if two or more different immunoreactants need to be detected in the same sample. Fig. 12.1 gives the structural formulas of haptens discussed.

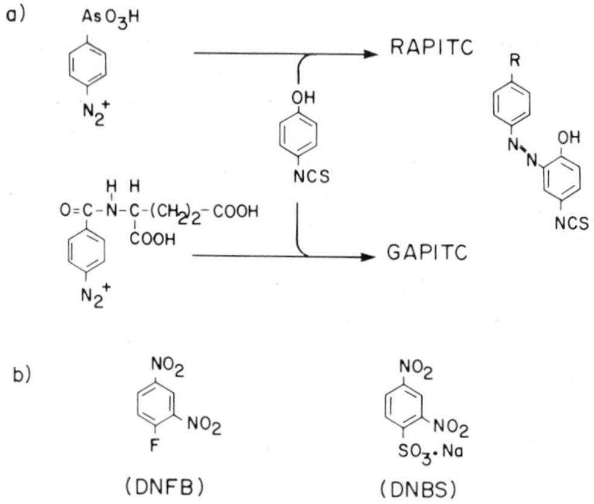

Fig. 12.1. Some active molecules used for the haptenation of antibodies. In (a) *p*-aminobenzenearsonic acid or *N*-(4-aminobenzoyl)-L-glutamic acid are diazotized (according to Table 12.4) and reacted separately with 4-hydroxyphenylisothiocyanate to yield ars-azo-hydroxyphenylisothiocyanate (RAPITC) and glut-azo-hydroxyphenyl-isothiocyanate (GAPITC), respectively, which differ in R. 2,4-Dinitro-1-fluorobenzene and 2,4-dinitrobenzene sulfonate are presented in (b).

A most common method of haptenation is dinitrophenylation and anti-DNP antibodies are commercially available (e.g., Miles). Reagents used for this purpose are 2,4-dinitrobenzene sulfonate (DNBS) or 2,4-dinitro-1-fluorobenzene (DNFB) which are reactive mostly with amino groups. DNBS is highly water-soluble, whereas DNFB is soluble in organic solvents (e.g., ethanol). Reactions with DNBS (Table 12.10) are better controlled because they are slower and, in contrast to DNFB, more restricted to amino groups. For the DNFB method, the protein should be present at a concentration of 10–20 mg/ml in 1 M sodium bicarbonate to which 0.05 ml of 1% DNFB (in ethanol) is added and vigorously mixed. Free DNFB and reaction by-products are removed by desalting chromatography on Sephadex G-25 or, if protein blots are directly dinitrophenylated (Section 16.3.1), by washing.

Another successful method is the haptenation of IgG with azoben-zenearsonate residues (Table 12.11). Ricardo and Cebra (1977) re-

TABLE 12.10

Dinitrophenylation of IgG using 2,4-dinitrobenzene sulfonate (Eisen, 1964)

1. IgG is suspended in distilled water or dissolved in PBS at a concentration of 20 mg/ml. K_2CO_3 is added to a final concentration of 20 mg/ml and the suspension stirred until complete dissolution. The subsequent procedures are shielded from light as much as possible, e.g., by wrapping the container in aluminum foil, since dinitrophenyl (DNP) derivatives are light sensitive.

2. Dinitrobenzene-sulfonate (DNBS) is recrystallized from ethanol by dissolving its sodium or potassium salt (15 g) in 950 ml ethanol at 70 °C with vigorous stirring. Norit A (2 g) is added, the mixture is stirred and then filtered rapidly through several layers of filter paper (Whatman No. 3) on a preheated funnel. Cooling causes the formation of small crystals. This procedure is repeated 2–4 times. The crystals (mp > 300 °C) are dried at 37 °C and stored at 4 °C in a dark container.

3. Recrystallized DNBS is added to the IgG in the proportion of 1 mg per mg IgG.

4. The mixture is stirred until the desired degree of haptenation is obtained. This can be determined by measuring the absorbance at 360 nm. For simplicity, this absorbance can be assumed to be due solely to DNP-lysine groups, the molar extinction coefficient of which is 17 530. Thus, the (moles of DNP)/(moles of protein) ratio can be calculated from the expressions (using the law of Lambert Beer; Section 9.2.3.4):

$$\text{moles of DNP} = \frac{A_{360\,nm,\,1\,cm}}{17\,530}$$

$$\text{moles of protein} = \frac{\text{concentration of protein (mg/ml)}}{\text{molecular weight of protein}}$$

5. The reaction can be stopped by rapid passage of the mixture over a small Sephadex G-25 column (10 times sample size). It is also possible to precipitate DNP–IgG by acidification, since DNP–IgG is usually insoluble at pH 4.

placed the diazonium compound by a bromoacetyl derivative to favor site-directed labeling.

Wallace and Wofsy (1979) prepared non-cross-reacting haptens (p-aminobenzoyl glutamic acid and p-aminobenzoyl glycine) which, after diazotization can be directly linked to carriers. IgG conjugated with the bifunctional reagent (methyl-4-hydroxybenzimidate) is used (Table 12.12). In the next step, however, an excess of hapten over

TABLE 12.11

Haptenation of IgG with azobenzene-arsonate (ars) residues (Wofsy et al., 1974)

1. Dissolve and diazotize arsanilic acid (Sigma Chemical Co.) as in Table 12.4.

2. Dissolve IgG (5 mg/ml) in 250 mM borate buffer, pH 8.5, and add slowly p-diazonium phenyl arsonate (to 4×10^{-4} M), while maintaining the pH at 8.5 with NaOH.

3. Incubate overnight at $4\,°C$ with gentle tumbling.

4. Quench unreacted diazonium groups with 4 mmole imidazole while stirring.

5. Purify as in step 5 of Table 12.9.

TABLE 12.12

Hydroxybenzimidate-mediated haptenation of IgG with p-aminobenzoyl glutamic acid or p-aminobenzoyl glycine (Wallace and Wofsy, 1979)

1. Diazotize either of the haptens (Sigma Chemical Co.). To prepare 12 ml of 250 mM diazonium solution, dissolve 3 mmol aminobenzoyl hapten in 9 ml 1 N HCl and add slowly 3 mmol $NaNO_2$ in 3 ml water.

2. For the preparation of the hapten-azo-crosslinker (30 mM hapten with respect to cross-linker), dissolve 0.6 mmol methyl-p-hydroxybenzimidate hydrochloride (HB; Pierce Chem. Co.) in 3 ml 340 mM sodium borate buffer, pH 9.8. Add slowly with stirring at $0\,°C$, 12 ml 250 mM diazoniumbenzyl hapten solution (maintain pH at 9.2 ± 0.2 with 2 N NaOH).

3. Warm mixture to room temperature after 20 min (when reaction is virtually complete) and allow reaction to continue for about 2 h (monitor pH).

4. Add 4 mmol imidazole with stirring and incubate for 1 h to quench unreacted diazonium groups.

5. Adjust pH to 8.6 with 2 N HCl and dilute to 20 ml (this reagent may be divided into aliquots and stored at $-20\,°C$ up to several weeks).

6. Haptenate IgG by mixing 2 volumes of the hapten-azo-HB solution with 1 volume of IgG (about 10 mg/ml) in 340 mM borate buffer, pH 8.6. Incubate the reaction mixture for 15–20 h at room temperature.

7. Purify conjugate by precipitation with $(NH_4)_2SO_4$.

cross-linker (molar ratio of about 5) should be used to ensure solubility of the IgG.

Simmonds et al. (1982) reported the synthesis of two non-cross-reacting 3-(substituted-phenyl)-azo-4-hydroxyphenylisothiocyanates (Fig. 12.1). These reagents haptenate rapidly Ig molecules. Loss of antigen-binding activity was found to be negligible. p-Aminobenzenearsonic acid (p-arsanilic acid) or N-(4-aminobenzoyl)-L-glutamic acid are diazotized and then reacted with 4-hydroxyphenylisothiocyanate giving ars-azo-hydroxyphenylisothiocyanate (RAPITC) and glut-azo-hydroxyphenylisothiocyanate (GAPITC) as presented in Table 12.13. The conjugation of these haptens with proteins is extremely simple (Table 12.13, part D) and requires mild conditions.

TABLE 12.13

The haptenation of IgG with two non-cross-reacting 3-phenylazo-4-hydroxyphenyl-isothiocyanate derivatives

---

A. *Preparation of immunogens for the production of anti-hapten antibodies*
Arsanilic acid and N-(4-aminobenzoyl)-L-glutamic acid are diazotized and coupled to KLH (0.05 mmol/100 mg) and to BSA (0.1 mmol/100 mg), respectively, according to the method given in Table 12.4. These preparations are used for the production of antibodies which can be purified by the methods given in Section 7.

B. *Synthesis of 4-hydroxyphenylisothiocyanate*
Preparation of 4-hydroxyphenylisothiocyanate is performed by the method of Dyson and George (1924), by treating 4-aminophenol with thiocarbonyl chloride. The product is purified by distillation (bp at 0.1 mm is 140 °C).

C. *Preparation of RAPITC and GAPITC (Fig. 12.3)*[a]
  1. Diazotize the appropriate substituted aniline (1 mmol) in 2.5 ml of 1 N HCl as described in Table 12.4.

  2. Add slowly 10 ml 340 mM borate buffer, pH 9.3, to a stirred solution of 4-hydroxyphenylisothiocyanate (151 mg = 1 mmol) in 2 ml DMF.

  3. Cool to 4 °C, add the diazonium solution dropwise while keeping the pH between 8.8 and 9.2 with 5 N NaOH and incubate for 40 min while monitoring the pH.

  4. Wash twice with ether (20 ml) and acidify to pH 1.0 with 2 N HCl.

  5. Wash twice with water (20 ml), suspend in water and lyophilize.

6. Dissolve crude product in 0.5 ml 100 mM borate buffer, pH 8.6, and chromatograph on a 1.5×112 cm column of Biogel P-2 (Bio-Rad Lab.), equilibrated with the same buffer.

7. Collect the second, major colored band, acidify and wash the precipitate as in step 5. Lyophilize and precipitate at $60\,^\circ$C over P_2O_5.

D. *Conjugation with RAPITC or GAPITC*

1. Dissolve the hapten derivative and protein in 340 mM borate buffer, pH 6.8 (protect from light). IgG should be at a concentration of about 10 mg/ml. Mix equal volumes of the two solutions and incubate for 20–24 h. About 1/5 of the hapten will be conjugated to IgG.

2. Purify the conjugate by gel filtration through a column (20 times larger than reaction volume) of Biogel P-6 (Sephadex is not satisfactory for this hapten).

[a] The molar extinction coefficient of RAPITC at 505 nm is 8900 $M^{-1}cm^{-1}$ and for GA-PITC 10900 $M^{-1}cm^{-1}$ at 520 nm, both at pH 13.

The immobilization of immunoreactants on solid phases

13.1. Relative merits of solid phases

The simple manipulations required to separate free antibody or antigen from immune complexes immobilized non-covalently on plastic solid phase is probably the most important reason for the rapid increase in popularity of EIA. Desired traits of the solid phase are: (i) high capacity for binding immunoreactants (high surface/volume ratio); (ii) possibility of immobilization of many different immunoreactants; (iii) minimal dissociation; (iv) negligible denaturation of immobilized molecule; and (v) orientation of immobilized antibody with binding sites towards the solution and the Fc to the solid phase (e.g., Section 13.2.2).

Plastic is by far the most popular solid phase, since it makes the procedures extremely simple. However, plastics may also have some important limitatons: (i) they are immunoreactant-consumptive, i.e. often require 10 times more reactants than particulate solid phases or membranes; (ii) the avidity of immobilized antibodies for large antigens decreases by 1–2 orders of magnitude (Zwolinski, G.; Josephson, L.; cited by Parsons, 1981), probably due to the wide spacing of epitopes or paratopes; (iii) the rate of antibody–antigen interactions is slower than in solution or with particulate solid phases (hours instead of minutes), due to the necessity of the free immunoreactant to diffuse to the solid phase (association kinetics is largely dictated by diffusion rate; Section 8.4); and, (iv) few suitable antibodies will be bound to plastic due to its low adsorption capacity per unit area, particularly if the fraction of high-avidity IgG is low. Nevertheless, plastic has proven extremely useful for EIA.

Nitrocellulose membranes are not yet widely used but should replace plastic in many investigations in which: (i) only the presence of an immunoreactant is to be established and not its quantity (though the latter is also possible); (ii) only very small samples (e.g., less than 1 µl) are available; and, (iii) ionic detergent-solubilized antigens are to be tested. Nitrocellulose binds close to 100% of most antigens or antibodies.

Particulate solid phases (agarose, cellulose, polyacrylamide, dextran) are very efficient since they may be dispersed throughout the reaction mixture and have a much higher ratio of surface area/volume. Moreover, the immunoreactant is covalently bound.

13.2. The use of plastics as solid phases

13.2.1. Nature of protein–plastic interaction

Non-covalent adsorption works generally well and is most frequently used. However, up to 68% of non-covalently adsorbed antigen may be desorbed during the test (Engvall et al., 1971; Hermann et al., 1979; Lehtonen and Viljanen, 1980b). This desorption is strongly influenced by the serum used (Dobbins Place and Schroeder, 1982). If no proper care is taken, a whole spectrum of binding, ranging from very tight to rather loose will be obtained. In each step, some of the loosely bound antigen detaches and competes for the immunoreactant added, leading to decreased detectability and increased variation. Two simple measures can be taken to minimize this problem: (i) to use the immunoreactant for immobilization at the appropriate concentration; and, (ii) to wash extensively after immobilization and after every subsequent step (Christensen et al., 1978; Lehtonen and Viljanen, 1980b). As many as 6 washes may be necessary instead of the usual 2 or 3 advocated in standard procedures for the complete removal of loosely bound immunoreactants. Though covalent linkage improves binding (Hendry and Hermann, 1980; Suter, 1982), this is not always accompanied by a similar increase in detectability.

In a recent study (Viscidi et al., 1984) desorbing activity (up to 60%) was linked to certain fractions in the sample (fecal) with a molecular weight of about 25000 having proteolytic activity since this effect could be reversed with protease inhibitors or a large excess of inert protein.

The non-covalent adsorption process is poorly understood, despite its widespread application. It has been investigated most extensively with respect to the introduction of synthetic materials into the cardiovascular system (Morissey, 1977). Protein adsorption to plastic surfaces is generally attributed to non-specific hydrophobic interactions and is independent of the net charge of the protein, although binding is different and characteristic for each protein (Cantarero et al., 1980). The unique adsorptive behavior of each protein to polystyrene is independent of its pI, charge and molecular weight. Partial denaturation of IgG increases its adsorption, presumably due to an increase in hydrophobicity which, compared to native IgG, increases its detectability in EIA about 5 times (Ishikawa et al., 1980; Conradie et al., 1983).

Up to a certain limit, a constant fraction of the proteins is adsorbed to plastic surfaces. For example, 80% of the IgM but only about 25% of BSA is adsorbed, with a limit of about 1.5 ng/mm^2 for both proteins, indepedent of the input. According to Butler (1981), the protein molecules at this limit become equidistantly distributed on the surface and the failure to exceed this coverage (about 1/3 of the surface) is due to steric hindrance.

With an excess of protein, more adsorption occurs than dictated by the binding capacity, due to the formation of multiple layers, stacked on the protein monolayer by protein–protein interactions. Such secondary interactions are not very stable and interfere in the EIA. Early studies of Oreskes and Singer (1961) on the interaction of human IgG with polystyrene indicated that adsorption occurred in two steps, characterized by different binding constants, corresponding to protein–plastic and protein–protein interaction. Maximum adsorption was observed at the pI of the proteins probably since the electrostatic repulsion between proteins is the lowest at this pH. Undesired multiple layers are also most difficult to remove at pH values near the pI (MacRitchie, 1972). However, the negative surface charge of the plastic does not interfere with the plastic–protein interaction, pointing to a non-electrostatic adsorption.

An important implication of these studies is that antigen present in a complex mixture binds in a non-competitive manner, up to a limit of about 1.5 ng total protein/mm^2, above which the binding is no longer representative of the concentration of the various antigens in the sample.

Among 11 different polystyrene microplates (from 4 different companies), Kenny and Dunsmoor (1983) distinguished essentially two types: one which adsorbs albumin poorly and the other which adsorbs it well; IgG is adsorbed well on both types. Plates which bind albumin well are best suited for mixtures of antigens; however, background staining also tends to be higher. A 100-fold excess of a non-specific protein during adsorption prevents the detection of the antigen (Kenny and Dunsmoor, 1983). Some brands of plates bind at least three times more antigen from a dilute solution than others (Signorella and Hymer, 1984). Protein desorption may result not only from disaggregation of multiple layers and proteolysis, but also from true desorption from the solid phase and some protein, such as fibrinogen, may even replace the adsorbed protein on some solid phase (Morissey, 1977).

Not only do plastic plates exhibit a significant variability among the various lots, but also among the wells of the same plate (Shekarchi et al., 1984). Irrespective of the origin of the plates, the coefficient of variation of absorbance can range from 5% for the wells of one plate to 30% of the other for the same lot (Kricka et al., 1980). Notorious is the 'edge effect' (Chessum and Denmark, 1978; Kricka et al., 1980): wells at the perimeters adsorb more proteins than those in the interior. Many investigators forego the use of almost 40% of the available wells for this reason. This edge effect has been attributed to differences in surface characteristics of the plastic (Burt et al., 1979) or to thermal characteristics (moulding temperature, cooling) different from those in the interior (Denmark and Chessum, 1978). A critical analysis of this edge effect (Oliver et al., 1981) indicated that thermal gradients during incubation may be responsible: polystyrene is a poor conductor and a thermal gradient may exist between the outer and central wells during an incubation period of 30 min, with initial and final temperatures of 20°C and 37°C, using a routine laboratory incubator. The use of a forced-air incubator may eliminate this edge effect, giving a much lower coefficient of variation and a higher reproducibility. Warming both the plate and the solution to the incubation temperature prior to the addition of the solution seems a simple alternative.

To test for reproducibility, essential for reliable EIA, a solution with a less than saturating concentration of conjugate can be adsorbed. The optical density and standard deviations of all wells of the same plate (perimeter and interior wells) or of different plates are compared. Shekarchi et al. (1984) found well-to-well variation to be of greater statistical significance than the edge effect. Plates are selected with respect to the antigen. Pretreatment of plates with cleaning agents has little effect unless an oily film is present, which can be removed by washing for 5 min with 25% acetone. Soaking of polystyrene in 6 N HCl for 2 h permits the reuse of plates (Shekarchi et al., 1984).

13.2.2. Non-covalent adsorption of antigens to plastic

The attachment of proteins to plastic by non-covalent bonds is often little affected by the buffer. Many different protocols can be indiscriminately used without any significant modification in the procedures. Some recent methods were designed to expose more of the hydrophobic regions of the proteins and seemed to have a beneficial effect on the end-results. The three most important variables for the adsorption of proteins on a solid phase are temperature, time and concentration.

The most widely used coating buffer is 50 mM carbonate, pH 9.6. Other buffers are 10 mM Tris–HCl, pH 8.5, containing 100 mM NaCl or PBS (10 mM sodium phosphate buffer, pH 7.2, containing 100 mM NaCl).

For a new assay it is recommended to investigate if one of the buffers is indeed the most appropriate. The frequent use of a given buffer is not necessarily a proof of its superiority. For example, Barlough et al. (1983) observed that the use of carbonate buffer for the coating with coronavirus antigens produced diffuse and non-specific color reactions both in viral and control experiments. This was primarily due to the high pH and not to the carbonate or the ionic strength. The use of PBS, 0.9% NaCl or deionized water as solvent gave superior results in this system. It is not clear from these studies whether or not the carbonate buffer promoted the stacking of multiple protein layers.

Non-ionic detergents (Triton X-100, Tween 20) should be avoided during coating since they compete strongly with the protein for the solid phase and prevent the formation of hydrophobic interactions.

The conditions most frequently chosen for incubation are overnight at 4°C, in a humid chamber. However, incubation may be shortened by increasing the temperature or the antigen concentration (Fig. 13.1 and 13.2). Adsorption of densonucleosis virus to polystyrene plates (Fig. 13.1), was shown to be optimal at about 10 μg/ml (2 μg/well) and at 37°C at least 4 times shorter sensitization times (less than 20 min) were required than at 4°C. In contrast, for purified IgG, the optimum coating concentration was 1 μg/ml but at least 60 min at 37°C were required (Fig. 13.2). The optimal concentration of antigens or antibodies for coating is commonly between 1 and 10 μg/ml (Engvall, 1980). Coating with complete antiserum (Fig. 13.2) is more complicated since a pronounced optimum is achieved at a dilution of 10^{-4}. A 10-fold change in this dilution lowers the detection limit by a factor of about 2, whereas at a 100-fold change (i.e., a dilution of 10^{-2} or 10^{-6}) the detectability is 20–30 times less. However, even at its optimum, the detectability with complete antiserum is about 4 times less than with purified IgG (Fig. 13.2).

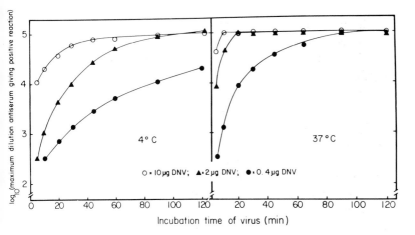

Fig. 13.1. Coating of polystyrene plates with densonucleosis virus (DNV) at different concentrations (0.2 ml/well) and incubation at 4°C or 37°C. The dilution of antiserum giving an optical density of 0.15 (cut-off value) after 30 min was plotted against the incubation period. For DNV, incubation at 37°C has the advantages that short incubation periods are needed (e.g., 20 min) and that relatively more virus is coated if present in low concentrations (from Tijssen et al., 1982; courtesy *Archives of Virology*).

In some cases, the detectability of EIA can be increased considerably by partial denaturation of the coating material: solid-phase coating was improved when the antibody was exposed to pH 2.5 (Ishikawa et al., 1980) or to other denaturants (urea, high temperature) prior to coating (Conradie et al., 1983) and an increase in the hydrophobicity of the proteins was proposed to be involved in this phenomenon. Since Fab is much more resistant to denaturation than Fc (Section 8.2) it is conceivable that these treatments expose more hydrophobic regions in the Fc region, which may then be preferentially adsorbed. The Fab segments may thus be more oriented towards the solvent, thus increasing the efficiency of antigen binding. In addition, Conradie et al. (1983) observed that more antibody becomes bound.

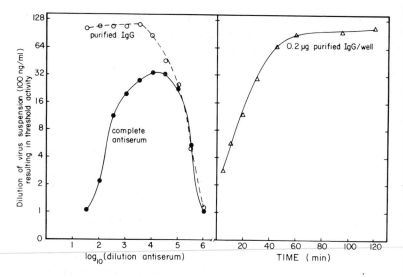

Fig. 13.2. Coating of polystyrene with purified IgG (5 mg/ml) or with complete antiserum in serial dilutions. With the latter a very pronounced optimum of dilution is found, whereas with purified IgG a slight 'hook effect' is observed when tested with the corresponding virus in a sandwich assay. However, the use of purified IgG produces higher detectability than that of complete antiserum for coating. Incubation time required for optimum IgG coating at 37°C was longer than for DNV (Fig. 13.1) (from Tijssen et al., 1982; courtesy of *Archives of Virology*).

Partial denaturation of IgG is carried out with samples containing 10 µg/ml in 50 mM glycine-HCl buffer, pH 2.5, containing 100 mM NaCl, incubated for 10 min at room temperature and neutralized with 500 mM Tris. The sample is then dialyzed against the coating buffer. Alternatively, IgG may be denatured in neutral buffer by the addition of an equal volume of 6 M urea and incubation overnight at room temperature, followed by extensive dialysis. Thermal denaturation is carried out for 10 min at 70°C for sheep antibodies or at 82°C for rabbit antibodies (Conradie et al., 1983). This treatment may be different for IgG preparations from other species.

The treatment of antigens with chaotropic agents (NaSCN, guanidine.HCl) prior to dilution with carbonate buffer and coating may enhance the detectability of EIA (Inouye et al., 1984). Conroy and Esen (1984) observed that proteins solubilized with 6–8 M urea or 60%-solutions of methanol, ethanol or acetic acid are efficiently coated on plastic. However, 6 M guanidine·HCl in the coating buffer was less suitable and 60% isopropanol or 0.1% SDS prevented binding to plastic.

Adsorption of lipid antigens (mycobacterial glycolipid, cardiolipin) to polystyrene (Reggiardo et al., 1980) is performed at a concentration of 2 µg/ml in a buffer containing sodium deoxycholate (1 mg/ml) for 3 h at 37°C. The addition of 10 mM $MgCl_2$ in the coating buffer (and in subsequent incubations at 20 mM) is beneficial for the coating of lipopolysaccharides (Ito et al., 1980).

Proteins separated by SDS-PAGE (Chapter 16) can directly be coated to plastic by diffusion from the gel following electrophoresis. The gel is incubated for 15 min in water at 37°C. The gel is cut into 1 mm slices which are incubated (in separate wells) with a 20–25-fold excess of carbonate buffer for 24 h at room temperature.

13.2.3. Covalent attachment of antibodies or antigens to plastic

While covalent coupling is obligatory for the coating of solid phases other than plastics, it may also be advantageous for plastics. Some of the methods for covalent linkage of proteins are quite undemanding and convenient for the large-scale preparation of immunoreactant-coated solid phases. Such methods are also necessary for the attachment of antigens which are poorly adsorbed on plastic, such as native DNA, small oligopeptides and haptens.

A simple method for the attachment of most reactants possessing free amino groups, i.e., oligopeptides and haptens (Weigand et al., 1981; Suter, 1982) is the pretreatment of polystyrene with GA (Barrett, 1977). Polystyrene is activated at a relatively low pH where GA has no strong tendency to react or to form polymers (Table 13.1). After the addition of the immunoreactant, the pH is raised to 8 or 9.5 with 100 mM carbonate (Dobbins Place and Schroeder, 1982), to increase the reactivity of GA. Either GA or ethylchloro-

TABLE 13.1
Pretreatment of polystyrene with glutaraldehyde for covalent linkage (adapted from
Weigand et al., 1981, and Suter, 1982)[a]

1. Pretreat polystyrene with 0.2% (v/v) GA in 100 mM sodium phosphate buffer, pH 5.0, for 4 h at room temperature

2. Wash twice with the same buffer.

3. Add the reactant to be coupled (2–10 μg/ml) in 100 mM sodium phosphate buffer, pH 8.0, and incubate for 3 h at 37°C.

4. Wash twice with 0.9% NaCl.

5. Add 100 mM lysine in sodium phosphate buffer, pH 8.0, for 1 h at 37°C.

6. Wash with several changes of PBS, containing 0.05% Tween 20.

[a] In another version of this method (Dobbins Place and Schroeder, 1982) the GA concentration is raised to 2% and, after coating the wells with antigen or antibody, the plates are post-fixed with 0.007% ethylchloroformate in PBS (pH 7.0) for 2 h at room temperature.

formate (ECF) can be used for the treatment of the plates, but the results are better when the two reagents are combined (Table 13.1). The mode of action of ECF is not well understood, but it may make the adsorbed reactant less polar and promote hydrophobic interaction. Microtiter plates thus treated can be stored for at least 4 weeks. Sera which produced strong desorption of non-covalently bound hepatitis antigens did not release the same antigens adsorbed on such treated plates.

Pretreatment of antibodies with GA prior to coating can also decrease their desorption and give a higher detectability in EIA (Parsons, 1981), in particular for plates not irradiated with ^{60}Co by the manufacturers (Beards et al., 1984). GA at 0.2% is mixed with 5 volumes of serum (diluted 2000-fold with 10 mM phosphate buffer, pH 6.0). The mixture is incubated for 20 min at 37°C, diluted with 1/5 volume of 400 mM sodium phosphate buffer, pH 8.5, and used for coating the plates for 1 h at 37°C.

Modified polystyrene beads are offered commercially (Pierce

Chemical Co.). Derivatized polystyrene beads may contain hydrazide groups, alkylamine groups or Sanger's reagent (about 3 μmole reactive groups per bead) (Fig. 13.3). A typical procedure to link covalently IgG to hydrazide beads is given in Table 13.2. Beads can also be used by the method of Inman (1974) or Sanger (1945).

Several other methods to link covalently antibodies to plastic were compared by Neurath and Strick (1981), such as coupling to partially hydrolyzed nylon with carbodiimides or GA (Hendry and Hermann, 1980), to diazotized polyaminopolystyrene (PAPS; Phillips et al., 1980), or to PAPS with GA (Reimer et al., 1978, Table 13.3); particularly the latter was suitable.

The method of Hendry and Hermann (1980; Table 13.4) is quite simple and attractive for large-scale preparation of antigen- or antibody-coated nylon beads, particularly for antigens which are generally poorly adsorbed. About 30 times more antibody is attached per surface unit of nylon than adsorbed non-covalently on polystyrene.

The increase in detectability of EIA is generally considerably less than the increase in the amount of the immunoreactant bound to the solid phase, possibly due to masking of epitopes.

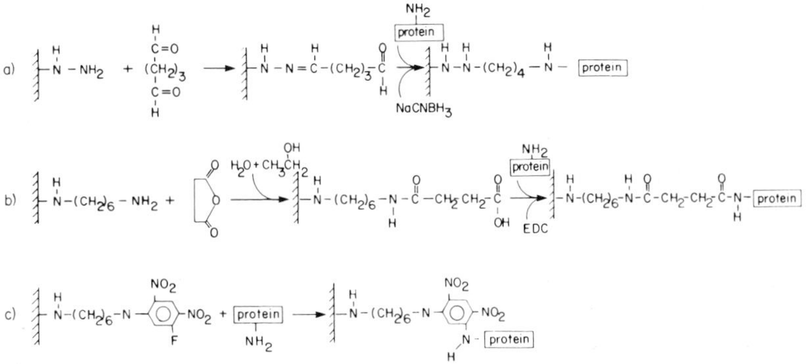

Fig. 13.3. Modified polystyrene beads for covalent binding of proteins. Proteins can be linked to hydrazide beads (a) with glutaraldehyde or to beads derivatized with alkylamine using succinic anhydride and carbodiimide or Sanger's reagent (Pierce Chemical Co.; Technical Information).

TABLE 13.2
Covalent linkage of IgG to hydrazide-derivatized polystyrene beads

1. Add 5 ml of 12.5% (v/v) GA in 50 mM sodium phosphate, pH 7.0, to 25 hydrazide-derivatized polystyrene beads (6.4 mm diameter; from Pierce Chemical Co.) and shake very gently for 2 h at room temperature.

2. Wash on Buchner funnel (without filter paper) with 100 ml water and with 20 ml 100 mM sodium phosphate buffer, pH 6.0.

3. Add GA-activated beads to 2.5 mg IgG dissolved in 5 ml of sodium phosphate buffer, pH 6.0.

4. Add 1 mg NaCNBH$_3$ (step advised by Pierce; may not be necessary).

5. Shake gently overnight at room temperature.

6. Wash beads with 100 ml 100 mM sodium phosphate buffer, pH 6.0, and then with 50 ml 100 mM NaHCO$_3$.

7. Block residual aldehydes with 5 ml 100 mM lysine for 1 h at room temperature.

8. Wash with 100 ml 100 mM Na$_2$CO$_3$ and with 100 ml water and dry beads with paper towel.

9. Store the IgG-beads dry at 4 °C.

13.2.4. Attachment of antigens or antibodies to plastic using bridging molecules

Antigens which bind poorly to plastic may be attached to the solid phase by a bridging molecule, e.g., a protein with a high affinity for the plastic to which poor binders may be conjugated by any of the methods discussed in Chapter 11. Positively charged compounds, such as protamine sulfate have been used to bind native DNA to polystyrene (see below).

Skurrie and Gilbert (1983) used BSA as the bridging molecule for the binding of rubella antigens. BSA (fraction V) in distilled water is added to the wells and the plates are dried in a water bath at 56 °C under a stream of air. An equal volume of ethanol–

TABLE 13.3

Covalent linking of antibodies to polystyrene plates (Neurath and Strick, 1981)

1. Fill in a well-ventilated hood the wells of the microplate with methanesulfonic acid and incubate overnight at room temperature.

2. Empty the wells, wash extensively with distilled water and dry.

3. Place the plates in a heating block (40 °C) and fill the wells with a mixture of glacial acetic acid and fuming HNO_3 (1:1).

4. Incubate for 4 h and wash with water until the pH of the wash is 6 or higher.

5. Place plates in the heating block (50 °C) and fill the wells with 0.5% $Na_2S_2O_4$ in 500 mM NaOH and incubate for 1 h.

6. Wash the plates extensively with water, fill the wells with 1% GA in 50 mM phosphate buffer, pH 8.5, and incubate for 2 h at room temperature and then for about 16 h at 4 °C.

7. Wash plates, fill each well with a solution of IgG (100 g/ml) in 50 mM phosphate buffer, pH 8.5, and incubate at 4 °C overnight.

8. Wash and treat the wells with 1 M glycine–100 mM borate buffer, pH 8.5, for 4 h at room temperature.

9. Wash with Tris-buffered saline (10 mM Tris–HCl, pH 7.2, containing 0.9% NaCl). The plates may be stored with the wells filled with the same buffer, containing 0.02% NaN_3.

acetone (4:1) is then added to each well and left for 30 min at room temperature, followed by three washings with distilled water and air-drying. For the conjugation of the antigen to the BSA coating, the wells are filled with a solution of 1-ethyl-3(3-dimethyl-aminopro-pyl)carbodiimide-HCl in distilled water (10 mg/ml), incubated for 30 min at room temperature, before the addition of the rubella antigens (25 times diluted from the preparation of Flow Laboratories; otherwise use 5–20 µg/ml) and incubated in a water bath at 45 °C for 4 h. The plates are then washed 6 times with water, rinsed with 1% BSA solution and with 7.5% (v/v) glycerol and stored at −70 °C or quick-frozen in ethanol/dry-ice prior to transfer to the

TABLE 13.4
Covalent linking of antibodies to nylon[a]

1. Hydrolyze nylon 6/6 (poly-hexamethylene-adipimide) balls with a diameter of either 3.2 or 6.4 mm (Precision Plastic Ball Co., Chicago, U.S.A., or other suppliers) with 3.5 M HCl for 24 h at room temperature.

2. Wash balls with distilled water, treat for 1 min with concentrated acetic anhydride, wash with distilled water and then with 100 mM carbonate buffer, pH 9.5 for 1 min.

3. Wash with PBS and react either with 4% (v/v) 1-cyclohexyl-3-(2-morpholinoethyl)-carbodiimide metho-p-toluene sulfonate (CMC) 10 min or with 8% (v/v) GA in distilled water (2 h; in the latter case treatment with acetic anhydride in step 2 is omitted).

4. Wash with distilled water and incubate with the solution of antibodies (100 μg/ml per 36 beads) or antiserum (dilution 1:3000) or the antigen preparation (equivalent molar amount) in PBS, pH 7.2, at room temperature for 4 h for the GA-activated nylon or 2 h at room temperature followed by 18 h at 4°C for the carbodiimide-activated nylon.

5. Wash with PBS and then with 2% (w/v) BSA in PBS for 1 h.

[a] The aldehyde concentration on the beads was found to be much more uniform when the beads were shaken when in acid and aldehyde baths (Perera et al., 1983). Background staining can be decreased significantly by treatments with 500 mM lysine and 5% BSA after coupling of the immunoreactant to the beads.

freezer. Most cross-linkers discussed in Chapter 11 may be used instead of the carbodiimide. In view of the variation in the affinity of polystyrene for albumin (Section 13.2.1), even within the same lot, other proteins may be more suitable.

In contrast to single-stranded DNA, native DNA adsorbs poorly to polystyrene (Engvall, 1976). This problem can be overcome by treating the polystyrene with a 1% solution of aqueous protamine sulfate for 90 min (Klotz, 1982), followed by three washes with distilled water and drying. Other polycationic substances, such as MBSA (Section 5.2.3.3, Ferrua et al., 1983) or poly-L-lysine (type VII B; Sigma), may also be used (Leipold et al., 1983). Poly-L-lysine is suspended in water at a concentration of 1 mg/ml (which may be lowered at least 10 times without harm) and incubated with the plastic for 2 h at room temperature. The wells are then washed 4 times with water and dried.

DNA may be adsorbed onto such pretreated plastic at a concentration of 10 µg/ml in 50 mM Tris–HCl buffer, pH 7.5, containing 10 mM EDTA and 10 mM EGTA for 60 min. Single-stranded DNA may interfere in the assay for antibodies to native DNA (Klotz, 1982) and may be removed, after washing with PBS for three times, by digestion with S_1 nuclease (100 units/ml; Sigma type III, in 50 mM sodium acetate buffer, pH 4.5, supplemented with 50 mM NaCl, 1 mM $ZnSO_4$ and 5% glycerol) for 1 h at 37°C. After digestion, the plates are washed with PBS-Tween (Section 14.2)

A variety of bridging molecules can be used to attach cells to plastic surfaces, e.g. antibodies, lectins (phytohemagglutinin), GA, or poly-L-lysine. The method of Heusser et al. (1981) is satisfactory (Table 13.5). The stability of attachment is quite similar with the different bridging molecules, but the cell monolayer should be fixed with GA if the plates are to be stored.

13.2.5. Forms of plastic solid phases

Separation of free immunoreactant from reactants immobilized on plastic is achieved simply by decanting, aspirating or retrieving the solution, in contrast to the often cumbersome techniques used in other systems (precipitation, chromatography, centrifugation, non-specific adsorption on charcoal, talc or dextran). This simplicity has a direct, positive effect on the reproducibility and sensitivity of the assay.

The forms of plastic supports for EIA may be varied: beads, discs, tubes, plastic-coated toothpicks, matchsticks, and even cocktail stirrers (Shekarchi et al., 1982). Undoubtably, many other utensils could be used for this purpose. However, the most common supports are polystyrene or polyvinylchloride (PVC) microtitre plates with 12×8 wells of 0.3 ml. Although PVC plates may adsorb IgG more

TABLE 13.5

Binding of cells to polyvinylchloride microtitre plates

1. Pretreat plates with GA (0.25%), or poly-L-lysine (10 μg/ml), or phytohemaggluti-nin (PHA)-P (20 μg/ml; Difco Laboratories) or anti-cell antibodies (20 μg/ml), us-ing as coating solution Dulbecco's PBS, for 1 h at 37 °C.

2. Wash the cells extensively with Dulbecco's PBS and suspend a concentration of 1–5 × 10^6 cells/ml (depending on cell size).

3. Add cell suspension to wells (shake often to prevent concentration differences) and centrifuge plates at 100 × g for 3 min.

4. Post-fix plates with 0.25% GA (if plates are to be stored) by gentle immersion in a 1 litre beaker containing 0.25% GA in Dulbecco's PBS at 4 °C for 5 min (prevent air trapping).

5. Wash by repeated immersions in PBS and gentle decanting.

6. Saturate unreacted sites with 1% BSA in Dulbecco's PBS. Incubate for 1 h and wash again. Use egg white (prepared by stirring chicken egg white in PBS for 1 h), followed by centrifugation at 10 000 × g for 15 min) in PBS (A_{280} of about 14) for blocking unreacted sites of PHA-coated plates.

efficiently, they also tend to give higher background levels and release little of the adsorbed immunoreactant (Zollinger et al., 1976). Frankel and Gerhard (1979) used PVC plates for the quantitation of hybrido-ma proteins.

Among the polystyrene plates, a variation exists in the quantity of additives (lubricants) used in their preparation which may account for some of the differences encountered. Special plates ('immulon') have very little of these lubricants. Nevertheless, it is necessary to establish for each antigen or antibody the most suitable lot. Signorella and Hymer (1984) found that immulon 2 binds three times more prolactin than immulon 1. Most plastics display a negative electrical charge (ζ potential) at their surfaces which is quite often modified during manufacturing by a treatment for a few seconds with an intense electrical field at the solid–solution interface. This potential gives rise to a diffuse double-layer of ions. The ζ potential is also affected by the adsorbed protein. All these physical parameters may have different but unpredictable effects on EIA (Section 9.2.2) and affect the accuracy of EIA.

The wells of the microtitre plates may have flat, U-shaped or V-shaped bottoms. The choice between these shapes depends on the method used for quantitation of the EIA: with a read-through photometer flat-bottomed wells give less variation, for visual inspection U-shaped wells are better. The microtitre plates have not been designed for the EIA but adapted for this purpose and equipment has been devised for these plates; possibilities for more optimal designs are obvious, e.g. by increasing the surface/volume ratio. Labrousse et al. (1982) used microwells (0.8 mm diameter, 0.8 mm depth) drilled in plexiglass plates with the top of the wells (0.2 mm depth) enlarged to a diameter of 1.5 mm. Such wells have a capacity of about 0.30 µl, in contrast with the 200-µl capacity of the regular plates; however, rapid desiccation poses serious problems. Solutions are added with suitably prepared capillary pipettes. The reduced volume of reagents lowers the limit of the number of molecules which can be detected (i.e. about 10^6 antibody molecules). The concentration limits for positive detection remain, however, largely unchanged since the surface/volume ratio is hardly affected. It is conceivable to increase this by a different well design. The reagents could then be more effectively used and the reaction product (enzyme signal) would become less diluted. This aspect remains to be explored.

Plastic tubes are also employed. Here, the choice of the plastic is also critical. Polypropylene is preferred over polystyrene, since it is easier to handle and is less breakable. It is mostly used in commercial kits. There is, however, little or no difference in the coating characteristics of the two plastics. The size of the tubes is $10–12 \times 70–75$ mm, and their form may be conical, round- or flat-bottom. Tubes generally require larger volumes (1 ml) than microtitre plates, but their surface/volume ratio can be increased by rotating almost horizontally in circular test-tube racks. Upon slow rotation, a relatively large surface is covered. Disposable polystyrene cuvets are used in some cases since they can be directly used with a common spectrophotometer. Volumes of such containers are quite large. Another often used form is beads. Placed in a round-bottom container only slightly larger than the beads themselves, they have a favorable surface/volume ratio. Beads have been popular in RIA and are used by some commercial suppliers.

Shekarchi et al. (1982) used stainless steel microsticks coated with carrier material. Alternatively, plastic microsticks are available from Dynatech Laboratories. Irrespective of their nature (steel, teflon, polystyrene), they may be coated with polycarbonate or nitrocellulose. The latter is applied as a thin film of colloidon diluted with 4 volumes of ether (laboratory grade). The microsticks are dipped in this solution, dried and arranged in a transfer plate designed for use in a microtitre plate. They can be cleaned with 6 N HCl after use.

13.3. Nitrocellulose membranes and paper

Nitrocellulose membranes have found wide application in nucleic acid research, but are also becoming very popular in protein blotting. The nature and requirements of these membranes will be discussed in Chapter 16.

The attractiveness of these membranes resides in the fact that very small amounts of immunoreactants are required, providing thus a method of choice for many experiments, e.g. monitoring column effluents, screening hybridoma clones, analysis of detergent-dissociated complexes. Minute drops (less than 1 μl, containing about 100 pg, or less if antigen is pure) are applied and dried on the membrane, limiting the binding of the antigen in a small area (diameter less than 1 mm). Other binding sites can then be saturated with an unrelated inert protein or other blocking agents. The subsequent immunoenzymatic revelation of the antigen produces an insoluble colored product which precipitates at the site of the enzyme and is viewed against a white background. The discriminatory power of this technique was claimed to be greater than that obtained in microtitre plates and various substances, such as proteins, nucleic acids, cell membranes, subcellular organelles, fungi, protozoa, bacteria and viruses, were all tightly bound to the membrane (Hawkes et al., 1982). Another advantage of these membranes is that antigens may be bound in the presence of detergents, although a lower efficiency of binding is observed when the concentration of non-ionic detergents (Triton X-100, Tween 80) exceeds 0.01% (Palfree and Elliott, 1982). Jahn et al. (1984) observed that for small proteins this was due to desorbing during washing and incubation steps. A fixation step (15 min in a solution containing 10% acetic acid and 25% isopropanol followed by rinsing in water) after dotting prevented this desorption, and a 7-fold excess of Triton was found to be beneficial if SDS is present in the sample (up to 7% Triton/1% SDS). The suitability of this solid phase is attested by the rapidly growing number of publications describing their use.

Dotting with small volumes may be done directly on the nitrocellulose sheet on which a rectangular grid (3×3 mm) has been drawn with a pencil (Hawkes et al., 1982; Rordorf et al., 1983). For large volumes (10–400 µl), discs (≈ 4 mm) punched from membrane sheets (Palfree and Elliott, 1982) are used. Alternatively, the nitrocellulose sheet can be inserted in a 'Hybridot' or similar apparatus (BRL; Bio-Rad) (Domin et al., 1984) or homemade devices (Smith et al., 1984). The disc method, designed for detergent-solubilized antigens, needs more antigen for detection than the dotting method.

Discs (with an indexing notch), on which several antigens or allergens are dotted separately, allow the simultaneous detection of antibodies against them from a small serum sample (50 µl; Walsh et al., 1984). This permits rapid screening, e.g. for allergens, by applying on the first disc several dots with different antigen mixtures, and detecting the antigens from a positive spot separately on a second disc. The use of 0.1–0.4% zwitterionic detergent in the blotting buffer was found (Mandrell and Zollinger, 1984) to restore partially the antibody-binding capacity of SDS-denatured antigens.

The enzyme of choice for these methods is POase, though APase may also be used. After reaction, the spots are examined visually for the presence or absence of a reaction. It is, however, also possible to quantitate such spots by reflectance densitometry with a thin-layer plate scanner. Variations can be expected to be high, though this may be reduced by the apparatus which ensures uniform dots. It is also possible, as for the disc method (Section 13.3.2), to use a substrate which yields a soluble product (such as OPD) and to perform the revelation reaction in the wells of a plate.

Paper may also be used as a support. This inexpensive solid phase has the advantage that large amounts of coated solid phase may be prepared.

13.3.1. Dot-binding of antigens to nitrocellulose

Antigens may be bound in small dots to nitrocellulose (Table 13.6), using micropipetting devices. With dilute solutions of antigen, the sample is applied in small successive doses at the same site, allowing the filter to dry between applications. Dry membranes are much more prone to breaks than wet membranes. The baking step in the dotting procedure is necessary to stabilize binding with nucleic acids (Southern, 1975; Thomas, 1980). Instead of blocking with an 'inert' protein, such as BSA or gelatin, Tween 20 at 0.05% can be used (Batteiger et al., 1982) in the solutions of the various immuno-reactants, preventing non-specific adsorption. This is particularly advantageous after transferring proteins from polyacrylamide gels (Chapter 16), since protein bands may be stained without the interference of blocking proteins.

Post-fixation with GA (Section 13.3.2) or acetic acid/isopropanol (Section 13.3) is generally not necessary but may be performed when required or if Triton X-100 is added to the immunoreactants.

13.3.2. Binding of detergent-solubilized antigens on nitrocellulose membrane discs

Palfree and Elliott (1982) used nitrocellulose discs to bind detergent-

TABLE 13.6
Binding of antigens in small dots on nitrocellulose

A. *Protein dotting* (Hawkes et al., 1982)

  1. Prepare the nitrocellulose sheet by drawing a rectangular grid (3 × 3 mm) with a pencil, wash with distilled water for 5 min and dry at room temperature.

  2. Place small drops (0.1–0.5 µl) of the sample containing 0.1–1.0 mg protein per ml. For less complex mixtures, the concentration may be reduced accordingly.

  3. Dry the filter thoroughly; the membrane may then be stored for several weeks.

  4. Place the membrane in the cold for 5–10 min and wash for 5 min with 50 mM Tris–HCl buffer, pH 7.4, containing 200 mM NaCl (TBS).

  5. Cut squares from wet membrane with a scalpel and ruler and place squares, face upward, into wells of a 96-well tray.
    (Alternatively, strips can be used and placed in appropriate containers).

  6. Block remaining active sites on the membrane with a 3% solution of BSA in TBS and shake gently for about 15 min. Tween 20 (at 0.05%) is also effective in preventing nonspecific adsorption.

B. *Nucleic acid dotting* (Rordorf et al., 1983)

  1. As in step 1 of method A.

  2. Apply spots as in step 2 of method A, using the nucleic acid (single- or double-stranded) solution at a concentration of 80 µg/ml in 20 mM Tris-HCl buffer, pH 7.8, containing 150 mM NaCl, according to Thomas, 1980.

  3. Air-dry membrane and bake for 2 h at 80 °C.

  4. Proceed as in steps 4 through 6 of method A, for the wetting, cutting and blocking of the membrane.

solubilized membrane glycoproteins. Triton X-100 or Tween 80 should not be used over 0.01%, whereas deoxycholate, taurocholate or octylglucoside can.

Small discs (≈ 4 mm) punched from the nitrocellulose membrane are floated on the surface of distilled water. The moist discs are then placed on absorbent filter paper and evenly soaked by the application of 10 or 20 µl samples. Gentle pressure is sometimes necessary to assure good contact of the discs with the filter paper. The discs are air-dried and incubated in microtitre trays (96-well, V-bottom) with 0.1 ml 3% BSA in TBS (Table 13.6, step 4) at 37°C for 1 h to block free binding sites.

For optimal fixation with GA, the discs are rinsed briefly with BSA and incubated with 0.1 ml 0.25% GA in 10 mM sodium phosphate buffer, pH 7.5, containing 150 mM NaCl (PBS), for 15 min at room temperature. The discs are then rinsed three times with PBS, the residual active GA groups are blocked with 0.1 ml 100 mM glycine (pH 7.5) and 0.1 ml 3% BSA in TBS for 60–100 min at 37°C and washed with the phosphate buffer. This fixation prevents desorption of proteins when Triton X-100 is used.

13.3.3. Covalent coupling to paper

The method of Ceska and Lundkvist (1972) as applied by Pauwels et al. (1977), Lehtonen and Viljanen (1980a,b) and Giallongo et al. (1982) is described here. The cellulose paper from Munktell Swedish Filter Paper or Whatman No. 52 yields about 400 and 330 discs of 6 mm diameter per gram, respectively.

Activation of paper discs with CNBr is not unlike that of Sepharose, as described in Section 7.1.9.2.2., and the same safety precautions should be taken. Activation of paper discs and subsequent coupling of antibodies or antigens is given in Table 13.7.

Lehtonen and Viljanen (1980b) compared the CNBr-activated paper method with non-covalent adsorption on polystyrene and nylon. A considerable desorption occurred both from polystyrene (30%) and nylon (60%) in all steps of the assay; however, very high concentrations of antigens were used for the adsorption (100 µg/ml) which could be responsible, at least in part, for the leakage (Section 13.2.1). With the CNBr-activated paper, 5–10 times more antigen was bound from the same antigen solutions and desorption during the EIA was only 13% of the mean surface concentration of the antigen, with a standard deviation 3–10 times smaller than for the other solid phases. The response ratio (positive/negative sera) with CNBr-

TABLE 13.7
Activation of paper with CNBr and subsequent covalent coupling of immunoreactants[a]

A. *Activation*
1. Punch paper discs of 6 mm diameter ($\approx$ 2.5–3 mg/disc).

2. Swell 20 g of discs in 200 ml distilled water for 3 min.

3. Add 600 ml of CNBr solution (20 g in 600 ml of distilled water. For precautions, see Section 7.1.8.2.2).

4. Raise immediately the pH to 10.5 and maintain this pH, by adding up to about 100 ml of 1 mM NaOH, for 30 min.

5. Wash discs with the following solutions:
   a. 500 ml 0.005 mM $NaHCO_3$ (12 times)
   b. 500 ml distilled water (twice).
   c. 500 ml (twice) in graded series of acetone (25, 50, 75%) and four times in acetone.

6. Air-dry at room temperature and store at 4°C.

B. *Covalent coupling*
7. Dilute 4 ml of purified antibody or the IgG fraction of the antiserum (or the same amount of the antigen preparation) in 40 ml 100 mM $NaHCO_3$ (4°C).

8. Add 1 g of activated discs to the solution and stir gently for 3 h at 4°C.

9. Wash at room temperature with:
   a. 100 ml 0.5 mM $NaHCO_3$ (twice for 10 min).
   b. 100 ml 50 mM ethanolamine in 100 mM $NaHCO_3$ (3 h with gentle stirring).
   c. 100 ml 0.5 mM $NaHCO_3$ (twice for 10 min).
   d. 100 ml 100 mM sodium acetate buffer, pH 4.0 (once for 30 min).
   e. 100 ml incubation buffer (twice: the incubation buffer used for the subsequent stages contains 50 mM phosphate buffer, pH 7.5, 150 mM NaCl, 0.1% Tween 20 and 0.1% gelatin).

10. Store discs, if not used immediately, in a small volume of the incubation buffer at −20°C.

---

[a] The punching of the paper discs may also be done after the covalent coupling of the protein (Lehtonen and Viljanen, 1980b). The use of PBS in the coupling was claimed to be as effective as the bicarbonate buffer.

activated paper was twice as high as with polystyrene, with half
the standard deviation of the latter.

Paper can also be activated with 1-(3-nitrobenzyloxymethyl)pyr-
idinium chloride (NBPC), according to the method of Alwine et
al. (1979). The nitrobenzyloxymethyl (NBM) paper thus prepared
is stable for at least one year and can be reduced to aminobenzyloxymethyl (ABM) paper. Treatment of ABM paper with nitrous
acid produces diazobenzyloxymethyl (DBM) paper to which antigens
(nucleic acids, proteins) can be covalently linked (Fig. 13.4). In this
reaction negatively charged molecules first interact electrostatically
with the DBM paper, followed by their essentially irreversible covalent interaction via the azo linkage. This paper is primarily used
for the transfer of proteins or nucleic acids from gels (Chapter
16). The preparation of this paper is given in Table 13.8.

13.3.4. Non-covalent dot-immunobinding on paper

Esen et al. (1983) described a method in which ordinary chromatography paper is used for binding of water-insoluble proteins. This
material is easier to handle than nitrocellulose, is very cheap, and
requires no particular pretreatment. It has, however, a lower detectability. Detection of spotted antigen is as in Table 16.12, but the

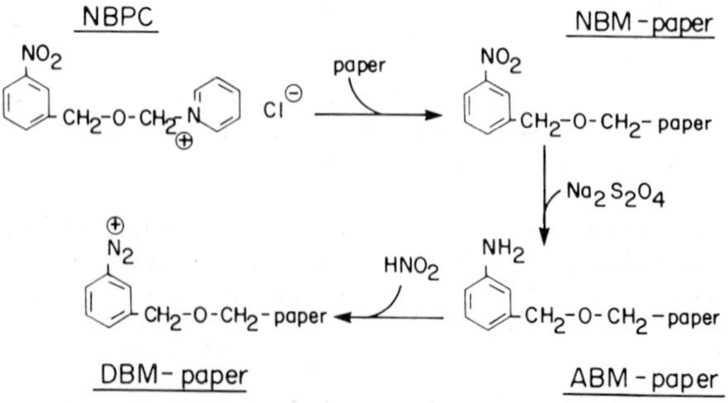

Fig. 13.4. Activation of paper with 1-(3-nitrobenzyloxymethyl)-pyridinium chloride
(NBPC) via nitrobenzyloxymethyl (NBM), aminobenzyloxymethyl (ABM) to diazobenzyloxymethyl (DBM)-paper to which antigens may be covalently bound.

TABLE 13.8
Preparation of diazobenzyloxymethyl paper

A. *Preparation of nitrobenzyloxymethyl (NBM) paper*

1.   Cut Whatman No. 540 paper to fit bottom of a container which is placed in a water bath of 60 °C.

2.   For each cm^2 of paper use a solution of 2.3 mg of 1-(3-nitrobenzyloxymethyl)-pyridinium chloride (Sigma) and 0.7 mg of sodium trihydrate in 28.5 μl of distilled water. Pour the solution evenly over the paper and push out any air bubbles (use rubber gloves).

3.   Rub solution evenly over the paper until dry. Dry further at 60 °C in an oven for about 10 min and then bake the paper for 30–40 min in an oven at 135 °C.

4.   Wash paper several times with water (total 20 min), and 3 times with acetone (20 min total) and air-dry.

5.   Paper can be stored for at least 1 year in refrigerator.

B. *Preparation of aminobenzyloxymethyl (ABM) paper from NBM paper*

6.   Incubate the NBM paper in a fume hood with 150 ml of 20% (w/v) solution of sodium $Na_2S_2O_4$ in water, for 30 min at 60 °C, with occasional stirring.

7.   Wash the ABM-paper several times with large volumes of water for a few min until no odor of hydrogen sulfide remains.

C. *Preparation of diazobenzyloxymethyl (DBM) paper from ABM paper*

8.   Wash the ABM paper with at least 100 ml of 1.2 mM HCl (for a 14 × 14 cm paper). Transfer the wet paper directly to ice-cold 1.2 N HCl, using 0.3 ml/cm^2. Add, with mixing, a solution of $NaNO_2$ (10 mg/ml) in water prepared immediately before use, in the proportion of 2.7 ml for 100 ml of HCl.

9.   Keep paper at least 30 min in this solution at 0–4 °C with occasional swirling (after 30 min, a drop of the solution should give a positive (black) reaction for nitrous acid with starch–iodide paper).

10.   Keep the DBM paper in acid until the gel is ready for the transferring of proteins or nucleic acids. Before use, wash quickly the DBM paper with ice-cold water and twice with ice-cold transfer buffer (total time 2–3 min).

antiserum is less diluted (100 to 500-fold) and shorter incubation periods (half of those in Table 16.12) are used. Blocking as for nitrocellulose is not required if antisera are diluted less than 1000 times.

The paper discs (diameter 1 cm), cut from Whatman No. 1 chromatography paper (wear gloves!), are placed in a polystyrene microplate so that the center of the discs and of the wells coincide. One to 2 μl of the protein solution (solubilized in 60% ethanol) is spotted (marked with pencil). After drying, the discs can be stored or used directly for EIA; detectability is 1–2 ng/spot.

13.4. Glass as the solid phase for enzyme immunoassays

Antigens or antibodies may be fixed to glass surfaces by heating, fixation with formaldehyde or coupling with GA to aminoalkylsilyl glass rods. Glass is not frequently used in EIA but may carry some advantages in particular situations.

Proteins may be coupled to glass (Robinson et al., 1971; Hamaguchi et al., 1976), details of which are given in Table 13.9. With this method the detectability in EIA, using BGase as marker, is about 30 amole (30×10^{-18} mole) of antigen per assay tube (1 ml), which is about 10 times better than with Sepharose 4B. The reproducibility of the technique is also greater.

Particulate or non-particulate antigens may be assayed quantitatively on slides by the method of Conway de Macario et al. (1983) which resembles the nitrocellulose dotting technique (Section 13.3.1). A 5-μl drop of the immunoreactant is applied on a circular glass surface (3 mm diameter) delineated by a thin layer of a hydrophobic material and fixed according to Table 13.9B. The immune reactions are then performed by successive incubations with drops of the reagents, with intermittent washings. After the application of the substrate, the enzymatic reaction is evaluated visually (e.g. with a microscope) or measured with a vertical beam spectrophotometer (e.g. Dynatech MR590 minireader). Many samples may be screened in a short time and background staining is very low.

TABLE 13.9
Fixation of antigens or antibodies on glass

A. *Coupling of antigens or antibodies to aminoalkylsilyl glass*

   1. Bake pyrex glass rods (diameter 3 mm, 5 mm long at 500 °C for 5 h).

   2. Immerse the rods for 24 h in a 2% solution of 3-aminopropyltriethoxysilane (Sigma) in acetone at 45 °C.

   3. Wash the rods with acetone and dry.

   4. Immerse the rods in 1% (v/v) aqueous GA for 1 h.

   5. Wash the rods with 250 mM sodium phosphate buffer, pH 7.5.

   6. Immerse the rods in a solution of the antigen or antibody in the same buffer (2 mg/ml) for 30 min.

   7. Wash the rods with the buffer used for EIA.

B. *Fixation of antigens as small dots on glass slides*

   1. Clean the glass slides (printed with circles of 3 mm diameter; e.g., from Flow Lab.) with 95% (v/v) ethanol.

   2. Apply the desired amount of antigen (in 5 μl) in each circle and fix as follows (with minimum amounts of antigens between parentheses):

      a. Viruses: 1 μg/circle; dry by evaporation.

      b. Archaebacteria: 1000/circle (prefixed in suspension with 1% FA in PBS); Eubacteria: 250/circle; apply drops to slide and heat back of the slide quickly with a Bunsen burner three times.

      c. Fungi: 5–10000/circle.

      d. Protozoa: 5000/circle; prefix as in b, and fix by drying.

      e. Mammalian cells: 5000/circle; air-dry and add a drop of chilled acetone.

      f. Nonparticulate antigens: 5 μg/circle; dry by evaporation and incubate for 30 min with Dulbecco's PBS.

13.5. Particulate solid phases for enzyme immunoassays

Particulate solid phases have originally been used for the separation of radiolabeled antibody–antigen complex from free labeled antibody in immunometric assays (Wide and Porath, 1966; Woodhead et al., 1974).

13.5.1. Agarose, cellulose, and Sephacryl solid phases

Linking of an immunoreactant to Sepharose, activated with CNBr (Section 7.1.9.2.2), has the advantage that the immunoreactant can be held in suspension by mild agitation but settles quickly in the sucrose separation procedure (Hunter, 1980) without centrifugation. Moreover, Sepharose 4B has large pores and, thence, has a high binding capacity: 10 µl of a Sepharose 4B immunosorbent suspension has about 5–40 times more antigen bound than a paper disc of 6 mm diameter and about 100 times more than a well of a microtitre plate (Giallongo et al., 1982). Non-specific adsorption levels are also low. However, CNBr has two important disadvantages: (i) it is toxic; and, (ii) as CNBr-activated paper (Section 13.3.3), leakage of bound proteins may occur (Corfield et al., 1979).

A useful alternative is the activation of Sepharose with $NaIO_4$ (Section 7.1.9.2.1; Guthrie, 1961). Agarose (and thus Sepharose) has no abundant vicinal diols and is, therefore, less reactive and binds less immunoreactant than Sephadex, cellulose or Sephacryl (Wright and Hunter, 1982). The structure of Sephadex, however, is quite easily disrupted by oxidation with $NaIO_4$. For these reasons Ferrua et al. (1979, 1980) and Wright and Hunter (1982) favor the use of Sephacryl or cellulose as particulate solid phase. Activation of cellulose with $NaIO_4$ has been discussed in Section 7.1.9.2.1. For the activation of Sephacryl (S300), Wright and Hunter (1982) used a lower pH (100 mM sodium acetate buffer, pH 5.0) and 5 mM $NaIO_4$ instead of the 60 mM used by Ferrua et al. (1979). For cellulose, IgG is used at a concentration of about 8 mg/ml, for Sephacryl at about 2 mg/ml and the amounts for various antigens are similar. The theoretical aspects of this coupling procedure were discussed in Section 11.2.2.

Sephacryl S-1000 may be suitable as solid phase, since this gel is more porous and may better accommodate larger complexes.

Large batches of activated beads may be stored at $-20°C$ without appreciable loss of activity over prolonged periods. For the immobilization of haptens or small antigens on a solid phase spacer molecules, are recommended (Section 7.1.9.2.3) to prevent the interference by the matrix.

Particulate cellulose may also be activated with NBPC by a method similar to that for the activation of paper (Section 13.3.3; Fig. 13.4). Gurvich et al. (1961) and Hales and Woodhead (1980) described a somewhat different method: 5 g cellulose are suspended in a Petri dish in a mixture of 0.5 g sodium acetate in 2 ml water and 1.4 g NBPC (BDH or Sigma) in 18 ml of ethanol. The slurry is dried in an oven at 70°C and subsequently for 40 min at 125°C. The pale brown nitro-derivative is washed on a sintered glass funnel 3 times with 200 ml benzene and sucked dry. The nitro groups are reduced as in steps 5–7 of Table 13.8. The resulting cellulose is dried and pulverized in a mortar.

For diazotization, 1.5 g $CuCl_2$ are dissolved in 5 ml water and 75 ml of freshly prepared 1 M NaOH are added with stirring. The blue precipitate is washed with water on two layers of filter paper until the pH of the wash is below 9.0. The precipitate is then dissolved in 40 ml NH_4OH (specific gravity 0.880) to form a saturated solution. Excess of $Cu(OH)_2$ is removed by centrifugation after at least 15 min of stirring. About 0.5 g of ABM-cellulose is added to this solution with continuous stirring. Any ABM-cellulose which does not dissolve after 15 min is removed by centrifugation, the supernatant is decanted into 1.5 l water and 10% (v/v) H_2SO_4 is added until the dark-blue solution becomes almost colorless (pH below 4). ABM-cellulose forms a white precipitate which is collected after 1 h and washed (by centrifugation) with water to remove all traces of copper. If difficulties arise in sedimenting the precipitate, a few drops of 1 M HCl should be added. The ABM-cellulose is then suspended in 50 ml of 2 M HCl, cooled in an ice bucket and 2 ml 1% $NaNO_2$ are added drop-wise. The presence of excess of nitrous acid is tested with starch-iodide paper (step 10 of Table 13.8). At the end of the reaction, i.e. after 20 min, about 5 g urea are added to the diazocellulose suspension until the starch-iodide test becomes almost negative. The diazocellulose is then washed by centrifugation (at 4°C!) 3 times with water and 2 times with 200 mM borate buffer, pH 8.2, and resuspended in this buffer to 10 mg/ml. A small aliquot of this diazocellulose should be tested with β-naphthol which should produce a bright orange color; in the absence of such a reaction, the preparation is not good and should be discarded.

The coupling of the protein to the pale yellow-green diazocellulose occurs almost instantaneously at high pH. The protein should be used at a high concentration (>10 mg/ml) in ice-cold 100 mM borate buffer, pH 8.2, even if it is available only in small amount. The reaction mixture is incubated at $4°C$. The color of the cellulose turns to a deeper yellow and only little washing is necessary to eliminate free proteins. Washing is also advised after a prolonged storage (at $4°C$).

Antigens bound in the interior of the cellulose are often inaccessible to IgG conjugates.

13.5.2. Protein A-containing fixed bacteria as solid phases

SpA-containing Staphylococci (Section 3.3), fixed with trichloroacetic acid (TCA) or formalin (Section 3.3.1), may also serve as immunosorbent for many mammalian antibodies (Table 7.1). Both fixation procedures are satisfactory but yield products with different properties. Fixation of Staphylococci with hot TCA (Lindmark, 1982) removes the negatively charged cell-wall polymer teichoic acid, producing an IgG-sorbent which can bind 1.4 mg human IgG per ml of a 10% (v/v) suspension of bacteria and is stable for about 5 months. Formalin-fixed bacteria (Kessler, 1976) bind 35% more IgG and are stable for at least 1 year. However, IgG can be eluted quantitatively from TCA-fixed bacteria but not from formalin-fixed bacteria, probably due to the interaction between IgG and teichoic acid, unless 80 mM $MgCl_2$ is included in the acid buffer.

The production of Staphylococci and their fixation with formalin has been described in Section 3.3.1. For the fixation of the bacteria with TCA, the bacterial suspension is heated in a boiling water bath for 2 min and an equal volume of hot 10% TCA is then added while swirling. The mixture is heated for 6 min at $90°C$

and rapidly cooled in an ice bath. The suspension is diluted with 1.2 volumes of cold potassium phosphate buffer, pH 7.4 and the fixed bacteria are collected by centrifugation (6 min $4000 \times g$). The bacteria are then incubated in PBS, containing 0.5% (v/v) Tween 20, for 15 min at room temperature and washed by centrifugation with the same buffer (Lindmark, 1982).

Teichoic acid may also be removed from formalin-fixed bacteria by alkaline hydrolysis (Roger and Garret, 1963).

13.5.3. Other solid phases

The preparation of immunosorbents by direct cross-linking of antigens is generally too costly to be practical (Section 7.1.9.2.5).

Other particulate solid phases include polyacrylamide gels (Dolken and Klein, 1977), bentonite clay (Cheng and Talmage, 1969) and possibly other supports. Generally, these rarely used solid phases are not very practical and find their application only in particular cases.

13.6. Separation principles for the various solid phases

Large solid phases (plastic, glass, membranes, paper) retain the attached specific immunoreactant while unbound and/or unreacted molecules are removed by aspiration or decanting. This simple separation procedure is probably responsible to a large degree for the wide application of these solid phases, despite their lower binding capacity.

Particulate solid phases with a high surface/volume ratio (consequently higher efficiency) give faster reactions since the solid phase is dispersed throughout the reaction mixture, but may suffer from the necessity of more involved separation techniques such as centrifugation, filtration or special procedures (Hunter, 1980). This also makes automation more difficult.

A possibility to circumvent these problems is the use of iron-containing particles and magnetic transfer devices (Hersh and Yaverbaum, 1975; Avrameas, 1977; Smith and Gehle, 1977; Anderson, 1978; Druet et al., 1982). The beads may contain magnetite (Magnogel 44, Industrie Biologie Française, Villeneuve la Garenne, France) or small iron cores (Smith and Gehle, 1977). These may be coated with a film of polycarbonate by immersing the beads in a 5% solution of methylene chloride, scattering them on slick paper and drying. Adsorption or conjugation of antigens or antibodies can then be performed as in Section 13.2. One bead per well is used in a microtitre plate.

CHAPTER 14

Quantitative enzyme immunoassay techniques

14.1. The choice of an EIA procedure

This chapter deals with the operational details of EIA. Many different designs can be found in the hundreds of publications which appear annually. The assays described here are general methods and might need modifications for individual systems.

The nature of the starting material and the type of results desired determine which design is most appropriate. In Chapter 2, the specificity and detectability of the different designs were compared. Though these parameters determine to a certain degree the reliability of the results, the true state of positivity (prevalence) is crucial for the selection of a test. At low prevalence, high specificity is required even if this is at the cost of detectability, whereas the contrary holds for high prevalence (Section 15.1). The consequences of modifying a test to obtain less false negatives at the cost of more false positives (and vice versa) have to be weighted for individual cases. Furthermore, designs also depend, on the method chosen for data processing, the particular enzyme selected (Section 10.1), and the type of conjugate (Section 11.1). Qualitative EIA are conveniently carried out on a solid phase, such as nitrocellulose, whereas for quantitative assays measurements of absorbance or fluorescence should be feasible.

The two bases of EIA, the immune reaction and the measurement of the enzyme activity, are discussed in two separate sections since they can be combined in different manners. For the sake of simplicity, the immunological interactions are divided into solid-phase or homogeneous designs and further separated into competitive or non-competitive assays. Some applications are mentioned to illustrate their potential. In addition to the basic details of the immune and enzyme reactions, various means to improve the detectability and specificity of these reactions and to accelerate the assay, as well as the use of novel or alternative approaches, equipment and automation procedures are discussed.

In the schemes in this chapter, x and y denote different animal species, H hapten, Ab antibody in general and AB antibody to Ig (anti-Ig), Ag antigen, E enzyme,]= is the symbol for solid-phase immobilization, covalent links are indicated by a stop (Ab·E, H·E), immunological or other non-covalent links (biotin–avidin, Ab–H, Ab–Ag, Ab–AB, SpA–Ab) are indicated by long hyphens and links in immune complexes, prepared prior to addition, by a colon (Ab:E).

14.2. Solid-phase enzyme immunoassays

In solid-phase EIA, one of the immunoreactants or some other molecule (complement factors, receptors, capture, etc.) is immobilized on the solid phase (Chapter 13), the sample is added, and the test substance retained is reacted with the corresponding immunoreactants, one of which carries an enzyme label. By measuring the extent of the enzymatic reaction the activity or concentration of the immunoreactant in the test sample is determined.

For some situations it might be necessary to heat-inactivate the complement in the sera (incubation for 30 min at 56°C) to eliminate interference (Yolken et al., 1980; Mehta and MacDonald, 1982). Sometimes, though relatively rarely, it may be necessary to post-coat the solid phase, e.g. with gelatin or another 'inert' protein. In all cases, however, extensive washing after the coating is important. Six washings are recommended, though three may sometimes suffice, to remove weakly immobilized immunoreactants (Section 13.2.1), to decrease cross-reactivity (Section 8.6) or to prevent carry-over of unbound immunoreactants since this would decrease the detectability. The buffers used for the washing and incubation steps should favor both the immunological and the enzymatic reaction and prevent non-specific interactions. The composition of the three most generally used buffers is given in Table 14.1. The use of NaN_3 (0.2 g/l) is not advised for POase-based assays. The washing buffer should be left in contact with the solid phase for a few moments (10 sec to 5 min) before its removal (decantation, aspiration or centrifugation, depending on the nature of the solid phase). The volumes used in EIA depend on the solid phase but should be small. For the widely used microplates, originally the total volume was 0.3 ml per well; now most investigators use only 0.2 ml and some even prefer 0.1 ml (Yolken et al., 1980).

Antibodies to the IgG of one species quite often cross-react with IgG of other species (Section 17.3.4.1). A powerful method to prevent

TABLE 14.1

Buffers used for dilution of immunoreactants and washing of coated solid phases[a]

PBS-T (pH 7.2)[b]		TBS-T (pH 7.4)[c]		PBS-GM (pH 7.0)[d]	
KH_2PO_4	0.2 g	Tris	2.4 g	NaH_2PO_4	0.84 g
$Na_2HPO_4 \cdot 12 H_2O$	2.9 g	HCl (1 N) to pH 7.4		Na_2HPO_4	0.85 g
NaCl	8.0 g	NaCL	8.0 g	NaCl	17.5 g
KCl	0.2 g	KCl	0.2 g	$MgCl_2$	0.01 g
Tween 20	0.5 g	Tween 20	0.5 g	BSA	1.0 g
				Gelatin	5.0 g

[a] All buffers made up to 1000 ml with distilled water. The addition of 0.5% gelatin was shown to be advantageous (Section 14.5.2.) for some assays (instead of, or in addition to Tween 20).

[b] The almost universally used buffer for all enzymes, even if it is not always suitable.

[c] Should be used for APase, irrespective of the fact that some solid phases may decrease the degree of inhibition of the enzyme by phosphate.

[d] Advised for EIA using BGase. Kato et al. (1980) obtained somewhat better results if gelatin is digested with a protease for about 10 min prior to use. Though gelatin is primarily used for background reduction, enzyme activity is sometimes increased. Gelatin, however, should not be used for washing of nitrocellulose if the wash is drawn by vacuum through the membrane (in commercial equipment) since this will cause clogging.

this cross-reaction is to use anti-hapten antibodies and to haptenate the appropriate immunoreactant (Section 12.5). By labeling these anti-hapten antibodies with an enzyme, a general reagent is obtained which can be used against any haptenated molecule. It is good practice to include both positive and negative reference samples in the tests.

The optimal time and temperature for the incubation steps have to be established for each system, but the general conditions given here will yield satisfactory results. Although EIA are quite often performed at 37°C, some antibodies have no strong affinity at this temperature (Section 8.2).

The optimal dilution of the conjugate should be determined by checker-board titrations. Alternatively, the Ig can be adsorbed on the solid phase and incubated with a series of dilutions of the labeled anti-Ig for 3 h at room temperature. Either the dilution giving an absorbance of 1.0 after 30 min (particularly for plate-readers), or the dilution which contains twice the amount of conjugate found in the highest dilution still giving an adsorbance at the plateau (excess of conjugate) can be used.

The problem often arises that only one antiserum (or only from the same species) is available and that no appropriate conjugates exist for that antiserum. Thus, indirect sandwich assays (Fig. 2.2) cannot be performed, even if conjugates of the anti-Ig were available since the conjugate would not discriminate between the antibody immobilized on the solid phase and the antibody reacting with the antigen retained by the immobilized antibody. De Jong (1983) circumvented this problem by preparing soluble complexes of the conjugated anti-Ig and the primary antibody by mixing 1:800 diluted primary antibody with an equal volume of 1:50 diluted commercial anti-Ig conjugate and incubating for 1 h at 37°C. To prevent non-specific staining, a same volume of 1:10 diluted normal serum (from the same species as the primary antibody) was added and incubated for another 30 min before using in EIA to prevent the reaction of the labeled antibody with the solid-phase antibody. Checkerboard titrations are necessary to optimize this system. This procedure allowed the detection of 4 ng enterotoxin within 30 min.

14.2.1. Non-competitive enzyme immunoassays in which antigen is immobilized on the solid phase

Three different procedures can be distinguished: (i) direct method; (ii) indirect method; and, (iii) bridge methods. The detectability and general applicability of the test increases from (i) to (iii) because the same conjugates can be used for different systems, but as they involve more steps, the number of controls also increases and specificity decreases.

14.2.1.1. Direct non-competitive solid-phase enzyme immunoassays
This approach is little used for quantitative investigations, but often in qualitative tests, e.g. for the detection of antigens on protein blots (Chapter 16) or in EIH (Chapter 17). For each epitope a corresponding labeled antibody is needed. The immobilized antigen ($]=Ag$) reacts directly with the conjugate (Ab·E):

$$]=Ag + Ab\cdot E \quad \rightarrow \quad]=Ag\text{--}Ab\cdot E$$

This method has the advantage that only one incubation is needed and controls are at a minimum, but it has the disadvantage that relatively high concentrations of antigen are needed for detection and it requires more antiserum.

Incubation is carried out with the conjugate at various dilutions (200–50000 times, depending on the quality of both the antiserum and the conjugation), using a buffer from Table 14.1. A 2- to 3-h incubation at room temperature in a humid chamber is generally sufficient, but it can be shortened with antisera which are equally reactive at 37°C.

14.2.1.2. Indirect non-competitive enzyme immunoassays with antigens immobilized on the solid phase   This widely used EIA is for the determination of antibody activity. Its principle is quite simple:

$$]=Ag + Ab_{test} + AB\cdot E \quad \rightarrow \quad]=Ag\text{--}Ab_{test}\text{--}AB\cdot E$$

The immobilized antigen captures the antibody from the test-sample which is then revealed by the enzyme-labeled anti-Ig. This method can be optimized using reference sera (positive, weakly positive and negative), according to the method of Table 14.2A. The test itself is described in Table 14.2B.

This method has, generally, about 10 times higher detectability than the direct method. The same conjugate can be used to detect antibodies (Ab_{test}) from the same species. Enzyme-labeled SpA may be employed for IgG antibodies of different species (Table 7.1), though caution is warranted if the primary antibodies belong to less reactive subclasses. Yolken and Leister (1981) described the use and the advantages of this method.

14.2.1.3. Bridge methods in non-competitive enzyme immunoassays with antigens immobilized on the solid phase   Three different bridge-methods in which the enzyme is attached to one of the immunoreactants by non-covalent linkage rapidly gain popularity: (i) the immunologically linked enzyme, (PAP complexes, also known as a-ELISA; Butler et al., 1980); (ii) the avidin–biotin complex; and, (iii) lectin-based bridging.

The use of immunologically linked enzyme–antibody complexes will most probably increase due to the advent of monoclonal antibodies. The preparation of such complexes is not only extremely simple (Section 11.3.2), but can be done with crude enzyme extracts. A bridging antibody (AB_{link}) is needed to link the enzyme–antibody complex (Ab:E) to the primary antibody (Ab_{test}):

$$] = Ag + Ab_{test} + AB_{link} + Ab:E \quad \rightarrow \quad] = Ag-Ab_{test}-AB_{link}-Ab:E$$

in which the two antibodies, Ab_{test} and Ab:E, are most often but not always from the same species. Compared to early direct conjugation methods, the detectability is increased, however, differences with the improved conjugates are small. Evidently, the additional incubation steps require more controls and AB_{link} should be in excess,

TABLE 14.2

Indirect non-competitive solid-phase EIA for antisera

A. *Determination of optimal test conditions in microplates*
    1. Make serial dilutions of the antigen and coat each well in the same row with 0.2 ml of the antigen solution at the same dilution (overnight at 4 °C, or 2 h at room temperature) in a humid chamber (overcoating may lead to enhanced nonspecificity).

    2. After washing (Section 14.2), add 180 μl serially diluted reference sera (positive, weakly positive or negative) to each well of one vertical row (starting dilutions of 1:100 to 1:10000, depending on antibody activity; 2 vertical rows, i.e. 16 dilutions) and incubate for 2 h at room temperature in a humid chamber.

    3. Wash again and add 200 μl conjugate diluted to 1:200 − 1:10000 (depending on its quality; commercial preparations usually 1:1000) and incubate for 3 h at room temperature (optimal conjugate concentration will produce an absorbance of 1.5–1.8 when incubated with 0.1 μg IgG directly coated in well).

    4. Wash again and reveal enzyme activity as described in Section 14.4. Measure absorbances after 30 min or 1 h. The dilutions giving the maximal ratio of absorbances of positive/negative sera while the absorbance for the negative serum remains below 0.2 is chosen. If microplate readers are used, the immunoreactant concentrations giving an absorbance of 1.0 with minimum background are often chosen since photometer efficiency is then maximal.

B. *Indirect test for the determination of antibody activity*[a]
    1. Perform coating with the optimal antigen concentration as determined in test A.

    2. Wash 6 times (Section 14.2).

    3. Dilute the test and reference sera (positive and negative) in accordance with the method of data processing chosen (Section 15.1.4), using simple or serial dilutions. Add 0.2 ml of each dilution to duplicate wells and incubate plates for 2 h at room temperature in a humid chamber.

    4. Wash 3 times and add conjugate (0.2 ml). Since conjugated antibodies react slower than free antibodies (Tijssen et al., 1982) incubation should be for 3 h in a humid chamber at room temperature.

    5. Reveal enzyme activity as described in Section 14.4.

[a] Lengths of incubation periods may be shortened considerably by modifying various experimental parameters (Section 14.5.3).

otherwise both of its two combining sites would react with the Ab_{test} and none would be able to bind Ab:E. SpA instead of AB_{link} makes the method more generally applicable (Yolken et al., 1980). The increase in detectability which is achieved depends largely on the method with which it is compared. A typical procedure using the PAP complex is given in Table 14.3.

Biotin can be covalently coupled to enzymes, other proteins or polysaccharides by simple methods (Section 3.2.2), often without changing the biological activity. The reaction sequence (bridged avidin–biotin method, BRAB; Guesdon et al., 1979) is:

$$] = Ag + Ab_{test} + AB \cdot biotin + avidin + E \cdot biotin$$
$$\downarrow$$
$$] = Ag–Ab_{test}–AB \cdot biotin–avidin–E \cdot biotin$$

This approach is more generally applicable than the method of immunologically linked enzyme since there is no species restriction. In addition, this method is more sensitive (Madri and Barwick, 1983), the biotinylated anti-Ig antibody is not needed in excess, is applicable when xenogeneic antisera cannot be used, e.g. for Ig allotype markers (Jackson et al., 1982; Section 6.3), and biotinylation does not change significantly the diffusion properties of macromolecules (Bayer and Wilchek, 1980). The direct labeling of enzymes with avidin (LAB method; Guesdon et al., 1979) eliminates to a large extent the advantages of the avidin–biotin interaction (Yolken et al., 1983). However, enzymes which are inactivated by biotinylation (APase) may be labeled with avidin. The preparation of soluble avidin–biotin·E complexes (ABC; Hsu et al., 1981) prior to use in the test increases 20 to 100-fold the detectability (titre of 2×10^7 instead of 1.5×10^5 with the indirect method; Kendall et al., 1983). This is due, at least in part, to the very low background levels of the ABC method. The often-made statement that this increase is due to the capacity of one avidin molecule to bind 4 biotin molecules is false, since the active sites on avidin are situated in pairs (reaction of one blocks the other site; Section 3.1) and avidin can only serve as a bridge between two biotinylated molecules.

TABLE 14.3

Non-competitive solid-phase EIA using immunologically linked enzyme–antibody complexes[a]

A. *Determination of optimal test conditions in microplates*[b]

1. Establish optimum coating conditions (protein concentration usually between 50 and 500 ng/well) and the optimal dilution of the primary antibody (positive, negative and moderately positive reference sera) as described in Table 14.2A. Subsequently use the primary antibody at a dilution of 1:5 of the optimal.

2. Establish the excess of bridging antibody or SpA required. For this purpose:
   a. coat each well with the same amount of antigen;

   b. after washing, add the reference serum in two-fold serial dilution, beginning at twice the optimum concentration determined in step 1, each dilution to one vertical row (one plate per reference serum). Incubate for 2 h at room temperature in a humid chamber;

   c. after washing, add two-fold serial dilutions of the bridging antibody or SpA (highest concentration about 10 μg/ml) to horizontal rows of wells. Incubate for 2 h at room temperature in a humid chamber;

   d. after washing, add an excess of enzyme-antibody complexes (e.g., 25 μg/ml) and incubate for 2 h at room temperature in a humid chamber;

   e. establish enzyme activity after washing of the plates (Section 14.4). Optimum is determined as in Table 14.2A, step 4.
3. Establish the optimum concentration of enzyme-antibody complexes:
   a. proceed as in steps 2a en b; in step c use only the optimum dilution;

   b. after washing, add two-fold serial dilutions of the enzyme–antibody complexes (e.g., highest concentrations 50 μg/ml) to horizontal rows of wells and incubate for 2 h at room temperature in a humid chamber;

   c. establish optimum dilution as in step 2e.

B. *Performance of the test*

1. Perform coating and subsequent washings as discussed in Chapter 13.

2. Apply the test and reference sera as described in Table 14.2B, step 3.

3. Apply the bridging molecule and the enzyme-antibody complexes, as determined in Table 14.3A, steps 2 and 3.

4. Reveal enzyme activity as described in Section 14.4.

---

[a] Lengths of incubation periods may be shortened by modifying various experimental parameters (Section 14.5.3).

[b] Optimization as described in step 3 may preceed that of step 2 if this would make testing cheaper. The test may also be condensed to some pilot dilutions to have some preliminary idea about optimum conditions.

It is essential (Kendall et al., 1983; Yolken et al., 1983) to biotinylate correctly the antibody or enzyme, since there is a pronounced optimum (Section 3.2.2). However, current avidin/biotin methods may have to be changed with respect to biotinylation procedures to attain their full potential. The optimal dilutions of the biotinylated antibody, biotinylated enzyme and avidin solutions have to be determined and the test performed as detailed in Table 14.4. It is essential to use incubation periods of about 20 min (pronounced optimum) for the reaction between the biotinylated proteins and avidin (Kendall et al., 1983).

In the ABC procedure equal volumes of 1:10 diluted biotinylated POase and 1:10 diluted avidin (molar ratio POase:avidin = 3:1 in PBS containing 0.06% Triton X-100) are mixed and incubated at least 10 min before use. No change in activity is noted with incubation periods of up to 5 h.

Although the ABC method is versatile and has high detectability, there are several limiting or interfering factors. The test samples may contain one or more biotin-containing enzymes. Avidin, which is a basic glycoprotein (Section 3.1), may react non-specifically, either through its ion-exchange properties or oligosaccharide moiety, with molecules in the test sample. Heggeness and Ash (1977) observed the selective binding of avidin to condensed chromatin. Streptavidin (Section 3.1) produces less non-specific interactions. It is also possible to succinylate avidin to decrease non-specific interactions (Table 14.5).

Lectins can also serve as bridging molecules (Guesdon and Avrameas, 1980). Con A is known to have a strong affinity for POase, so that Ab·Con A conjugates prepared by the GA method, may serve as receptor for POase:

$$]=Ag + Ab \cdot Con\ A + POase \rightarrow]=Ag\text{–}Ab \cdot Con\ A\text{–}POase.$$

TABLE 14.4

Non-competitive solid-phase enzyme immunoassays based on the avidin–biotin system for the determination of antibody activity in sera[a]

A. *Determination of optimum test conditions with microplates*
  1. Perform step 1 of Table 14.3A (e.g., 0.3 μg antigen/well, and primary antiserum diluted 1:2000).

  2. Add to each well with immobilized antigen and primary antibody a constant amount of biotinylated anti-Ig antibody (e.g., 1 μg/ml) and incubate for 2 h at room temperature in a humid chamber.

  3. After washing, add 4-fold dilutions (e.g., 1:50 to 1:3200) of avidin (1.5 mg/ml) to horizontal rows of each reference serum. Incubate for 20 min at room temperature in a humid chamber.

  4. After washing, add three-fold serial dilutions of biotinylated enzyme, starting at 1:50 of a solution containing 1 mg/ml, to the vertical rows of each reference serum and incubate for 20 min at room temperature in a humid chamber.

  5. Establish the combination of optimum dilutions as in Table 14.2A, step 4.

  6. Establish optimum dilution of biotinylated anti-Ig antibody for step 2 using the optimum conditions established in step 5.

B. *Standard procedure for the performance of the test* (concentrations of reagents as established in A)
  1. Coat the plates with the antigen, eventually post-coat with 0.5% gelatin, and wash according to procedures described in Chapter 13.

  2. Add the sample(s) to be tested in the appropriate dilution or in serial dilutions, depending on the method chosen for data processing (Chapter 15). Incubate for 2 h at room temperature in a humid chamber and wash.

  3. Add biotinylated anti-Ig antibody, incubate for 2 h at room temperature in a humid chamber and wash.

  4. Add avidin and incubate for 20 min at room temperature in a humid chamber and wash.

  5. Add biotinylated enzyme and incubate as in step 4.

  6. Reveal enzyme activity as described in Section 14.4.

[a] With avidin-labeled enzyme or non-covalent avidin/biotin complex, the method is essentially similar; steps 3 and 4 of protocol A and 4 and 5 of protocol B become combined into one step. Covalently linked avidin is incubated for 2 h instead of 20 min.

TABLE 14.5
Succinoylation of avidin
(adapted from Finn et al., 1980)

Avidin may give high background staining due to its high pI (17 lysine or arginine residues/subunit). The reduction of this background by succinoylation of avidin is a relatively cheap alternative to the use of streptavidin.

1. Dissolve 50 mg avidin in 1.5 ml 0.1 N HCl.

2. Add 73.5 ml 200 mM borate buffer, pH 9.0.

3. Cool to 0 °C.

4. Add 0.9 ml peroxide-free dioxane containing 30 mg succinic anhydride and stir for 1 h at 0 °C.

5. Dialyze against 10% acetic acid (2 × 1 litre) overnight.

6. Lyophilize and redissolve in 2 ml 100 mM ammonium bicarbonate and desalt on Sephadex G-25 in same solvent.

7. Pool appropriate fractions and lyophilize. An average of 6–7 succinoyl groups per avidin subunit will be incorporated.

It is necessary, however, to incubate the Ab·lectin conjugate with an excess (200 mM) of the sugar specific for the lectin (Section 11.2.2.3) to prevent its non-specific adsorption to immobilized antigens. After the immunological reaction, the sugar should be removed by washing before the enzyme is added. This method offers no significant advantages over other bridging methods and has less detectability.

14.2.2. Non-competitive enzyme immunoassays with antibodies or receptor molecules immobilized on the solid phase

14.2.2.1. Non-competitive assays with antibodies immobilized on the solid phase   Immobilization of antibodies or their F(ab')$_2$ on the solid phase is widely and primarily used to quantitate antigens in the test sample ('immuno extraction'). It is also possible to use this system for the titration of antisera. Immobilized antibodies may also serve to trap antigens from crude extracts or antigens which are not easily immobilized by other means. A prerequisite of this technique is that the antigen or hapten should have at least 2 epitopes.

Variants of this technique can be illustrated as:

A. $] = Ab_x–Ag–Ab_x \cdot E$

B. $] = Ab_x–Ag–Ab_y–AB_x \cdot E$

C. $] = Fab_x–Ag–Ab_x–AB_y \cdot E$

D. $] = Fab–Ag–Ab–SpA–IgG \cdot E$

E. $] = Ab_x–Ag–Ab_y–AB_x–IgG_y \cdot E$

F. $] = Ab_x–Ag–Ab_x \cdot biotin–avidin–E \cdot biotin$

G. $] = Ab_x–Ag–Ab_y–AB_x \cdot biotin–avidin–E \cdot biotin$

H. $] = Ab_x–Ag–Ab_x \cdot H–Ab_x–H \cdot E$

Crook and Payne (1980) compared the direct (Section 14.2.1.1), indirect (Section 14.2.1.2) and the 'double-antibody sandwich' methods (variant A) for their ability to detect and discriminate between several granulosis viruses. The indirect method was the most sensitive (1 ng/ml), the direct method was the least sensitive (15 ng/ml) and method A had an intermediate detectability (10 ng/ml).

There are, however, some specific characteristics and limitations for these variants. When anti-Ig antibodies are used, they should not be reactive with the immobilized antibody, i.e., for the more sensitive indirect methods (variants B, E and G) primary antisera from two different species should be available. This is not always practical or feasible and various ways have been developed to circumvent this problem (De Jong, 1983; Section 14.2). In variants C and D, the solid phase is coated with Fab or $F(ab')_2$ and the complete antibody is applied in the third layer, together with enzyme-conjugated anti-Ig antibodies (C) or enzyme-labeled SpA (which is Fc specific; D) (Barbara and Clark, 1982; Koenig and Paul, 1982). Although this variant requires strictly Fc-specific antibodies, most anti-IgG antibodies, produced against complete IgG, are rather Fc-specific. If this is not the case, the anti-IgG serum could always be absorbed with an immunosorbent prepared with Fab or $F(ab')_2$. In variants F and G biotinylated antibody and biotinylated enzyme are used in the third layer, whereas in variant H both the antibodies and enzyme are haptenated, which are then linked by avidin or anti-hapten antibody, respectively.

A side-effect noted when microplates are coated with $F(ab')_2$ is a narrowing of the specificity of the antiserum in heterologous reactions against a series of serologically related viruses (Koenig, 1981; Rybycki and von Wechmar, 1981; Koenig and Paul, 1982). Cross-reactions observed among plant viruses with whole antibodies in indirect EIA were not, or only barely, detectable with variant C (Koenig and Paul, 1982).

All these methods differ only slightly in their methodology from those discussed in Section 14.2.1. For optimal results, coating of the solid phase should be carried out with purified IgG or antibody preparations at the optimum concentration indicated in Sections 13.2–13.5. It is good practice to include a negative reference serum for the coating of some wells. Solutions of known concentrations of the antigen (0.01–1000 ng/ml, depending on the detectability of the test) to be titrated should be included to obtain valid dose–response curves. The antigen solution is diluted with PBS-T, PBS-GM or TBS-T and incubated for 2 h at room temperature in a humid chamber. For titration of sera these assays can be used if the antigen cannot be coated directly to the plate (e.g., not pure, no affinity for the plate) and the same concentration of antigen is then used for each well.

14.2.2.2. Non-competitive assays with complement immobilized on the solid phase   Immobilization of C1q on the solid phase can serve for the trapping and quantitation of immune complexes. C1q can be prepared by the simple method of Pohl et al. (1980). Briefly, C1q is precipitated from fresh frozen human plasma at a relative salt concentration of 0.04 and redissolved in 300 mM NaCl and 10 mM EDTA, at pH 7.5. The crude preparation is further purified by affinity chromatography on rabbit IgG-Sepharose 4B. The adsorbed C1q is eluted with 100 mM Tris–HCl buffer, pH 8.6, containing 1.0 M NaCl, 50 mM EDTA and 10% sucrose and dialyzed against 10 mM phosphate buffer, pH 7.5, containing 1.0 M NaCl. The solution is chromatographed on a protein A-Sepharose column to remove contaminating IgG. C1q binds selectively to antigen–antibody complexes (Calcott and Müller-Eberhard, 1972) and C1q immobilized on a solid phase is efficient in measuring complexes involved in tissue deposition (serum sickness) which should provide a valuable tool to study this disorder (Pohl et al., 1981). The immune complexes bound to the C1q-coated solid phase can be detected with enzyme-labeled anti-IgG. C1q-coated solid phase can also be used for immune complexes prepared in vitro (Yolken and Stopa, 1980) (Table 14.6). This system requires fewer incubation steps and is applicable to many different Ag–Ab systems, but it has a lower detectability than some of the other methods, particularly if circulating immune complexes are present in the serum (Gabriel and Agnello, 1977). This method, however, obviates the necessity of antisera from two species as would be required in other assays.

Many other capture molecules could also be used (e.g., receptors, lectins); the principles of such methods do not differ from those discussed here.

TABLE 14.6
Non-competitive assays with C1q immobilized on the solid phase

1. Coat solid phase with C1q (about 2 μg/ml; Chapter 13) and store desiccated at 4°C until used in step 3.

2. Prepare serial dilutions of the antigen in the wells of a hard microtitre plate (Dynatech 223-24) and add to each well an equal volume of antiserum in the appropriate buffer (Table 14.1). Incubate for 3 h at room temperature or 2 h at 37°C (depending on the reactivity of the antibodies at these temperatures).

3. Transfer the immune complexes to the wells of the plate prepared in step 1, after washing the latter 6 times. Incubate for 2 h at 37°C in a humid chamber.

4. Wash the plate 5 times with the appropriate buffer.

5. Incubate with enzyme-labeled anti-Ig (Table 14.2) or use the method described in Table 14.3, Table 14.4 or Section 14.2.2.1.

6. Reveal enzyme activity as described in Section 14.4.

14.2.2.3. Immunoglobulin class capture methods   Class capture methods are designed to recognize the Ig class of the antibodies, e.g., to differentiate acute from chronic infections. As discussed in Section 5.2.1., IgM antibodies appear first in an infection, followed by an increase in IgG during a second infection. Conventional EIA for this purpose are based on the competition between IgG and IgM for the available antigen:

$$] = Ag + IgM \rightarrow] = Ag–IgM + AB_{anti-IgM} \cdot E \rightarrow] = Ag–IgM–AB_{anti-IgM} \cdot E$$

$$] = Ag + IgG \rightarrow] = Ag–IgG + AB_{anti-IgG} \cdot E \rightarrow] = Ag–IgG–AB_{anti-IgG} \cdot E$$

Rheumatoid factors (Section 6.1.6.3) or an excess of IgG may interfere with this reaction. Moreover, IgM often have lower affinity for the antigen. An improvement of this method (Yolken et al., 1980), in which excess of IgG is removed from the test serum with SpA, is still not satisfactory. The elegant class capture methods can be illustrated for IgM as:

$$] = AB_{anti-IgM} + serum + Ag\,(later) \quad \rightarrow \quad] = AB_{anti-IgM}–IgM–Ag$$

The immobilized anti-IgM antibodies extract ('capture') the IgM from the test sample. If this IgM contains antibodies, Ag is bound and quantitated by methods discussed in Section 14.2.2.1. The antibody activity due to IgM can then be compared to that of IgG established by a similar IgG class capture method.

14.2.3. Competitive solid-phase enzyme immunoassays

Competitive solid phase EIA primarily quantitate antigens. As with the non-competitive EIA, these procedures can be divided into two types, according to the immunoreactant immobilized on the solid phase.

14.2.3.1. Competitive enzyme immunoassays with antibody immobilized on the solid phase   These methods are based on the competition of enzyme-labeled antigen with the antigen present in the test sample for the antibody on the solid phase:

$$]=Ab + Ag \cdot E \quad \rightarrow \;]=Ab–Ag \cdot E \qquad \text{('zero dose')}$$

$$]Ab + Ag \cdot E + Ag \rightarrow \; \begin{cases}]=Ab–Ag + Ag \cdot E & \text{(test} \\ & \text{or} \\ ]=Ab–Ag \cdot E + Ag & \text{standard)} \end{cases}$$

Two approaches may be taken to determine [Ag]: (i) the quasi-equilibrium saturation method (scheme above); and (ii) the sequential saturation method (Ag·E added later; two extremes shown):

$$]=Ab + Ag \quad \rightarrow \quad]=Ab–Ag + Ag \cdot E \quad \rightarrow \;]=Ab–Ag$$
$$+ \text{ unbound } Ag \cdot E$$

and (if no Ag is present),

$$]=Ab \quad \rightarrow \quad]=Ab + Ag \cdot E \quad \rightarrow \quad]=Ab–Ag \cdot E$$

The theoretical background of these approaches has been discussed in Section 8.8. Sequential saturation has high detectability but lowered specificity (Section 2.3). Both methods reveal the presence of the Ag by a decrease in enzyme activity, compared to the calibration. The decrease, however, is more pronounced in the second method, particularly if the large-scale exchange of Ag by Ag·E is prevented using high-affinity Ab and a short second incubation period (otherwise the system approaches equilibrium). An example of this method is given in Table 14.7A. A practical application is illustrated by the detection of insulin at picomole levels (Albert et al., 1978).

A variant of the sequential method (Belanger et al., 1976; Van Weemen et al., 1978), which is routinely used for human placental lactogen and oestrogens, is as follows (3 steps):

step 1: Ag (sample) + Ab (small excess) → Ab–Ag + Ab

step 2: add Ag·E → Ab–Ag + Ab–Ag·E

step 3: add]=AB to mixture of step → $\begin{cases}]=AB–Ab–Ag \\ ]=AB–Ab–Ag \cdot E \end{cases}$

TABLE 14.7

Sequential competitive assay procedures on immobilized antibodies

A. *Variant A*[a]

1. Coat solid phase with antibodies (Chapter 13). Optimum conditions for various steps are determined as described in Table 14.8.

2. Test in preliminary experiments the concentration range of the labeled antigen which will provide an excess for the available immobilized antibody.

3. For the test, dispense in the antibody-coated wells of a microplate different dilutions of the test sample (diluting buffers: Table 14.1), as well as various standards for the calibration curve. Incubate overnight at 4°C or for 2 h at room temperature.

4. Wash three times.

5. Add an excess of enzyme-labeled antigen (established in step 2) to determine the amount of antibody still free after the test sample had the possibility to saturate these antibodies. Incubate for 2 h (optimum time should be established) at room temperature in a humid chamber.

6. Wash three times.

7. Reveal enzyme activity (Section 14.4) and construct calibration curve as discussed in Section 15.1.5. The sample dilution giving about 50% of the maximum activity is often the most reliable.

B. *Variant B*

1. Incubate 0.5 ml sample, at the appropriate dilution (determined in preliminary tests), with 0.1 ml antiserum for 30 min at room temperature.

2. Add 0.1 ml antigen–enzyme conjugate and incubate for another 30 min at room temperature (determine in a preliminary test the amount of conjugate required to saturate 0.1 ml antiserum).

3. Add anti-Ig antibodies immobilized on a particulate solid phase and shake for 2 h at room temperature.

4. Centrifuge at low-speed, discard supernatant, wash pellet, centrifuge again and discard supernatant.

5. Reveal enzyme activity (Section 14.4) by resuspending the pellet in 2 ml substrate.

[a] If the affinity of the antibody is not high, it is sometimes possible to improve the detection limit of the assay by reducing the number of washing steps.

The solid phase in this case is particulate (e.g. microcrystalline cellulose) and the activity (complexed Ag·E) is measured in the pellet after centrifugation. This activity is inversely proportional to the amount of antigen present in the sample since unreacted Ab (due to the absence of Ag) is quantitated. Although this method is more laborious than the first variant of sequential saturation, it has a wider applicability (Table 14.7B). These methods require highly purified antigens in sufficient amounts for labelling.

The quasi-equilibrium saturation method on solid phase is less frequently employed than emphasized in review articles. The antigen present in the test or calibration sample and the enzyme-labeled antigen compete simultaneously for the available antibody on the solid phase. The enzymatic reaction in the various wells is then inversely proportional to the amount of the unlabeled antigen present. Evidently, it is essential to prepare calibration curves. This method is more useful for the assay of small molecules for which sequential incubation does not increase detectability, in contrast to that of larger proteins, probably because small molecules diffuse much faster than the conjugates. For this reason, the technique in Table 14.7 (A or B) is applied with the difference that the addition of the antigen (test or calibration sample) is immediately followed by the addition of the conjugate. Alternatively, for a better approach of the equilibrium conditions, a known amount of enzyme-labeled antigen is mixed with the sample (test or calibration) and the mixture is then exposed to the antibody-coated solid phase (Borrebaeck et al., 1978). A possible problem in this technique is that antibodies or Ig in samples of body fluids may interfere.

14.2.3.2. Competitive enzyme immunoassays with antigen immobilized on the solid phase   This technique is based on the inhibition of the reaction of enzyme-labeled antibodies with the immobilized antigen by free antigen present in the test or calibration sample:

$$] = Ag + Ab \cdot E \quad \rightarrow \quad] = Ag\text{--}Ab \cdot E \qquad \text{('zero dose')}$$

$$] = Ag + Ag_{sample} + Ab \cdot E \rightarrow \begin{cases}] = Ag\text{--}Ab \cdot E & (Ag_{sample} \text{ absent}) \\ ] = Ag & (Ag_{sample}\text{--}Ab \cdot E \text{ unbound}) \end{cases}$$

The amount of enzyme immobilized on the solid phase is inversely proportional to the amount of free antigen present in the incubation mixture. This approach has been used both in the equilibrium and sequential technique (Tijssen and Kurstak, 1981). The technical procedures are similar to those in Table 14.7 and its quasi-equilibrium variant with the modifications that Ag is coated on the solid phase and Ab·E is used.

In a variant of this method, Ag is not incubated directly with Ab·E but with Ab and the captured antibody is quantitated with enzyme-labeled anti-Ig antibodies. At the two extreme cases:

Ag absent in sample:

$$]=Ag + Ab \rightarrow]=Ag{-}Ab + AB \cdot E \rightarrow]=Ag{-}Ab{-}AB{\cdot}E$$

Ag present in sample:

$$]=Ag + Ab{-}Ag \rightarrow]=Ag + AB \cdot E \rightarrow]=Ag$$

This method was applied by Altschuh and van Regenmortel (1982) for the study of the antigenic composition of tobacco mosaic virus (Table 14.8). The virus was immobilized on the solid phase and

TABLE 14.8
Indirect competitive enzyme immunoassay procedure using antigen-coated solid phase

---

1. Use the indirect noncompetitive solid-phase EIA for antisera (Table 14.2) as basic procedure.

2. Determine absorbance with different combinations of coated antigen (1 : 2 dilutions in columns, e.g., 6.4 μg to 50 ng/well) and antiserum (1 : 3 dilutions in rows, e.g., starting at 1 : 100) using the optimal concentrations of conjugate (Table 14.2A, step 3).

3. Among the combinations giving 0.8–1.3 absorbance, each antiserum (two-fold higher concentration of that combination) is incubated overnight with an equal volume of serially diluted competing antigen, and added to the correspondingly coated wells.

4. A standard curve is obtained for each antibody concentration and the best are selected with respect to sensitivity, detectability, and reproducibility (Section 15.4; Tijssen, 1985).

---

was detected by the sequential addition of Ab and AB·E. Analysis of the inhibitory activity of various peptides obtained after tryptic digestion of the viral protein revealed that T protein has 7 epitopes. As in other competitive methods, it is essential that the competing immunoreactant should not be in an excess (Section 2.2).

Another interesting application is the analysis of the specificity of monoclonal antibodies, i.e., whether they recognize different epitopes on the antigen (Friguet et al., 1983). After coating the antigen, two monoclonal antibodies are added, either to separate or to the same well and the amount of bound antibody is quantitated with enzyme-labeled anti-mouse IgG. Additivity of enzyme activity is observed when the monoclonal antibodies bind to distinct epitopes. The additivity index (AI) for a pair of antibodies is then defined as:

$$AI = \frac{A_{1+2} - (A_1 + A_2)/2}{A_1 + A_2 - (A_1 + A_2)/2} \times 100 = \left(\frac{2A_{1+2}}{A_1 + A_2} - 1\right) \times 100$$

in which A_1, A_2 and A_{1+2} are the absorbances obtained with the antibodies separate and together. This method is only reliable if avidities of both antibodies are similar or above the threshold where the effects of washing are negligible.

14.3. Homogeneous enzyme immunoassays

Both non-competitive and competitive assays are found in this group, though the latter is the most common. These assays are generally used for the quantitation of small molecules. In contrast to RIA and solid-phase EIA, homogeneous EIA do not require separation steps because the immune reaction influences the enzyme activity. This approach is not complicated by the possibility of non-specific adsorption on the solid phase and by limitation of the antibody concentration imposed by the area of the solid phase (Yolken, 1982). The small size of the molecules studied by these methods insures an intimate interaction between the antibody and the enzyme within the complex, producing a modulation of the enzyme activity. It is more difficult to achieve this effect with large antigens, such as proteins. The proximal linkage method is a potentially powerful homogeneous EIA for large antigens but has not yet been fully exploited (Section 2.5.2). The enzyme-channelling immunoassay designed by Litman et al. (1980) resembles this proximal linkage procedure in that two different enzymes are brought into each other's vicinity so that high concentrations of the product formed by the first enzyme occur locally which is then used by the second (indicator) enzyme to produce a measurable product.

14.3.1. Competitive homogeneous enzyme immunoassays

Five types of competitive homogeneous EIA can be distinguished (Section 2.5.3), depending on which component of the assay is labeled.

14.3.1.1. Competitive homogeneous enzyme immunoassays using enzyme–hapten conjugates
The prototype of these assays (Rubenstein et al., 1972) was used to detect morphine (detection limit 1×10^{-9} M). Among the various enzymes, lysozyme and GPDase are the most often used for the detection of drugs in urine and serum, respectively. Lysozyme, which has a large substrate (*Micrococcus luteus*), is conjugated to morphine and added to the test sample, together with a certain amount of anti-morphine antibodies (sequential saturation principle, Section 8.8), giving the extreme cases:

$$\text{absence of H: Ab} + \text{H} \cdot \text{E} \quad \rightarrow \quad \text{Ab–H} \cdot \text{E}$$

$$\text{presence of H: Ab} + \text{H} \quad \rightarrow \quad \text{Ab–H} \xrightarrow{\text{H} \cdot \text{E}} \text{Ab–H} + \text{H·E}$$

In the first reaction the conjugate reacts with the antibody, which thus modulates the enzyme activity (often a decrease but sometimes an increase; see below), in the second reaction the free hapten present in the test sample occupies the antibody sites, leaving, depending on the [H], H·E unchanged. The original method of Rubenstein et al. (1972), which takes only a few minutes to perform, is given in Table 14.8A. A problem with these methods, compared to solid-phase EIA, is the possible interference by factors in the body fluids, an advantage is the rapidity of the result.

Rowley et al. (1975) investigated some important parameters of these assays using MDase, haptenation of which decreases only moderately enzyme activity, if the extent of substitution is less than 16 per enzyme.

Thyroxine–MDase conjugates are peculiar in that they are enzymatically inactive but become activated by the binding of anti-thyroxine antibodies (Ullman et al., 1975). It seems that the conjugated thyroxine inhibits the enzyme by hindering its active site, whereas the antibody reactivates the enzyme by pulling the thyroxine away from the active site. Although this mechanism is not clearly understood, inhibition appears to be due to an increase in the K_m (Van Lente and Galen, 1980). Many of these assays are marketed under the trade name 'EMIT' by Syva Co. Enzyme activities are measured as discussed in Chapter 10.

Information on the major interactive variables of the EMIT tests is scanty (Mulé et al., 1974; Osterloh and Butrimovitz, 1982). Antibodies used for the inhibition or reactivation of the enzyme are heterogeneous and the later-bound (lower-affinity) antibodies differ in their effect on the enzyme. The V_{max} may change due to different antibody populations or to allosterism (Osterloh and Butrimovitz, 1982). The antibodies in commercial kits are often heterogeneous on purpose to obtain a wider specificity.

Similar methods have also been developed for large antigens. In the method of Gibbons et al. (1980), a macromolecular substrate is sterically excluded from the enzyme–antigen conjugate if the antigen is complexed with the corresponding antibody. In this study, o-nitrophenyl-β-galactoside was linked to dextran. Though labeling of BGase with up to 7 large antigen molecules did not change substantially its activity for unimolecular substrate, it had, unexpectedly, a higher activity for the dextran-linked substrate than the native enzyme. The addition of antibodies to the conjugated antigen increased the K_m with the polymerized substrate but not with the unimolecular substrate. The method is presented in Table 14.9B.

TABLE 14.9

Competitive homogeneous immunoassays using enzyme-labeled hapten or antigen

Three basic protocols can be distinguished for haptens: 'stat', 'batch', and 'endpoint'. Protocol A is representative for the stat method and is analogous to sequential addition in radioimmunoassays in that the sample reacts briefly with the antibody before the conjugate is added and enzyme activity is determined kinetically in less than 1 min. Calibration curves are usually stable within a working day. The batch method (e.g., for thyroxine) is used when higher detectability is required. This method requires larger samples, longer incubation periods for antibody and kinetic measurement, and a calibration curve for each batch (hence its name) of samples. These requirements for an initial reading and precise incubation period (15–30 min) are eliminated with the endpoint method. In this method (e.g., for digoxin) a blank tube is used for each sample and a reagent is added to quench the enzyme after 1.5–2 h of incubation. Pretreatment of the samples is sometimes necessary to liberate drugs from binding proteins or to destroy enzyme activity. For example, for T-4 treatments with 500 mM NaOH (1:1 v/v) to release T-4 from thyroid binding globulin and β-cyclodextrin (a fatty acid sequestering agent) to prevent interference by fatty acids are included (1-anilino-8-naphthalenesulfonic acid used in radioimmunoassays interferes with enzyme activity determinations).

A. *Original method of Rubenstein et al. (1972) for haptens*
  1. Label lysozyme with carboxymethyl-morphine (e.g., with the mixed anhydride method, Section 12.3.1).

  2. Add, at 37°C, the sample (e.g., 50 μl urine) to 200 μl substrate (suspension of *Micrococcus luteus,* see Section 10.4.1.4).

  3. Add 50 μl of hapten antibody.

  4. Add 50 μl of enzyme-labeled hapten.

  5. Measure the enzyme-catalyzed reaction over a 40-sec period (*A* is measured and compared with standard curve, Section 15.1.5); a longer period of measurement produces a 30-fold improvement of the detection limit.

B. *Assay for enzyme-labeled antigen*
  1. Preparation of the macromolecular substrate: Dextran (Pharmacia, with an average molecular weight of 40000) is carboxymethylated with sodium chloroacetate in 1.25 M NaOH to give about 0.2 groups/glucose residue. *N,N'*-Bis-(3-

aminopropyl)piperazine is coupled to the carboxymethylated polymers using 1-ethyl-3-(3-dimethylaminopropyl)-carbodiimide at pH 4.8 and the resulting amino dextran is acetylated with the NHS ester of 3-carboxy-6-nitrophenyl-β-galactoside.

2. Incubate the antigen-containing samples (test or calibration) for 1 h at room temperature with 13 pmol of antibodies in 50 μl of 10 mM sodium phosphate buffer, pH 7.0, containing 128 mM NaCl, 1 mg/ml BSA and 0.05 mM magnesium acetate.

3. Add BGase-antigen conjugate (50 μl of a 19.4 mM solution) and incubate for an additional hour.

4. Assay by diluting a 50 μl aliquot of the mixture to 1 ml with the buffer of step 2, in the presence of 0.4 mM dextran-linked substrate. Measure the change in optical density at 420 nm at 37 °C for 30 sec.

14.3.1.2 Homogeneous enzyme immunoassays using avidin–ligand conjugates   Interaction of avidin (or haptenated avidin) with pyruvate carboxylase (EC 6.4.1.1), which has biotin as coenzyme, inhibits the enzyme reaction. The method of Bacquet and Twumasi (1984) is based on inhibition of this interaction by antibody to the hapten (Fig. 2.4; Section 14.6.8). The presence of free hapten (5,5-diphenylhydantoin) in the sample prevents the antibody from reacting with the haptenated avidin. Details are given in Table 14.10.

14.3.1.3. Homogeneous competitive enzyme immunoassays using substrate-labeled antigen   The method of Ngo et al. (1981) to quantitate IgG is equally applicable for other large antigens. It is similar to the EIA described by Burd et al. (1977a) for the detection of small molecules using hapten-labeled substrate. IgG is covalently labeled with 6-(7-β-galactosyl-coumarin-3-carboximido)-hexylamine (galactosyl umbelliferyl; GU) (Ngo et al., 1981). The galactoside residue of GU-IgG is hydrolyzed by BGase and followed by the increase of fluorescence. The presence of antibody to IgG lowers the amount of substrate available for the enzyme and, thus, lowers the activity. On the other hand, if IgG is present in the test sample, it will compete for the anti-IgG antibody, leading to an increase

TABLE 14.10
Homogeneous enzyme-immunoassay with avidin-ligand as enzyme modulator

Pyruvate carboxylase (EC 6.4.1.1; from *Bacillus stearothermophilus*), which is not present in significant amounts in human body fluids, is grown and purified as described by Bacquet and Twumasi (1984). In the following assay, 5,5-diphenylhydantoin (DPH) is used as the ligand.

A. *Conjugation*

Avidin (2 mg/ml) is dialyzed against 160 mM borate, pH 7.9, containing 130 mM NaCl. Biotin-binding sites are blocked by titration with 10 mM 4-hydroxyazobenzene-2-carboxylic acid as described by Green (1965). For conjugation, 5 mg/ml N^3-(5,5-diphenylhydantoin) acetic acid (*N*-hydroxysuccinimidyl ester) in dimethylacetamide is added with constant stirring at 4°C to a 21-fold excess. After 15 min it is brought to room temperature and stirred for another 30 min. The conjugate is purified on Sephadex G-25.

B. *Measurement of enzyme activity*

The reaction mixture (1 ml of 100 mM Tris-HCl buffer, pH 8.0) contains 5.0 μmol MgCl$_2$, 0.1 mmol KHCO$_3$, 3.3 μmol sodium pyruvate, 0.1 μmol acetyl coenzyme A, 1.7 μmol adenosine 5'-triphosphate, 0.1 μmol dithiobis(2-nitrobenzoic acid) (DTNB) and 1.0 U of citrate synthase. The activity of pyruvate carboxylase is determined after adding the enzyme from the initial increase in absorbance due to the reduction of DTND by coenzyme A (molar extinction coefficient DTNB at 412 nm is 14150 $M^{-1}cm^{-1}$).

C. *Assay*

20 μl of 1:2 diluted anti-DPH antiserum, 100 μl of serial dilutions of DPH or sample, and 30 μl of DPH-avidin (0.2 mg/ml) are incubated for 10 min at 23°C and assayed by adding 50 μl of pyruvate carboxylase (12 U/mg; 0.02 μg/ml).

---

in enzyme activity, giving the extreme cases:

absence of Ag:

$$Ab + Ag\cdot GU \rightarrow Ab - Ag\cdot GU \xrightarrow{BGase} \text{no fluorescence}$$

presence of Ag:

$$Ab + Ag \rightarrow Ab - Ag; \quad Ab - Ag + Ag\cdot GU \xrightarrow{BGase} \text{fluorescence}$$

The GU substrate is synthesized as described by Ngo et al. (1981)

and Burd et al. (1977) and is coupled to IgG (or to other proteins or haptens) as follows: 8.5 mg substrate (18 µmoles) in 2 ml distilled water are mixed with 10 mg dimethyladipimidate·2HCl (40 µmoles; Pierce, Rockford, IL) and 40 µl of triethylamine. The solution is stirred for 10 min at room temperature and 40 mg IgG in 100 mM pyrophosphate buffer, pH 8.5, are then added. After stirring for 2 h, the unreacted substrate is separated from IgG on Sephadex G-25 (3×50 cm) equilibrated with 100 mM sodium phosphate buffer, pH 7.0. The fractions with an absorbance ratio 280 nm/340 nm > 1 are pooled and dialyzed extensively (first against the column buffer with 1 M NaCl, then against the column buffer). Immediately before use, IgG·GU is diluted with 50 mM Bicine [N,N-bis(2-hydroxy-ethyl)glycine buffer, pH 8.2, containing 0.1% NaN_3]. The absorbance values indicate the relative content of IgG (at 280 nm, 0.1%; $A = 1.4$/cm) and of GU (at 340 nm, 1 mM; $A = 20.5$/cm). The test is described in Table 14.11.

A method similar in concept was described by Burd et al. (1977b) using haptens coupled via an ester bond to umbelliferone. Hydrolysis of the ester by porcine liver esterase is followed by the liberation of the fluorescent umbelliferone. This hydrolysis, however, is prevented or sharply reduced by the presence of antibody to the hapten: free hapten present in the test sample competes for the available antibody and more hydrolysis is produced by the enzyme.

14.3.1.4. Homogeneous competitive enzyme immunoassays using antibody–enzyme conjugates   Phospholipase C acts on phospholipids and hemolyses erythrocytes (RBC). Wei and Reibe (1977) conjugated antibody to this enzyme and showed that the enzyme becomes much less active when the antibody is complexed with a large antigen:

absence of Ag: → Ab·E + RBC → hemolysis

presence of Ag: → Ag–Ab·E + RBC → less hemolysis

In their study the antigen was IgG. The method is described in Table 14.12.

TABLE 14.11

Competitive homogeneous enzyme immunoassays using substrate-labeled antigen

Both tests are performed at 25°C.

A. *Determination of the concentration of large antigens (Ngo et al., 1981)*
   1. Prepare standard antigen solutions by serial dilution.

   2. Dilute the test sera 100-fold with 50 mM Bicine[a] buffer, pH 8.2. (Samples with very high or very low antigen concentrations are diluted accordingly.)

   3. Pipet into plastic cuvets suitable for fluorimetry, 0.1 ml diluted sample and 3 ml of the solution containing 0.28 nmole GU-Ag[b] in 50 mM Bicine.

   4. Add 100 μl of antiserum (10 × diluted in Bicine buffer).

   5. Mix and add 100 μl of the BGase solution containing 0.005 units of enzyme.

   6. Measure after 30 min fluorescence intensities with spectrofluorometer.

B. *Determination of the concentration of small antigens* (Burd et al., 1977).
   1. Mix BGase (25 ng/ml) and sufficient amounts of antiserum to decrease the reaction by about 25% in a total volume of 2 ml of 50 mM Bicine buffer, pH 8.2.

   2. Add to the mixture 1 μl of standard or test sample.

   3. After mixing, add 5 μl of GU-labeled hapten (about 0.125 absorbance units at 245 nm), and monitor the increase in fluorescence over 2–3 min.

---

[a] Bicine = N,N-bis(2-hydroxyethyl)-glycine.
[b] GU = β-galactosyl-umbelliferone   label   (= 6-(7-β-galactosylcoumarin-3-carbox-amido)-hexylamine.

14.3.1.5. Homogeneous competitive enzyme immunoassays using cofactor-labeled antigen   When an indispensable cofactor is conjugated with a hapten, reaction with the anti-hapten antibody prevents enzyme activity (Carrico et al., 1976; Schroeder et al., 1976). Carrico et al. (1976) conjugated a hapten (Ag) to nicotinamide-6-(2-amino-ethylamino) purine dinucleotide (aeNAD$^+$), a derivative of NAD$^+$, which is active with several dehydrogenases. The cycling sequences (Section 9.2.3.3) are:

TABLE 14.12

Homogeneous competitive enzyme immunoassays using antibody–enzyme conjugates

1. Pellet erythrocytes (RBC) by low-speed centrifugation and suspend in 30 volumes of PBS.

2. Incubate 50 μl of enzyme-labeled antibody with various amounts of antigen (50 μl) for 30 min at 37 °C.

3. Add 0.5 ml of diluted RBC suspension and incubate for 30 min at 37 °C with occasional stirring.

4. Centrifuge to sediment intact cells.

5. Carefully remove supernatant, mix with 1 ml of cyanomethemoglobin reagent (Hycel Inc., Houston, Texas) and measure absorbance at 540 nm against a blank containing a mixture of 1 ml cyanomethemoglobin reagent and 0.5 ml of incubation mixture without enzyme-labeled antibody.

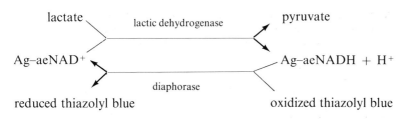

In this reaction sequence thiazolyl blue is measured since Ag-ae-NAD$^+$ concentrations are small compared to the K_m for NAD$^+$. Malic or alcohol dehydrogenase may also be used with Ag-aeNAD$^+$, with a considerably higher cycling speed than the combination above. The detectability may be improved with bacterial luciferase (Schroeder et al., 1976):

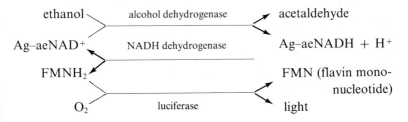

The light is generated within a few seconds after the formation of NADH and disappears shortly afterwards. However, various problems may arise in this assay (non-specific binding, degradation of NAD^+) and sensitive equipment for the measurement of bio-luminescence is needed.

14.4. Measurement of enzyme activity in enzyme immunoassays

14.4.1. Measurement of enzyme activity in solid-phase enzyme immunoassays

Interference with enzyme activity by sample constituents as encountered in homogeneous EIA is generally absent in solid-phase EIA, due to washing prior to revelation. Moreover, the integrity of the antibody–antigen interaction is not essential in the latter and pH can be raised (e.g. to 9.8, the optimum of APase), since disruption of the bonds between antibody and antigen at this point will not change the amount of enzyme present in the sample. On the other hand, the solid phase may influence the parameters of the immobilized enzyme (Section 9.2.2). It is hardly possible to give general rules for the optimum conditions, not only because of the large variety of solid phases in use, but also because of the substantial variation between or within the various lots of the same solid phase (Section 13.2.3). A preliminary test to establish the optimum conditions for a certain batch is simple and highly recommended. The conditions presented here may often serve as a guideline.

Most quantitative tests are designed so that after a short incubation period (e.g. 30 min), the build-up of colored product is suitable for measurement. Only few assays use enzyme kinetics for the estimation of enzyme concentrations, probably because such methods are less sensitive. Methods based on product build-up require the stopping of the reaction for all samples at the same time.

14.4.1.1. The preparation of substrate solutions and measurement of activity of horseradish peroxidase   The usefulness of POase is attested by its wide use. It is much cheaper than other enzymes, particularly if prepared by the fast and simple method (Section 10.1.1.2), it is easily conjugated and its activity is easily detected.

The substrate generally used for this enzyme is H_2O_2 which is unstable in stock solutions, but its concentration can be readily established from the optical density (Section 10.1.1.5). This is important since H_2O_2 is not only substrate but also inhibitor for POase. Therefore, optimal results are obtained only in a limited concentration range (Fig. 14.1). Though this effect is obvious for POase in solution, it should be investigated for POase immobilized on the solid phase used since it may significantly shift the optimum concentration (Section 9.2.2). Fig. 14.2 shows such a test for solid-phase EIA on polystyrene. Generally, little attention is paid to this fact and in most studies 2–4 times more substrate is used than needed for optimal reaction. The decrease in enzyme activity due to excess of H_2O_2 is more pronouced for the immobilized enzyme than for

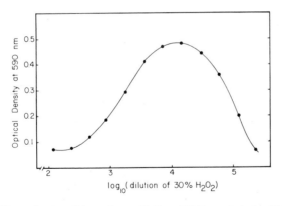

Fig. 14.1. Determination of the optimum dilution of H_2O_2 as substrate with horseradish POase C with DMAB/MBTH as H-donor. High dilutions as well as high concentrations of the substrate decrease the detectability of the enzyme. The optimum is around 0.0025–0.003% H_2O_2 (reproduced from Tijssen et al., 1982; courtesy of *Archives of Virology*).

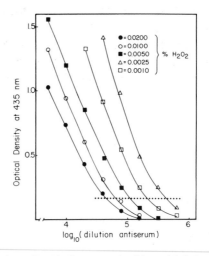

Fig. 14.2. Solid-phase EIA (indirect assay) with purified 5-aminosalicylic acid as H-donor and different concentrations of substrate. Best results are obtained with 0,0025% H_2O_2. Courtesy *Archives of Virology*.

the free enzyme (unpublished observation). If the concentration of the 30% H_2O_2 stock solution is indeed 30%, dilution by a factor of 10000–12000 is often optimal for the substrate. Care should be taken that this dilution is indeed obtained, since large pipetting errors may occur (a drop on the pipet tip may increase considerably the concentration due to the small amounts needed). Metal microsyringes should not be used; in fact solutions used for POase should be free of metal ions. H_2O_2 is diluted immediately before use.

The preference for any of the different chromogenic H-donors depends largely on individual laboratories. In general, the most commonly used donors are quite satisfactory. In EIA both the substrate and the product should have an adequate solubility to keep light scattering at a minimum. In contrast, in immunoblotting and EIH 4-chloro-1-naphthol (Chapter 16) and 3,3'-diaminobenzidine (Chapter 17) are preferred as substrate, yielding an insoluble product which precipitates at the location of the enzyme. The most commonly used H-donors in EIA are 5-aminosalicylic acid (5-AS), *o*-dianisidine

(ODA), 2,2′-azino-di-(3-ethylbenzothiazoline-6-sulfonate) (ABTS), *o*-toluidine (OT), *o*-phenylenediamine (OPD), 3,3′,5,5′-tetramethylbenzidine (TMB), and the MBTH–DMAB pair [MBTH: 3-methyl-2-benzothiazolinone hydrazone; DMAB: 3-(dimethyl-amino) benzoic acid]. The preparation of the most suitable H-donors is given in Table 14.13.

TABLE 14.13

Preparation of hydrogen donor solutions for solid-phase enzyme immunoassays using peroxidase[a]

A. *Preparation of substrate solution from commercial (95% pure) 5-aminosalicylic acid (5-AS)*
1. Dissolve 80 mg of 5-AS in 100 ml distilled water and heat at 70 °C for about 5 min with stirring.

2. Cool solution to 20 °C and adjust the pH to 6.0 with a few drops of 1 M NaOH.

B. *Preparation of substrate solution from pure 5-AS*
1. Purify commercial 5-AS according to Section 10.1.1.4.

2. Store the purified preparation in a desiccator in the dark.

3. Dissolve 1 g in 1 litre of 10 mM phosphate buffer, pH 6.0, containing 0.1 mM EDTA.

4. Store in convenient aliquots (e.g., 20 ml) at −20 °C.

5. Before use, bring to room temperature to dissolve white precipitate appearing just after thawing, under the hot water tap.

C. *Preparation of 2,2′-azino-di(3-ethylbenzthiazoline-6-sulfonic acid) (ABTS)*
Dissolve 40 mg ABTS in 100 ml 100 mM phosphate-citrate buffer, pH 4.0.

D. *Preparation of o-phenylenediamine (OPD)*
Dissolve just before use 200 mg OPD in 100 ml 100 mM sodium citrate (pH 5.0) and shield from light. OPD from Merck gave 3 times higher absorbance than from Sigma (Gallati and Brodbeck, 1982). However, this may, at least partially, be due to the use of the HCl form of the OPD from Sigma. This OPD·HCl at the concentrations used by these authors decreases considerably the pH and lowers thus the activity (adjust pH after dissolving OPD·HCl!). The commonly used concentration of 0.4 mg/ml is considerably suboptimal.

E. *Preparation of o-dianisidine*
   1. Dissolve *o*-dianisidine in methanol (10 mg/ml).

   2. Just before use, dilute 0.9 ml of this solution with 100 ml 100 mM phosphate-citrate buffer, pH 5.0.

F. *Preparation of 3-methyl-2-benzothiazoline hydrazone (MBTH) and 3-(dimethyl-amino)benzoic acid (DMAB)*[b]
   1. Prepare 30 mM DMAB in 100 mM phosphate buffer, pH 6.5, and store in tight-ly closed amber bottles at 4°C.

   2. Prepare 0.6 mM MBTH in 100 mM phosphate buffer, pH 6.5, and store as in step 1.

   3. Just before use, mix 7 volumes of 100 mM sodium phosphate-citrate buffer, pH 6.0, with 1 volume of the MBTH and 1 volume of the DMAB solutions.

G. *Preparation of o-tolidine (OT)*
   1. Dissolve 21.2 mg OT (dihydrochloride salt) in 1 ml DMF.

   2. Add 200 mM sodium acetate buffer, pH 3.7, to 100 ml and adjust the pH to 3.7.

H. *Preparation of 3,3′,5,5′ tetramethylbenzidine (TMB)*
   1. Dissolve 5 mg TMB in 2.5 ml absolute ethanol (heating to 40°C may be neces-sary).

   2. Prepare 200 mM acetate buffer, pH 3.3, and add 5 ml to 92.5 ml distilled water containing 100 mg nitroferricyanide.

   3. Mix the two solutions and peroxide just before use. Containers should be free of oxidizing agents since TMB is readily oxidized (TMB should remain pale red-dish brown).

---

[a] H_2O_2 should be added just before use and the optimum concentration should be deter-mined for the individual test conditions (0.003% H_2O_2 is generally satisfactory). Tem-perature of the reaction should be controlled to have meaningful results: in solid-phase EIA, POase is less active at temperatures above 20°C. Porstmann et al. (1981) recom-mend the addition of Tween 20 (0.05%) to the solutions to prevent inactivation of the enzyme.
[b] An alternative method for POase detection using modified MBTH has been reported (Capaldi and Taylor, 1983) but not yet applied in EIA.

Bullock and Walls (1977) evaluated 5-AS, ODA and 3-amino-9-ethylcarbazole (AEC) and found 5-AS the most satisfactory. Saunders et al. (1977) compared 5-AS with ABTS, using 414 nm for ABTS and 500 nm for 5-AS, and found ABTS more satisfactory (stronger absorbance, higher stability of stock solutions, availability of substrate in pure form). Voller et al. (1979) compared ODA, 5-AS, ABTS, OT and OPD; they noted the limited solubility of ODA and 5-AS and preferred OPD over the others. OPD is mutagenic (Voller et al., 1979), and although it gives the highest absorbance values, background levels (with negative reference sera) are also higher. Recently, Al-Kaissi and Mostratos (1983) compared ABTS, 5-AS and OPD and found that they were equally satisfactory.

5-AS is a most convenient H-donor, despite some contrary reports cited above. Two important considerations, one or both of which were ignored in these comparative studies, should have been taken into account: none of these studies used pure 5-AS (commercially not available) and all but the study of Al-Kaissi and Mostratos (1983) monitored the oxidation of 5-AS at a suboptimal wavelength. Commercially available 5-AS preparations are brown-purple and poorly soluble whereas the purified product is white, soluble, stable in stock solutions and yields considerably lower background staining. Purification of 5-AS is very simple (Section 10.1.1.4.2). ABTS is commercially supplied in a pure form. However, the initial supposition that it is not dangerous to health is contradicted by recent reports (Section 18.2). OPD is a convenient H-donor (Section 10.1.1.4.2) and generally yields the highest absorbance, though it is quite photosensitive. Full advantage of OPD can be taken only if the cut-off level of absorbance (Section 15.2.3), above which the color development is considered indicative of the presence of enzyme, can be chosen sufficiently high since background levels tend to be significant.

Oxidative coupling of MBTH and DMAB (Section 10.2.1.4.2) has been applied successfully for EIA (Tijssen et al., 1982; Geoghegan et al., 1983). The detection limit for POase is about 2 fmoles and both detectability and background levels are higher than with 5-AS

(Tijssen et al., 1982) (Fig. 14.3). Geoghegan et al. (1983) found large differences among the buffers used with these H-donors: 100 mM phosphate–citric acid, pH 6.0 was as satisfactory as HEPES, but much cheaper. MBTH and DMAB are poorly soluble below pH 5.5–5.8, but higher pH or lower ionic strength increases the absorbance of the blanks. The reaction should be stopped (by enzyme inhibition) after 20–30 min. Both DMAB and MBTH are photo-sensitive and the blanks develop color when exposed to light.

The presence of non-ionic detergents (Tween 20, Triton X-100) in the substrate solution is uncommon, but may have a beneficial effect on enzyme activity (Section 10.1.1.4.2). These detergents delay inactivation of the enzyme and increase the optimum temperature

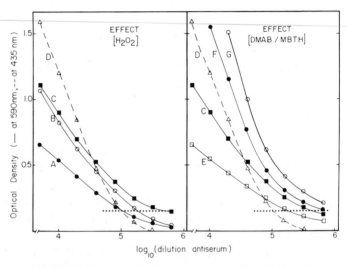

Fig. 14.3. DMAB/MBTH as H-donor and the effect of H_2O_2 as compared to 5-aminosalicylic acid (D). In the left frame various concentrations of H_2O_2 namely 0.03% (A), 0.0003% (B) and 0.003% (C) were used with the standard concentrations of DMAB (25 mg/100 ml) and MBTH (0.75 mg/100 ml). The response could be increased (right frame) by increasing the DMAB/MBTH concentration two-fold (F) and four-fold (G), whereas a two-fold dilution decreased the detectability (E), the H_2O_2 concentration being kept constant (0.003%). The DMAB/MBTH system gave, however higher backgrounds. Courtesy *Archives of Virology*.

(from 15 to 20°C) and this effect is H-donor dependent (activation ranging from 20% for ABTS to 90% for ODA).

Determination of POase activity in solid-phase EIA is different from that of free POase in solution (Section 10.1.1.5). The amount of chromophore produced during a certain period (20 min, 30 min, 1 h, etc.) is determined from the absorbance [5-AS at 492 nm; ABTS at 415 nm; OPD at 492 nm if acidified with HCl (pH 1.0), at pH 5.0 the peak is at 445 nm (usual filter 436 nm); ODA at 400 nm; DMAB/MBTH at 590 nm (usual filter, 620 nm)]. To obtain the exact color development in each sample, it is necessary to stop the reaction after identical periods. Color development with ABTS and 5-AS can be stopped with 0.2 volume of 37 mM NaCN (poison!), oxidation of OPD is blocked with 0.5 volume of 4 M H_2SO_4 or HCl and the reaction with MBTH/DMAB is arrested with 0.1 volume of 1M H_2SO_4 or HCl (the blue-purple color changes to blue, but the absorption at 590 nm remains virtually unchanged).

The ubiquitous catalase may sometimes interfere (Geoghegan et al., 1983), because it is a strong competitor for H_2O_2. NaN_3 may be used for the pH-dependent selective inhibition of catalase without affecting POase (Lenhoff and Kaplan, 1955).

14.4.1.2. The assay of β-galactosidase on the solid phase   BGase is often used with a fluorogenic substrate for ultrasensitive solid-phase EIA (Section 14.5.1.1.1). Absorption methods for the determination of BGase are based on the release of NP (absorbing at 405 nm) upon hydrolysis of *o*-nitrophenyl-β-D-galactoside (*o*-NP-G) by the enzyme (Section 10.1.2.3).

Substrate solution is prepared by dissolving 70 mg (2.3 mM) *o*-NP-G per 100 ml 100 mM potassium phosphate buffer, pH 7.0, containing 1mM $MgCl_2$ and 10 mM 2-ME. It is not advised to assay the enzyme over prolonged periods at temperatures exceeding 30°C because of possible spontaneous hydrolysis of the substrate (Section 10.1.3.5). At a fixed period after the addition of the substrate, catalysis is stopped with 0.25 volumes of 2 M Na_2CO_3. The absorbance is measured at 405 nm, after calibration of the spectrophotometer or microplate reader with known amounts of o-NP (prepared as in Section 10.1.3.6).

14.4.1.3. The assay of alkaline phosphatase on the solid phase
The different substrate solutions for the bacterial and the intestinal mucosal enzyme are prepared as in Table 14.14. In the case of the intestinal mucosal enzyme, diethanolamine (DEA) buffer should be used, because of the poor buffering capacity of the glycine buffer (sometimes used) at pH 10.0. However, $MgCl_2$ does not activate the enzyme in DEA buffers as noted for other buffers (Section 10.1.3.4). The reaction is traditionally stopped after a predetermined incubation period with 0.25 volumes of 2 M NaOH. Enzyme activity can also be stopped with metal-chelating products (Section 10.1.3.4). Brauner and Fridlender (1981) arrested color development for at least 1 day with cysteine and EDTA or EGTA at final concentrations of 1 and 5mM, respectively. Yolken and Leister (1982) studied the effect of the incubation time on the detection limit of antigens and found that about 640 pg of antigen was detectable after 10 min and about 10 pg after 240 min. This corresponds to the minimum amount of antigen detectable with a fluorogenic substrate but in

TABLE 14.14
Preparation of substrates for bacterial and intestinal alkaline phosphatase immobilized on the solid phase[a]

A. *Bacterial APase*
Dissolve 1 mg p-nitrophenyl phosphate in 1 ml 100 mM Tris-HCl buffer, pH 8.1, containing 0.01% $MgCl_2$, just before use.

B. *Intestinal mucosal APase*
1. Mix 97 ml diethanolamine (DEA) with 1 l 0.01% $MgCl_2$ solution, adjust the pH to 9.8 with 1 N HCl. The solution, 10% (w/w) DEA buffer, can be stored at room temperature in an amber bottle if NaN_3 (0.2 g/l) is added.

2. Dissolve p-nitrophenyl phosphate in the buffer to a final concentration of 1 mg/ml, just before use.

[a] Reaction is stopped after predetermined period by adding 0.1 volume of 10 mM cysteine.

a much shorter time (≈ 10 min). Detectability in this system seems, therefore, to be limited by the ability of the antigen to bind to the antibody on the solid phase.

14.4.1.4. The assay of glucose oxidase on the solid phase   The catalytic properties of GOase have been discussed in Section 10.1.4.3. Among the different assays of GOase, both fluorometric (Section 10.1.4.4) and spectrophotometric (Section 10.1.4.3) techniques are popular in EIA. GOase converts glucose to D-glucose-δ-lactone while producing H_2O_2 (Section 10.1.4.3). The addition of an excess of POase and a suitable H-donor serves as an indicator system for the GOase activity. A problem with GOase is that the concentration of oxygen is usually not much higher than its K_m and mixed-order kinetics can be expected (Section 9.1.2). The substrate solution is prepared by dissolving glucose to 280 mM in 67 mM phosphate buffer (pH 5.6), adding a suitable H-donor (Table 14.13) and POase (25 μg/ml). Commercial preparations of GOase often contain catalase which interferes (Section 10.1.4). Therefore, GOase-conjugates should always be tested for catalase activity and POase should be used at a large excess.

14.4.1.5. Titration with urease on the solid phase   Urease is used for titration only since its utility is based on the shift of pH due to the hydrolysis of urea (production of ammonia) which is detected with an indicator (bromocresol purple), added to the substrate solution (pK of 6.3). A change from yellow to purple indicates the positive samples. The preparation of the substrate is given in Section 10.1.5.

14.4.2. Measurement of enzyme activity in homogeneous enzyme immunoassays

Homogeneous assays are not subjected to separation steps and the assay mixture may contain many substances (introduced with the sample) such as inhibitors, activators, contaminating enzymes, etc., in addition to the essential components.

Enzyme activity is established under optimum conditions, as discussed for the various enzymes in Chapter 10, unless contraindicated in Section 14.3. However, these conditions should not be to the detriment of the antigen–antibody interaction, i.e., the pH should be close to neutrality and the ionic strength suitable. Homogeneous systems with assay conditions different from those described in Chapter 10 are given in Section 14.3.

14.5 Improvements in the detectability, specificity, and speed of enzyme immunoassays

Although the various parameters of EIA are interrelated: i.e., higher specificity is often associated with a lower background staining but may be at the cost of detectability, which in turn may affect the incubation period, they are discussed separately.

Almost all studies designed to increase detectability were centered on a single aspect of the assay: efforts are generally concentrated on one particular parameter. However, much can be gained from the systematic improvement of each variable of the assay. An example, taking several factors into account, was recently given by Imagawa et al. (1982).

14.5.1. Improvements in detectability

The most obvious factors determining the detection limit in EIA are the absorption of the specific reagent to the solid phase (e.g., the use of polyclonal sera with only low levels of antibodies decreases detectability), the ratio of the surface of the solid phase to the volume of the sample, the stability of the interaction with the solid phase, the avidity of the antigen–antibody reaction, the quality of the conjugate and the chromogenic property of the substrate.

The design of the EIA may also be modified to improve the detection limit, as was discussed with the direct, indirect and bridge methods (Section 14.2.1.3).

Improvements in the adsorption of the immunoreactant on the solid phase and in the preparation of the conjugates have been amply discussed (Chapter 13; Chapter 11). Here, methods will be given to lower the detection limits of the enzymes and to increase the ratio of the enzyme molecules to the initially adsorbed immunoreactant in the complex.

14.5.1.1. Lowering of the detection limit of the enzyme   There are two critical factors limiting the detectability of enzymes: the assay conditions of the enzyme and its inherent specific activity. The former limit can be improved by using optimum assay conditions; the latter, by employing the enzyme with the highest specific activity, as illustrated for POase (Section 10.2.1.2). For example, BGase from *Escherichia coli* is 50–100 times more active than the same enzyme from *Aspergillus oryzae* (Ishikawa and Kato, 1978). Similar differences have been noted for other enzymes (APase, POase, etc., Chapter 10).

Another critical factor limiting the detectability in EIA is the amount of product which should accumulate before reliable measurements can be made. A fluorogenic, chemiluminescent or radioactive substrate may lower significantly the detection limit, but it may also require more sophisticated equipment.

14.5.1.1.1. Fluorogenic substrates   Extraneous fluorescent material may be present in ordinary distilled water, making filtration necessary.

Widely used fluorogenic substrates for APase and BGase are the 4-methylumbelliferyl derivatives which, upon hydrolysis, yield 4-methylumbelliferone (4-MU), detectable at a 100-fold lower concentration than NP. Using such substrates, Shalev et al. (1980) detected antigen at a concentration of about 5×10^{-15} mg/ml, i.e., 25000 molecules of IgG. This increase in detectability may not be achieved if, as is often the case, other factors are limiting (Section 14.4.1.3). Nevertheless, fluorogenic substrates may allow the detection of femtomolar (10^{-15}) or even attomolar (10^{-18}) levels of BGase (Ishikawa and Kato, 1978) or POase (Puget et al., 1977). The failure to enhance detectability using one of these substrates indicates that other assay conditions should be improved. The preparation of fluorogenic substrates is given in Table 14.15.

BGase is the most often used enzyme if high detectability is required. The hydrolysis of 4-methylumbelliferyl-D-galactopyranoside yields fluorescent 4-MU. The wavelength used for excitation and emission analysis are 360 and 440 or 450 nm, respectively. Although

TABLE 14.15
Preparation of fluorogenic substrates

A. *4-Methylumbelliferyl-D-galactopyranoside (4-MU-Gal)*
  1. Prepare 10 mM sodium phosphate buffer, pH 7.0, containing 100 mM NaCl, 1 mM $MgCl_2$, 0.1% NaN_3 and 0.1% BSA.

  2. Prepare a 0.1 mM 4-MU-Gal solution in the buffer. This is achieved by diluting 0.34 ml of a 1% solution of 4-MU-Gal (in DMF) with 100 ml of the buffer.

  3. The 'stop-buffer', used to terminate the reaction after a predetermined period (e.g., 60 min) by adding 0.5 volume, consists of 1.0 M glycine-NaOH, pH 10.3.

B. *4-Methylumbelliferyl-phosphate (4-MU-P)*
  1. Prepare buffer according to the enzyme, as in Table 14.14.

  2. Add 4-MU-P to a final concentration of 0.1 mM, immediately before use.

C. *3-(p-Hydroxyphenyl)propionic acid (HPPA)*
  1. Prepare 100 mM sodium phosphate buffer, pH 8.0 and add 5 g HPPA per litre (pH becomes 7.0).

  2. Add to solid-phase immobilized POase (washed prior with 100 mM sodium phosphate buffer, pH 7.0).

  3. After 5 min at 30 °C, add 1/5 volume 0.03% H_2O_2 and continue incubation for desired period (10–100 min; Table 10.2). It might be useful to determine the optimum peroxide concentration for a particular system.

  4. Stop the enzyme reaction and the generation of fluorescence by adding an equal volume of 200 mM glycine–NaOH, pH 10.3.

  5. Use 320 nm as the excitation wavelength and 405 nm as the emission wavelength (1 mg/l of quinine in 0.1 N H_2SO_4 can be used as a standard to adjust a scale to 100).

for quantitative investigations a spectrofluorometer is required, it is possible to use a UV lightbox for simple titrations (Forghani et al., 1980) or for the fast screening of a large number of samples. For spectrofluorometric determinations, an aliquot (e.g. 0.3 ml) is transferred from the microplate well to fluorescence cuvettes and diluted to 1 ml with distilled water (Konijn et al., 1982). Labrousse et al. (1982) described an accessory for the spectrofluorometer for the measurement of the fluorescence on thin layer chromatograms.

Essentially the same principles apply for APase, where also 4-MU is measured (produced by hydrolysis of 4-methylumbelliferyl phosphate, 4-MU-P). The fluorescent product can be measured within the range of 20–200 pM, whereas the chromophore, NP, is detectable only at 1000-fold higher concentrations (Shalev et al., 1980). The K_m of 4-MU-P is about 20000 times lower than for NPP (2.5×10^{-6} vs. 4.8×10^{-2} M) but the V_{max} for 4-MU-P is about 16 times lower than the V_{max} for NPP (Shalev et al., 1980). These Michaelis parameters were determined from the Lineweaver–Burk plot (Section 9.1.2). The V_{max}/K_m ratio (a measure of the preference of the enzyme for a substrate) is about 3000 times higher for 4-MU-P than for NPP. Other advantages of this system are the much shorter reaction time (maximum detectability is obtained after 15 min instead of 10 h since the substrate is not the limiting factor), the savings in the cost of the substrate (35 times less substrate is needed) and the wide range of detection offered by modern spectrofluorometers (channels with 1000-fold light multiplication). Compared to BGase, the APase system has the disadvantage of producing reagent blanks which are about 50-fold higher, due to the spontaneous degradation of the substrate (Neurath and Strick, 1981).

Zaitsu and Okhura (1980) described a sensitive fluorometric assay for POase using 3-(p-hydroxyphenyl) propionic acid, HPPA, (Aldrich), with which POase activity as low as 8 U could be detected (excitation wavelength 320 nm; emission wavelength 404 nm). This fluorogenic method, in contrast to the assays with BGase of APase, has not yet been used on a large scale. The K_m for HPPA and for H_2O_2 were 9.8 mM and 0.43 nM, and the V_{max} 20 mM and

1.3 mM, respectively. These measurements were carried out at relatively high pH (Table 14.17C) where the most intense fluorescence was obtained (pH higher than 9.0 induces more background fluorescence). It is known, however, that POase is more active at a lower pH (Section 10.1.1.5). An experiment, performing the reaction at a lower pH and measuring the fluorescence at a higher pH, was not reported.

14.5.1.1.2. Chemiluminescence   Analytical luminescence has a considerable potential but requires a special light-measuring device (e.g., liquid scintillation counter with the coincidence disconnected). With this method, quantitative estimation of IgG and herpes virus has about 100 times lower limits than absorptiometric EIA (Pronovost et al., 1981). POase catalyzes the oxidation of isoluminol by H_2O_2 and the reaction is accompanied by a measurable emission of light ('chemiluminescence').

The assay is performed at room temperature at high pH (10.5) in the dark. Polystyrene beads are used as the solid phase. At the end of the immune reaction, the beads are added to 1.24 ml distilled water, followed by the addition of 0.3 ml 1 mM EDTA and 30 µl isoluminol (0.1 mM in 1.0 M glycine–NaOH buffer, pH 10.5). The emitted light is measured immediately after the addition of 1 ml 0.3 mM H_2O_2. The blank contains no enzyme.

An alternative chemiluminescence method for EIA is based on the reduction of POase compounds I and II (Section 10.2.1.3) by eosin and EDTA (de Toledo et al., 1980). This method may overcome some of the difficulties encountered with luminol (hard to purify, rather poor reproducibility).

Chemiluminescent substrates have also been developed for luciferase (Neufeld et al., 1965), GPDase (Haggerty et al., 1978), catalase (Neufeld et al., 1965) and BGase (Puget et al., 1977).

14.5.1.1.3. Radioactive substrates   Radioactive substrates have also been used to enhance the detectability of EIA. Such methods generally require a step for the separation of the substrate from the product. This may be performed by ion-exchange methods (Harris et al., 1979; Yolken et al., 1980), as for APase with [³H]AMP as substrate (10 μCi/ml; 3.7×10^5 disintegrations/sec in 10% DEA buffer, pH 9.0 containing 1 mM $MgCl_2$). A positively charged ion-exchange resin (e.g., DEAE-cellulose) retains the negatively charged AMP or phosphate while the neutral adenosine flows freely through. This method is capable of detecting fmol levels of antigen.

Fields et al. (1981) eliminated the separation step by using glutamate decarboxylase which converts (in a scintillation vial) L-[^{14}C]-glutamic acid to $^{14}CO_2$ which is released from the aqueous phase. Detectability is about 100-fold higher than with RIA.

14.5.1.2. Increasing the enzyme/antigen ratio   The number of enzyme molecules per antigen molecule can be increased by simple changes in the design of the assay (Section 14.2.1.2 through Section 14.2.1.3). At the end of the actual assay, further amplification steps may also be introduced. If antigens are initially immobilized and antibodies are assayed, enzyme-coupled SpA in the last assay step followed by enzyme-coupled anti-SpA antibodies can amplify the reaction (Holbeck and Nepom, 1983).

Bovine serum albumin (BSA)–antibody conjugates in the last step of the EIA, followed by anti-BSA antibodies conjugated with enzyme can also be used (Guesdon et al., 1983).

14.5.2. Improvements in specificity

Non-specific reactions in EIA can be due to a variety of mechanisms, many of which are discussed in detail elsewhere (Section 6.1.6.3, Section 8.6, Section 17.3.4). Non-specific reactions enhance background levels ('noise of experiment') and have, therefore, a direct impact on the detectability.

Antibodies prepared against a crude antigen give positive reactions with antigens other than the target antigen. Absorption of the antibody preparation with the contaminating antigens (if available) or the production of monoclonal antibodies can eliminate this problem. Interference can also be prevented by the addition of normal serum to the antiserum. Hogg and Davidson (1982) identified thus 10% of positive sera as false positives.

Excessive background levels may be due to the presence of endogenous enzymes. Enzymes of microbial origin not occurring in mammalian cells, e.g., GOase, neutral BGase, β-lactamase (Citri, 1971), can overcome this problem. High background levels may also arise if only a small fraction of the antibodies is specific and a large excess of enzyme is needed for their detection.

Schuit et al. (1981) investigated the specificity of 29 fluorochrome-conjugated antisera against human IgG and found half of these commercial preparations unsatisfactory, indicating the frequent absence of adequate quality control. The adequacy of the antiserum should, therefore, be established by strict testing.

A most common reason for the occurrence of non-specific reactions is due to the presence of rheumatoid factors (RF; Section 6.1.6.3). These auto-antibodies react specifically with IgG, and may give a false-positive reaction when IgG is already in the complex. RF have variable species specificity and may be found also in sera and synovial fluids of normal subjects or of individuals with other diseases (Palosua and Milgrom, 1981). Several EIA have been developed to detect RF of the IgM- or IgG-type (Gripenberg et al., 1979; Palosua and Milgrom, 1981; Faith et al., 1982). IgM RF can be recognized by incubating the test serum directly with the IgG-coated solid phase in the absence of antigen and revealing with enzyme-labeled anti-IgM antibodies. For the IgG RF (Faith et al., 1982), the test serum is first diluted (1:50) with an acetate buffer (100 mM, pH 4.4) containing 10 µg/ml pepsin, incubated for 20 h at 37°C and neutralized with 250 µl of Na_2HPO_4 (80 g/l containing 0.05% Tween 20); 5 µl of this sample are then added to the IgG immobilized on the solid phase. After appropriate washings, IgG RF are detected with enzyme-labeled anti-Fab antibodies.

One or several of the following approaches may be taken to eliminate or reduce interference by RF: (i) use of F(ab')$_2$ (RF reacts only with the Fc of antibodies); (ii) removal of RF with an excess of Fc of the species used as antibodies (Winchester, 1980); (iii) addition of an excess of normal IgG or heat aggregated IgG (0.3 mg/ml) (Millan and Stigbrand, 1981); this method is very simple but can only be used if the normal IgG contains no antibodies towards the antigen tested; (iv) adsorption with beads coated with Fc (this immunosorbent may be regenerated with acid; Section 7.1.9.2.5); and, (v) reduction of the polymeric IgM RF in the test serum with 2-ME or N-acetylcysteine (Yolken and Stopa, 1979) (not suitable if the antigen to be tested is affected by reduction). In some cases RF do not cause false positive results unless anti-nuclear antibodies are also present in the test system (Naot et al., 1981). In this case the use of $F(ab')_2$ for the preparation of conjugates prevents non-specific reactions.

A simple method to reduce non-specific interactions between serum factors is to change the composition of the buffer (Kato et al., 1980), as for the prevention of non-specific interaction between the serum and plastics in the preparation of sections for EIH at the ultrastructural level (Section 17.4.3). This is achieved by raising the ionic strength (with 300 mM NaCl) and by adding 0.5% gelatin. However, gelatin increases considerably the viscosity of the buffer, particularly at lower temperatures. This effect can be corrected by digesting a 10% solution of gelatin in 50 mM sodium phosphate buffer, pH 8.0, containing 2 mM calcium acetate, with protease T (2 mg/ml) at 50°C; digestion is stopped after 20 min by boiling for 20 min.

Non-specific reactions may also follow from cross-reactivity among Ig of different species which may be so strong that assays may be based on it (Section 17.3.4.1). Such cross-reactivity is eliminated by haptenating the immunoreactant and using anti-hapten antibodies (Section 12.5).

It is a good practice, although time-consuming and costly, to confirm positive reactions with blocking tests (reaction of the antigen with antibodies from an independent source, prior to the addition of the test serum) or neutralization tests (treatment of the test serum with antigen, prior to the addition to the antigen-coated solid phase). If available, pre-infection sera should also be tested, as well as non-immune sera, as controls.

14.5.3. Shortening of the length of the assay

A systematic investigation of the various experimental parameters should reveal the minimum time required for the best and fastest results. This could reduce considerably the assay time required. Coating of the solid phase is generally achieved much faster at room temperature or at 37°C, than under the commonly used conditions of 16 h at 4°C. This reflects not only the higher diffusion rate and, therefore, higher collision rate of the particles with the solid phase, but also an increased hydrophobic interaction (Tijssen et al., 1982).

Immune reactions can be accelerated considerably in the presence of polyethylene glycol (PEG) 6000 (Hellsing and Richter, 1974). This method has been applied successfully for EIA (Salonen and Vaheri, 1981; Tijssen et al., 1982; Konijn et al., 1982). Several important conclusions of these studies should be considered (Fig. 14.4).

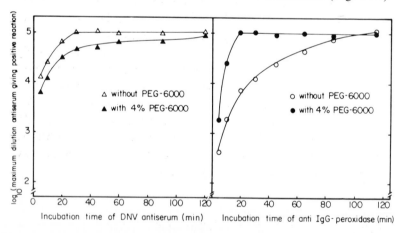

Fig. 14.4. Indirect EIA with or without polyethylene glycol (PEG) 6000. Virus was immobilized and antiserum was added with or without PEG 6000 (left frame) and detected subsequently with peroxidase-conjugated anti-IgG antibodies (right frame) with or without PEG 6000. The threshold activity obtained after various incubation periods of the solutions was determined. It can be seen that PEG 6000 has no beneficial effect on the first reaction, in contrast to the subsequent reaction(s).

Courtesy *Archives of Virology*.

Increasing the PEG 6000 concentration, both accelerates the reaction and increases the detectability but above 6% the background also increases. Therefore, 4% PEG 6000 is a good compromise. There is no acceleration and we even observed a negative effect, if PEG 6000 is included in the solution of the immunoreactant added to the coated solid phase. However, a very considerable acceleration (at least 3-fold) is obtained in all subsequent steps. In the indirect method 30 min incubation at 37°C with the conjugate suffices largely, instead of the 2–3 h otherwise used. PEG should not be included in stock solutions and sera, since it is detrimental to the shelf-life.

Another short-cut may be achieved by the use of two different monoclonal antibodies directed against two distinct epitopes. One antibody is adsorbed on the solid phase and the enzyme-conjugate of the other monoclonal antibody is added together with the assay antigen (Uotila et al., 1981). There is, however, a pitfall with this technique at high antigen concentrations (Nomura et al., 1983): the labeled antibody tends to mask the antigen which then fails to react with the immobilized antibody. Two considerably different concentrations of antigen yielded similar results and very high, but clinically expectable, concentrations of antigen gave false-negative results. Yolken and Leister (1982) used polyclonal antisera ('multiple-determinant EIA') with the modification that antigen (50 µl) was added to the immobilized antibodies 10 min before the conjugate (50 µl). The plates were washed 10 min later, incubated with the substrate for 10 min and the absorbance measured. The same problems may also be encountered with this assay as above.

14.6. Novel or alternative approaches to enzyme immunoassays

14.6.1. Cycling systems in enzyme immunoassays

Many enzymes yield more than 10^5 product molecules per enzyme molecule per min. However, it may take a long time to accumulate measurable amounts of product, during which the background may also increase and enzyme activity decrease. For some systems, enzyme cycling may be used to enhance the signal: the small amount of substrate, after its conversion to products, is immediately regenerated from one of the products. Harper and Orengo (1981) employed amyloglucosidase conjugated to antibodies by $NaIO_4$ method (Section 11.2.2). The basic feature of this amplification is that the concentration of the first substrate (glucose) is well below the overall K_m of the cycle, so that it obeys first-order kinetics (Section 9.1.2). Therefore, under appropriate conditions only time limits the detectability of the assay: femtomoles (10^{-15} M) may be measured in 3–5 min, but the limit of detection may be lowered by several orders of magnitude, simply by prolonging the incubation.

14.6.2. Thermometric enzyme immunoassays

This method is based on the measurement of heat evolved during an enzyme-catalyzed reaction (Mattiasson and Borrebaeck, 1980). A schematic presentation of this very rapid assay (12 min for solid-phase EIA) is given in Fig. 14.5. The heat generated during the catalytic reaction is measured with an enzyme thermistor unit. Sepha-

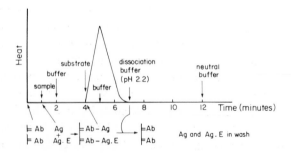

Fig. 14.5. Thermometric EIA. Antibody is immobilized in a small column in a thermistor unit. To these antibodies subsequent reactants are added as indicated in the bottom, the reaction is measured in terms of heat generated. Including the regeneration of the column, the total cycle takes about 12 min. This representation is modified from Mattiasson et al. (1977).

rose with the immobilized antibody is packed in a small glass or teflon column. A mixture antigen (test or calibration) and catalase-conjugated antigen is passed over such a column, substrate is added, the heat pulse measured. The column is regenerated by an acid wash. The thermistor was described by Danielsson et al. (1979).

14.6.3. Affinity chromatography-based enzyme immunoassays

As in the thermometric assays, affinity chromatography may serve to separate bound from free reactants (Terouanne et al., 1980). Instead of measuring heat as in Section 14.6.2., the product is measured in the effluent.

14.6.4. Immunocapillary migration systems

These approaches are very useful for field use since no laboratory equipment is required and are fast, though the concentration at the detection limit is rather high (150 ng/ml; Glad and Grubb, 1978, 1981). One is based on capillary migration of the antigen on immunosorbent strips (5 × 70 mm, cellulose acetate, with covalently linked antibodies). Each strip is marked at 60 mm from the end, placed in a cup containing the sample and capillary migration is allowed to proceed to the mark. The strips are washed briefly with buffer, incubated for a few minutes with the POase conjugate and, after another wash, the presence of conjugate is revealed with 4-chloro-1-naphthol (Section 16.3). The height of the staining is indicative of the antigen concentration and can be compared to calibration curves. Another system was devised for detection of different antigens.

Glass capillary tubes are internally coated with antibodies (Chandler and Hurrell, 1982) and tubes with antibodies of different specificity are joined and connected to a small (1 ml) syringe by silicone rubber tubing. The procedure then consists of simply drawing in and expelling the reagents in the order of test sample (10 min), washing buffer (three times), urease-conjugated antibodies (10 min), washing buffer, substrate solution (bromocresol, Gurr, London, UK; Section 14.4.1.5).

14.6.5. Enzyme immunoelectrodes and potentiometric enzyme immunoassays

The sensitive part of an electrode is covered with a membrane on which the enzyme is immobilized in immunocomplexes. The enzyme-catalyzed reaction takes place near the sensor (Mattiasson and Nilsson, 1977). The method is as fast as the thermometric assay but less sensitive. Electrode-based EIA using urease conjugates have been reviewed by Meyerhoff and Rechnitz (1980). This method has reasonably low detection limits. These promising potentiometric EIA are discussed by Boiteux et al. (1981) and Gabauer and Rechnitz (1982).

14.6.6. Diffusion-in-gel enzyme immunoassays (DIG-EIA)

The advantages of DIG-EIA over conventional EIA are its simplicity (undiluted serum is tested as such), economy (simple Petri dishes are used), easy standardization and versatility.

The principle of this method (Elwing and Nygren, 1979) is simple and resembles in some respects the single radial immunodiffusion of Mancini et al. (1965) (Fig. 14.6). The bottom of a plastic Petri dish is coated with the antigen, overlayered with agarose and a well is punched in the gel. The sample is placed in the well, from which it diffuses into the agarose. The agarose is then removed and an enzyme-labeled anti-IgG is reacted with its antigen. The substrate is added in hot agarose and poured over the bottom. The diameter of the reaction zones is proportional to the amount of immunoreactant present in the sample. This method is applied increasingly (e.g., Elwing et al., 1980; Nygren and Stenberg, 1982; Cursons, 1982).

14.6.7. Enzyme channeling immunoassays

In this method an appropriate enzyme (e.g., GPDase) and the antigen are co-immobilized on a solid phase. Hexokinase-labeled antibody produces an accelerated conversion of glucose, ATP and NAD^+ since the enzymes are in each other's vicinity.

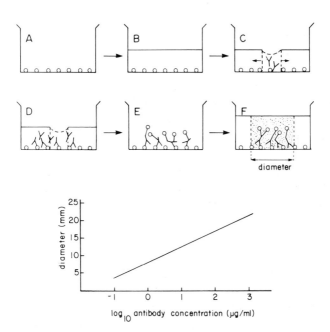

Fig. 14.6. Diffusion-in-gel EIA. The bottom of a Petri dish is coated with antigen (A), overlayered with agarose (B), and antibodies are allowed to diffuse from a well punched in the agarose (C, D). The agarose is removed and antibody is detected with enzyme-labeled anti-immunoglobulin (E). Substrate is added in hot agarose and the diameter of the stained zone (F) is measured and plotted in a standard curve against the antibody concentration.

14.6.8. Some other approaches to enzyme immunoassays

Ngo and Lenhoff (1980, 1981) reported some new approaches to EIA which they called AMETIA ('antibody masking enzyme tag immunoassay'; solid phase) and EMMIA ('enzyme modulator mediated immunoassay'; homogeneous). In the solid-phase method, a tag (e.g., biotin) is linked to the enzyme of an enzyme–ligand (antigen or hapten) conjugate, whereas on the solid phase a receptor to that tag (here avidin) is immobilized. Antibody to the ligand masks the tag and prevents the enzyme from being immobilized on the solid phase. Increased competition with free ligand produces more immobilization of the enzyme. In contrast to other competitive EIA, the conjugates bound to the solid phase are the free conjugates (not complexed with antibodies) and standard curves have positive slopes.

In the homogeneous assay, an enzyme modulator (antibody, inhibitor or receptor for the enzyme) is covalently linked to the ligand which competes with free ligand from the test sample for the available antibodies. The activity of the indicator enzyme depends on the amount of free modulator. As the amount of hapten increases, less hapten-modulator is bound by the antibody and the activity of the indicator enzyme (which is not conjugated) is more modulated (inhibited, e.g., avidin for biotin-dependent enzymes (Section 14.3.1.2), or activated, e.g., antibody to wild-type BGase with an inactive mutant of this enzyme, Section 10.2.2.1).

14.7. Equipment and automation in enzyme immunoassays

Though solid-phase EIA can be performed manually quite easily, mechanization and automation is necessary for their performance on a large scale. Mechanization of practically all steps proved to be feasible. Commercial equipment was reviewed by Sever et al. (1983).

Ruitenberg et al. (1976) and Ruitenberg and Brosi (1978) described an on-line system for macro-ELISA (EIA in disposable polystyrene tubes, 50×11 mm) for the daily processing of 4000 samples. Details on automation can be found in the reviews of Ruitenberg and Brosi (1978) and of Carlier et al. (1979).

Microplate EIA have also been automated. These systems consist in microplate carriers, dilution and dispenser devices for multiple samples, washers and shakers, photometer (through-the-plate reading) and a processor for multiple reading (desk-top calculator or microcomputer interfaced with the measuring equipment). Compared to other systems, EIA requires less sophisticated equipment for reliable results, available from various commercial sources.

14.7.1. Equipment for semi-automated enzyme immunoassays

For most purposes, semi-automated systems are the best compromise between cost and efficiency. Dilution and dispensing aids, such as the multichannel Finn-pipette as well as washing devices are offered by general laboratory suppliers (e.g., Flow, Dynatech, Fisher). Alternatives have been proposed by Park (1978, 1981), such as through-passage receptacles as the solid-phase support in which 24 receptacles are assembled into one tray. For washing, these trays are placed on a waste container overlaid with a 'wash box' to which a predetermined column of washing solution is connected. Conradie et al. (1981) designed a washing device for microplates which consists of 3 parts: (i) a 'shower', i.e., a tank with 96 needles to deliver the washing solution; (ii) a sump to collect washing fluid; and, (iii) a sliding base plate to position the plate correctly. With this device the plates are washed in less than 1 min and it can be built for a fraction of the cost of commercially available plate-washing machines. Plates may be dried by spin-drying centrifugation. Other washing equipment is based on magnetic transfer devices (Smith and Gehle, 1980) and a fully automated system is offered by Technicon Instruments Co. (Tarrytown, NY).

Several commercial through-the-plate readers are available (Titertek Multiskan, Flow Lab; Microelisa Autoreader, Dynatech Lab., Inc. Alexandria, VA), as well as inexpensive home-made readers (Ruitenberg et al., 1980; Rook and Cameron, 1981; Ackerman and Kelley, 1983). In a comparative study Genta and Bowdre (1982) evaluated the two commercial photometers for the linearity and reproducibility of the measurements. Their findings confirmed the earlier report of Ruitenberg et al. (1980) that photometric inaccuracy was minor in comparison to dispensing errors. Unlike in common photometers, the length of the light path is not fixed by cuvette dimensions. Microplate readers which measure simultaneously at two wavelengths may correct automatically for some causes of variability (e.g., scratches on plastic). An exhaustive evaluation of the performance of spectrophotometers was reported by Haeckel et al. (1980).

The home-made device of Rook and Cameron (1981) is inexpensive and easy to build, but is about 10 times slower (about 15 min per plate) than the commercial readers. This instrument has the disadvantage that the tip of the reading device has to be immersed into the liquid, but variations due to differences in the length of the light path can be minimized. An alternative probe colorimeter was constructed by Ackerman and Kelley (1983), based on a photometer of Brinkmann Instruments Inc., equipped with a fiber optic probe. The probe transmits phase-shifted modulating light generated by an alternating current through a fiber optic light-guide into the reaction liquid. A mirror is placed under the microplate which returns the transmitted light to the instrument through another light-guide in the same probe. An electonic chopper synchronized with the light source negates the effects of extraneous or ambient light.

Fluorometers have also been adapted for semi-automatic measurements (Section 14.5.1.1.1). It is also possible to use UV-light boxes (Forghani et al., 1980) but they are much less precise.

14.7.2. Equipment for homogeneous enzyme immunoassays

A great number of partially and fully mechanized analytical systems have been described for homogeneous EIA (Oellerich, 1980). The design of these EIA is favorable to mechanization. Many mechanized procedures for the determination of enzymic activity can be directly adopted to homogeneous EIA. Such arrangements consist in photometers equipped with thermally regulated flow-cells, in combination with suitable dispensers and dilutors or centrifugal analyzers.

CHAPTER 15

Processing of data and reporting of results of enzyme immunoassays

Results of EIA may be given in two forms: (i) expressing the activity of the antiserum in some arbitrary or relative units; and, (ii) expressing the concentration of the antigen or hapten (often in mg/ml).

The frequent homogeneity of haptens or antigens contrasts with the heterogeneity in affinity and concentration of antibodies in the antisera and results in fundamental differences in the nature of the dose–response relations for antibodies and for antigens.

An essential element in quantitative assays is the setting of the positive/negative discrimination level (cut-off value). The term negative is used as indicating the absence of specific antibodies or antigens above the background noise.

Various mathematical models can improve the precision of curve fitting, particularly for hapten dose–response curves, to obtain accurate results with less data required for the standard curve, saving both time and cost. This is particularly valid in situations where programmable calculators or microcomputers can be interfaced with microplate readers and printers.

15.1. Concepts for evaluation of results of enzyme immunoassays

The general use of standard deviation (SD) is, strictly speaking, not valid since EIA values for negative reference sera are distributed with a positive skew (i.e., a longer tail is observed toward higher values). Due to this skewness, false positives occur with a significantly higher frequency than expected from a normal distribution. The number of false positives can, therefore, be significant. For example, Cremer et al. (1982) noted that, for 115 sera tested, three gave false positives with a cut-off at the level of mean plus three SD, whereas one was observed at the cut-off of mean plus four SD. Non-parametric methods, which could be more accurate, are hardly used in EIA since they require larger sample sizes (Section 15.2.4). The SD of a limited number of results (< 30; otherwise $n-1$ becomes n) is determined by the formula:

$$SD = \sqrt{\frac{\Sigma(x_i - m)^2}{n-1}}$$

in which n is the number of results, x_i the respective results with the arithmetic mean m. The estimate for SD is prone to a significant error, even if the SD were estimated from large numbers of replicates (e.g., 100; Mainland, 1971). Results are often expressed as the mean with the corresponding SD, or mean with the relative scatter. The coefficient of variation (CV) expresses the SD as a percentage of the mean:

$$CV(\%) = \frac{SD}{mean} \times 100$$

Reproducibility is generally expressed by testing the samples in duplicate and the SD calculated by the equation:

$$SD = \sqrt{\frac{\Sigma(d)^2}{2N}}$$

in which d is the difference between duplicate absorbances and N the number of paired samples (Section 15.4). To reduce bias it is necessary to distribute randomly the duplicates in the test.

SD (or CV) is generally employed but their practical use is rather limited. More replicates in the assay will only increase the reliability of the estimate for SD, but the spread of the individual remains in principle unchanged. A more practical alternative, however, is to estimate the interval (e.g., 95% confidence interval) of the arithmetic mean obtained from replicates. More replicates produce a smaller interval since the extreme results are cancelled by averaging (calculated mean closer to the real mean). The SD_m for the distribution of means is $SD/\sqrt{n}$ (n is number of replicates; with large n, SD_m is small). The confidence intervals can be expressed with standardized deviates ('z statistic' for normal distributions). For a normal distribution the interval determined by a z statistic of, e.g., 2 is mean $\pm 2 \times SD$ (probability 4.55% of obtaining result outside this interval; Tables in statistics textbooks) or for a 95% confidence interval the z statistic is 1.96. The results of EIA are not normally distributed. However, the means are normally distributed (Central Limit Theorem), irrespective of the original distribution. For small sample sizes, the normal distribution is replaced by the t-distribution which has a relatively greater spread (more area in the tails). A larger number of replicates (or degrees of freedom, df $= n-1$) produces less area in the tails and the t-distribution resembles more a normal distribution (e.g., at df > 30). In analogy to the z statistic used for normal distributions, the t statistic expresses the number of estimated standard error of means ($SD/\sqrt{n}$) necessary to make a mean statistically different from the mean with which it is compared:

$$t_{\mathrm{df}=n-1} = \frac{\text{difference in means of two distributions}}{SD/\sqrt{n}}$$

Tables with critical levels of significance for t can be found in statistics textbooks.

Detectability of the assay is the lowest concentration of antigen exceeding the zero-dose precision. The difference of the mean of the absorbance values at the detection limit can be estimated by the t-distribution (one-tailed, since the curve here only increases):

$$t = \frac{\text{Absorbance}_{\text{detection limit}} - \text{Absorbance}_{\text{zero dose}}}{SD/\sqrt{n}}$$

For example, if the mean of 8 values (df $= n-1 = 7$) is 0.12

with an SD of 0.043, then the one-sided $t_{0.95;df=7}$ value (i.e., that 95% of the means of zero-dose samples are below the detection limit) is 1.895. The significance level (cut-off) is then at an absorbance of:

$$\text{Absorbance}_{\text{zero dose}} + \frac{t_{0.95} \times \text{SD}}{\sqrt{n}} = 0.12 + \frac{1.895 \times 0.043}{(8)^{1/2}} = 0.149$$

On the other hand, the $t_{0.95}$ statistic would be 2.920 (one-sided, df = 2) for 3 replicates and the absorbance at the detection limit would be 0.195 if the same mean and SD are obtained.

In Chapter 1 sensitivity has been defined as the responsiveness of the assay to changes in concentration of the substance tested, i.e., dR/dC. Therefore, on a sigmoid dose–response curve, sensitivity decreases at either end of the curve. As evident from Fig. 15.1, the interval of confidence for the concentration obtained can be defined by the ratio:

$$\Delta C = \frac{\text{standard error of response}}{\text{sensitivity at this response}} = \frac{\Delta R}{dR/dC}$$

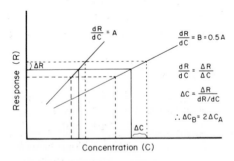

Fig. 15.1. The relation between sensitivity (dR/dC) and error in dose (ΔC). In this example, slope B is $0.5 \times$ slope A and the error in response (ΔR) would then cause an error, ΔC_b, which is twice that of slope A. The flattering part of the sigmoid curve has, therefore, an increasingly larger error in the estimation of the dose. Detectability reflects the confidence with which it can be stated that a certain response is larger than this error.

Though this ratio is usually defined as precision of concentration, imprecision (ΔC) would be a better term since the larger this ratio, the larger the imprecision of concentration. The precision of an assay can be expressed as:

$$C \pm \frac{\Delta R}{\mathrm{d}R/\mathrm{d}C} = C \pm \Delta C$$

The response error (ΔR) is not constant (heteroscedastic) so that the highest precision does not necessarily coincide with the highest sensitivity (Section 15.4).

The reliability of a positive or a negative result from an assay depends to a very large degree on the prevalence of the specific antigen or antibody in the population. This can be shown easily with Bayes' Theorem, but requires the definition of some parameters. The detectability index of positives, $DI(+)$, is defined as the ability of a test to give a positive result for positive samples (in the literature this is generally referred as 'sensitivity'; e.g., Papasian et al., 1984) and the detectability index of negatives, $DI(-)$, as the ability to give a negative finding for negative samples (in literature, 'specificity'). The reliability of positivity ('predictive value') is the likelihood that a sample giving a positive result actually is positive, whereas the reliability of negativity is the likelihood that a sample giving a negative result is truly negative. These concepts are defined as:

$$DI(+) = \frac{\text{true positives}}{\text{true positives} + \text{false negatives}} \times 100$$

$$DI(-) = \frac{\text{true negatives}}{\text{true negatives} + \text{false positives}} \times 100$$

$$\text{reliability of positivity} = \frac{\text{true positives}}{\text{true} + \text{false positives}} \times 100$$

$$\text{reliability of negativity} = \frac{\text{true negatives}}{\text{true} + \text{false negatives}} \times 100$$

To show the impact of prevalence on the reliability of results, two theoretical situations are considered for which the indices are the same (90%), but in one situation the prevalence is 2% and in the other 30% (e.g., respective prevalence of antibodies to hepatitis HBsAg in young adults of North America and some developing countries; Deinhardt and Gust, 1982). With the 2% prevalence, 20/1000 subjects are positive. However with a DI(+) of 90%, only 18 will be detected and 2 will be falsely negative. On the other hand, with a DI(−) of 90%, 882 of the 980 negative subjects are recognized as such, and 98 would be falsely positive. Among all positive test results (18 + 98) only 18 are truly positive, i.e. the reliability of positivity is 15.5%, and the reliability of negativity (= 100 × 882/(882 + 2)) is 99.8%. In the case of 30% prevalence, but similar indices (same test), the reliability of positivity increases sharply to 79.4%, whereas the reliability of negativity decreases slightly to 95.5%. At a prevalence of 90% the reliability of negativity would be only 50%. These considerations suppose that the exact prevalence and DI are known or can be estimated, e.g. as established by other methods or with testing groups of known positivity or negativity. Fig. 15.2 shows the effect prevalence has on the reliability of the results.

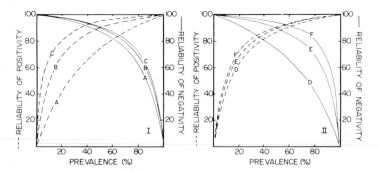

Fig. 15.2. The variation, while using exactly the same assay, in reliability of positive or negative results as a function of prevalence. In frame I the DI(+) is kept at 90%, while the DI(−) is 70% (A), 90% (B), or 95% (C), whereas in frame II the DI(−) is kept at 90% and DI(+) is 70% (D), 90% (E), or 95% (F). It can be seen that with low prevalences increasing the DI(−) has the greatest impact (A → C; e.g., achieved by using AM-type instead of AA-type assays), while at high prevalences the increase of DI(+) is a priority (D → F). These frames are mirror-like and suggest that a certain optimum (Fig. 15.4) can be found between DI(+) and DI(−).

15.2. Processing of data and reporting of results of activity-amplification assays

Relatively little attention has been paid to the handling of the results of AA-type EIA, despite the obvious importance of an objective evaluation of the data for the presentation, rationalization and standardization of EIA and for the improvement of the reproducibility of the test (De Savigny and Voller, 1980).

The most common methods, titration (highest dilution still giving a positive reaction) or the measurement of absorbance, suffer from important inconveniences (Section 15.2.4). The relative merits of various alternatives will be discussed. No matter how accurate the technique may be, the presentation of the results is only useful if communicated in a meaningful form.

Due to the large differences in antibody concentrations in sera, long dilution series may be required to find the exact titre or a reasonably precise absorbance value. The response curves are sigmoidal, the most sensitive part of which (i.e., the steepest part) has a relatively small range. The measurement of a single or of only a few dilutions is obviously ideal, but may carry serious limitations, particularly for the determination of antibodies.

15.2.1. The use of absorbance values for dose–response curves

Visual inspection is still widely used for titration. This method is very simple, but relies heavily on the skill of the operator due to subjectivity. Results of this nature are at best semi-quantitative and generally acceptable only for qualitative investigations.

In quantitative determinations usually the optical density of the product is measured. Absorbance values, obtained for different dilutions of the antibody or antigen of known concentration, mostly yield sigmoidal calibration dose–response curves. Although this procedure seems rather simple and straightforward, it is not. Enzyme kinetics may be influenced by any of the factors discussed in Chapter 9. Correlation of absorbance with sample dilution beyond the linear limits of enzyme–substrate reactions, a common practice in EIA, is not justified (Barlough et al., 1983). Moreover, chromogen color shifts may continue even after stopping of the reaction (Bullock and Walls, 1977). Kinetics-based solid-phase enzyme assays may be of help, particularly to eliminate type I errors (false positives), and, since the enzyme–substrate reaction rate is directly proportional to the quantity of the immunoreactant in the sample, they eliminate the need of performing the test at a series of dilutions (Barlough et al., 1983). Virtually all solid-phase EIA use much longer incubation periods (e.g., 1 h) than studies of enzyme kinetics. The optimum reaction period has been established in very few reports. For example, McLaren et al. (1978) followed the color development of a positive reference serum and stopped the reaction at various absorbance values (from 0.25 to 1.25). Optimum results were obtained when the absorbance of the reference serum reached 0.75 (after about 15–25 min). However, these important aspects of solid-phase EIA have not yet been adequately examined.

After prolonged reaction periods, dose–response curves for solid-phase EIA become steeper, although the detection limit remains virtually unchanged. After the optimum sensitivity has been reached, a steeper slope rapidly increases the coefficient of variation of the response $(=\Delta C \times dR/dC)$, and so decreases the span within which reliable results may be obtained.

15.2.2. Difference between dose–response curves for antigens and for antibodies in activity amplification assays

Concentration of the antigen can be readily determined from a standard dose–response curve. The range of antigen concentration rarely exceeds two $\log_{10}$ dilutions and is, therefore, much smaller than for different antisera. Microcomputers or desk-top programmable calculators, interfaced with microplate readers, may help to linearize rapidly the dose–response curves and to transform the values obtained for the test-samples into concentrations. In contrast, dose–response curves for antibodies are complicated by a variety of factors:

their range is generally much larger and often exceeds 4–6 $\log_{10}$ dilutions; the dose–response curves for various antisera are rarely parallel, i.e. cross-overs of the curves are observed, due to the differences in the concentration and affinity of the antibodies (Gripenberg et al., 1978; Sedgwick et al., 1983). A curve obtained from a single reference serum cannot take both parameters into account and is, therefore, hardly representative for other sera. Another problem may be the presence of antibodies in different Ig classes (De Savigny and Voller, 1980) which could cause a prozone effect (Section 8.7.2)

In solid-phase EIA the antibody activity is measured rather than its avidity or concentration (Chapter 8). The avidity of the bound antibodies is, in turn, influenced by the density of the antigen on the solid phase (Lehtonen and Eerola, 1982). Low dilutions (e.g. 1:100) of the antiserum favors the binding of high-affinity antibodies (affinity $> \approx 10^7 \, M^{-1}$) and this effect is enforced by a high density of the antigen on the solid phase. In contrast, end-point titers at high dilutions tend to correlate with a wider range of affinities. This problem has still not been solved satisfactorily.

Characteristics for the ideal form of presentation of the results, particularly for serological tests, are listed in Table 15.1.

15.2.3. The problems with setting the positive/negative discrimination level

An unfortunate, widespread practice in EIA is the inclusion of a number of negative serum samples at a single dilution to establish mean and SD of background staining, whereas the test samples are serially diluted. The assumption that non-specific binding (observed with negative sera) is constant, irrespective of the dilution factor violates the law of mass action. Serial dilutions should, therefore, also be used with the negative sera.

The selection of a suitable cut-off value is important to minimize false responses. This level can be moved upwards or downwards to incur more of the type I (false positive) or type II (false negative) errors, depending on which adjustment has less grave consequences.

TABLE 15.1

Characteristics required for the ideal reporting of data from serological EIA

Requirements
- Easy comprehension by those not familiar with the test.

- Clearness of qualitative information (positive or negative, reactive or non-reactive, above or within normal range).

- Linearity of the quantitative indication, preferably on a numerical and stepless (i.e., continuous) scale.

- Reproducibility of the data processing.

- Evaluation of the test should not assume normal distribution patterns or parallelism.

- Adequacy of the results for further processing (e.g., for epidemiologic analysis).

Some features which may obscure information or introduce errors
- Transformation of response curves (compression of errors with apparent improvement of data)

- Linear interpolation between points on curve or assumption of linearity.

- Subtraction of a constant value for background based on the assumption that nonspecific binding is constant over the complete range; this assumption is not valid since the law of mass action for nonspecific binding is ignored. Without subtraction the same results are obtained; however, a limit should be set to discriminate between a positive result and background staining (Section 15.1.3).

Some desirable factors
- Inclusion of controls for reagents, assay parameters and non-specific binding.

- Methods which minimize change in assay parameters (quality control methods, Section 15.3).

Results in this intermediate area may be classified as doubtful (Fig. 15.3; Heck et al., 1980). Samples giving doubtful results can be re-assayed in more replicates to decrease the cut-off value while retaining the same confidence.

The problem of setting the level to discriminate between positive and negative responses has been approached in several ways. This

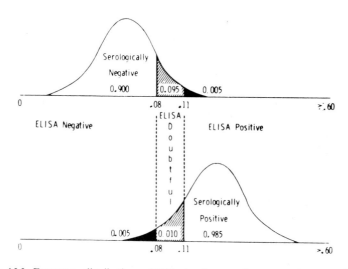

Fig. 15.3. Frequency distributions of EIA-absorbances of sera negative or positive for anti-*Brucella abortus* antibodies (Heck et al., 1980). Cut-off values were determined with the *t* test (Section 15.1; one-tailed confidence limit of 99.5%; positive sera (64): mean absorbance of 0.2797 with an SD of 0.0764; negative sera (32): mean absorbance of 0.0534 and an SD of 0.0198) for both the positive ($0.0768 = 0.2797 - 2.656 \times 0.0764$, since the $t_{0.995;df = 63} = 2.656$) and the negative sera (0.1077; $t_{0.995;df = 31} = 2.744$). Sera, for which values are obtained between these cut-off values, are classified as doubtful. The proportion of these doubtful results can be estimated by calculation of the *t* statistic corresponding to these cut-off values (assuming normal distribution). For example, the cut-off value of 0.1077 from the negative sera corresponds to the mean $- 2.251 \times SD$ in the distribution of the positives. A $t = 2.251$ (df = 63) corresponds, in turn, to a confidence limit of 98.6%. Therefore, the doubtful area is 0.9%. Similarly, 11.3% is obtained for the doubtful area of the negatives (the slightly different values in this Figure are obtained after rounding the cut-off values of 0.0768 and 0.1077 to 0.08 and 0.11, respectively). Courtesy Dr. F.C. Heck and *Journal of Clinical Microbiology*.

cut-off level is sometimes set at two or three times the mean of the results with sera from the negative group (Malvano et al., 1982), or at the mean + two or three SD of the mean if a large number of normal reference sera is available (Cremer et al., 1982; Richardson et al., 1983), or sometimes arbitrarily at 0.15 or 0.20 absorbance (Halbert et al., 1983). Fig. 15.4A shows some of these approaches compared with the cut-off values obtained with the method discussed

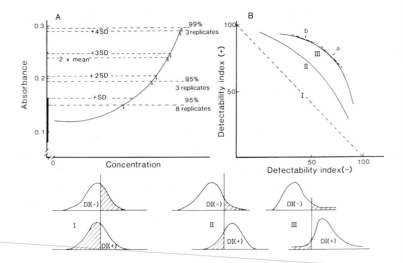

Fig. 15.4. A. Some examples of cutoff values reported in the literature and their reliability (in this example, mean of negatives is 0.12 with an SD of 0.043). For example, a cut-off value of mean + 2 SD approximates 95% confidence if 3 replicates are used to calculate the mean. B. The DI(+) and the DI(−) are inversely related and moving (as shown in frames I-III) the cut-off value to other absorbance levels (abscissae, frequency in ordinates) will increase one DI at the expense of the other. If no difference exists in the mean and distribution of the positive and negative sera (I), a straight line will be obtained in B. More curvature is indicative of more difference between the positive and negative sera distributions. The relative importance of DI(−) and DI(+) determines at which point on the curve the optimal combination is found (Section 15.2.3; at a both are equally important, whereas at b 3 × more weight is attached to DI(+)).

in Section 15.1 (with mean = 0.12 and SD = 0.043). The DI(+) and the DI(−) are inversely related (Fig. 15.4B). If, e.g., two antigens with shared reactivity, of which the common epitope reacts with the monoclonal antibody used in the assay, are tested a straight line is obtained since DI(+) + DI(−) = 100 irrespective of the cut-off value. For assays with higher specificity (i.e., a difference in the affinity of antibody for the specific and cross-reacting antigen; Section 8.6) an optimum cut-off value can be established. If the DI(+) and DI(−) are of approximately equal importance, the optimum cut-off value is where the tangent of the curve is 1. If some relative weight is attached to the two indices, the cut-off is chosen where the first derivative (i.e., the tangent) of the curve equals the inverse of the relative weights (W):

$$\frac{d(DI[+])}{d(DI[-])} = \frac{W_{DI[-]}}{W_{DI[+]}}$$

These relative weights depend on such factors as ease of assay and cost. The latter is directly related by the prevalence to the reliability of the results (e.g., cost of treatment of false positives versus benefits). Prevalence may, however, be less constant than commonly assumed and clustering (epidemics; genetic predisposition) may occur. Clustering patterns are recognized with the Poisson distribution (e.g., time, space; Section 5.4.3.2).

Various shortcuts have been proposed to determine the daily variations in a particular system. In one such procedure (van Loon and Van der Veen, 1980) the mean + 3 SD of a group of 44 normal sera corresponded to 40% of the absorbance of the reference serum. Therefore, in the subsequent tests only this reference serum was included as an internal standard to calibrate the cut-off level of the test system. Another way to normalize the tests is to include both a standardized positive serum pool and a standardized negative serum pool (Cremer et al., 1982). A simple, non-parametric, method is to assay many negative sera and to set the cut-off value at a level so that, e.g., 95% of all absorbances for negative sera are below this value. Critical reference sera are included in subsequent tests.

Methods were also proposed to eliminate a cut-off value altogether. One such method is based on the use of a positive reference serum and expresses the activity of the sample as a percentage of the absorbance of the reference serum. It remains, nevertheless, necessary to decide at which stage a response is to be considered positive.

15.2.4. Modes of expression of the results of serological activity amplification assays

15.2.4.1. Semi-quantitative tests
These methods are based on visual inspection and are, therefore, subjective. They are primarily used for qualitative results, such as in the screening for the presence of monoclonal antibodies by immunodotting (Section 13.3.1). These methods, however, are of limited value for many clinical situations. Nevertheless, they are very simple and many samples may be rapidly processed.

15.2.4.2. Titration method
The antiserum to be tested is diluted serially to establish the limit at which enzymic reaction can no longer be detected. Visual inspection is possible (about similar detectability as absorptiometry). The concept is simple and the test is quantitative for the antibody activity. The definition of the titre, however, may be confusing since with one method the titre may be much larger than with another for the same serum. Titrations generally are work-intensive and costly. It is difficult to establish by visual inspection the dilution (e.g. 1:512, or reciprocals, e.g., 512) at which the real end-point occurs. Thus, reproducibility may easily be one two-fold dilution difference from the accurate value. Therefore, a titre of, e.g. 1:4096 implies a false sense of accuracy (Section 1.3). Titration by visual inspection yields a discontinuous scale of results.

Some of these disadvantages may be circumvented by measuring the optical density which yields quantitative values and enables the determination of the cut-off value. The intersection of the dose–response curve with the cut-off level produces the titre. This value is thus on a continuous scale. The subjectivity factor is also eliminated and the cut-off value may be calibrated for every test by the inclusion of a suitable internal standard.

The relation between the results obtained by other calculation methods and titres is given in Fig. 15.5.

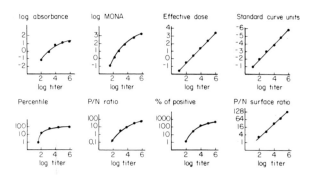

Fig. 15.5. Relation of titres (expressed in $\log_{10}$) of antisera to results obtained by other calculation methods (Sections 15.2.4.3 through 15.2.4.8). Only a few have approximate linear relationships. Sometimes, however, the surface ratio increases, while the titre remains the same (non-linear). This reflects a steeper curve (higher sensitivity) and is, therefore, a more reliable measure for seroconversions.

15.2.4.3. The Effective Dose (ED) method

Leinikki and Passila (1977) devised the ED method to assess the difference in activities of two sera. A positive reference serum is used to construct a dose–response curve to which the dose–response curves of the test sera are then compared. The major distinction between the ED and the titration method is that the difference between two sera is expressed by the log of the difference in the dilution at the linear part of the sigmoidal curves where sensitivity is maximal instead of at the flattening part of the curve (Fig. 15.6). Subsequently, Leinikki et al. (1978) refined this method by using a positive reference serum of known concentration of antibodies.

Advantages of this method are the improvement in the reproducibility of the test, which renders possible the detection of subtle seroconversions, and the linear proportionality between the ED results and the titres. Disadvantages of this method are the considerable work and the amount of reagents involved and the uncommon way of expressing the results, i.e. in Brigg's logs (e.g., for acute phase serum, ED = −80; for convalescent phase serum ED = 1.07). This method also assumes parallelism of the dose–response curves.

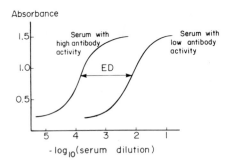

Fig. 15.6. Concept of Effective Dose (ED). Dose–response curves are compared at maximum sensitivity since, as shown in Fig. 15.1, errors will be lower at this point than at the cut-off value. The difference is expressed in Brigg's logs.

A similar approach was adopted by Soula et al. (1982) except that the titre was expressed as ELISA (50%), obtained after transformation of the sigmoidal curve into a linear response curve (according to the methods discussed in Section 15.2.5).

15.2.4.4. Expression of dose–response curves in standard units

Dose–response curves are constructed for a large group of sera, ranging from negative to strongly positive, and the titres determined at the intersection of these curves with the cut-off level. With each serum, the absorbance is then determined at a given working dilution (e.g. 1:1000). Plotting the absorbance of each serum at the working dilution against its titre produces a sigmoidal standard curve (Fig. 15.7). The standard curve is then linearized, as in Section 15.2.5. Carefully selected reference sera can be used as internal standards for subsequent assays to control assay differences.

This method (De Savigny and Voller, 1980) has the advantages that the absorbance values are transformed into quantitative units on a continuous scale, that the sera are tested at a single dilution and that the results are proportional to the titres. However, as with all absorbance-based methods, it is not valid at high absorbance values. Furthermore, a rigorous quality control is required and the dose–response curves are assumed to be parallel.

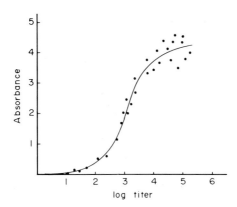

Fig. 15.7. Standard curve obtained by plotting the titre of various sera against their absorbance at a predetermined working dilution (e.g., 1:1000). Linearization of this curve allows the transformation of absorbance values into quantitative antibody activity units on a continuous scale.

A variant of this method was described by Malvano et al. (1982): standard unit response curves are constructed with aliquots of a highly positive serum diluted with a negative sample. This approach is based on the assumption that dose–response curve parallellism eliminates the necessity to employ many different sera for the calibration curve. This positive serum is then calibrated against a WHO standard serum and the antibody content of the positive serum is expressed in international units (IU). Calibration samples of the positive serum diluted with a negative serum are included as internal markers for between-run, between-laboratory and between-method normalizations to provide analytical consistency to the measurements.

15.2.4.5. The absorbance method   Results of solid-phase EIA are most commonly expressed in absorbance values, when a chromogenic substrate is used, or in arbitrary fluorescence units when a fluorogenic substrate is used. If a suitable dilution is chosen, a single measurement is sufficient and no processing of the data is required.

Though a continuous scale of absorbance values may be obtained, it is not very reliable outside the 0.2–0.8 range and the coefficient of variation tends to increase significantly outside this range. The absorbance values are not linearly proportional to the titres.

15.2.4.6. Ratio methods by comparison to a reference serum

Different ratio methods have been developed, such as the positive: negative (P/N) ratio, the ratio of the areas under the dose–response curves of the test serum and of a reference serum, and the percent of positive method.

P/N ratios (Locarnini et al., 1979) are often used. Normal or reference sera serve to establish the absorbance of the negative group (N value), whereas the sample serum at the same dilution yields the P value. The sample sera are usually considered positive with P/N ratios greater than 2 or 3. This method carries several advantages: it is easily understood, the use of negative sera in the test serves directly as an internal control and only a few, or even a single, dilutions are required. However, important disadvantages result from the use of low absorbance values which may vary significantly from test to test. Also, the P/N ratios are difficult to reproduce, may depend on the choice of the negative sera, are not linear with the titres since they are based on absorbance and the method is insensitive if the absorbance of the positive sample exceeds about 1.0.

In an attempt to circumvent some of these problems, Sedgwick et al. (1983) devised the method of the ratio of the areas under the dose–response curves of the test serum and of a reference serum. The area under the dose–response curve can be calculated by the simple midpoint estimate procedure for approximating the integral function the working formula of which is:

$$\text{area} = \frac{X \cdot (n-1) \cdot [2(\Sigma A_{\text{md}}) + \Sigma A_{\text{fd}} + \Sigma A_{\text{ld}}]}{4r}$$

in which A is the net absorbance at different dilutions (md = middle dilutions, fd = first dilutions and ld = last dilutions), $n-1$ is number of intervals (*n* dilutions) and *X* is the orbit ray interval used on the graph paper and *r* the number of replicates. Although several dilutions (6–8) can be made, it suffices to use the first, middle and last dilutions. For example, if for serial dilutions the 6 net absorbances obtained are 1.40, 1.00, 0.65, 0.35, 0.20, and 0.10, respectively and the orbit ray is 10 mm, then the area is 21.25. Sedgwick et al. (1983) calculated for each test the areas under the curve of pools of sera which were linearly proportional to the antibody concentration (at least over the 64-fold range tested). Advantages are that the cross-over effects, which may complicate some of the other methods, are taken into account and that the test sera are compared to a reference serum. However, serial dilutions are required (costly and work-demanding).

The percent of positive method expresses the absorbance of the test-sample as a percentage of that of a positive reference serum, measured simultaneously. This method is, therefore, quantitative and quite simple, does not require a cut-off value and fluctuates less than the P/N ratio method. However, the choice of the positive reference serum is very important, since a reference serum with a very high activity (i.e. high absorbance) will decrease the percentage of apparent positive sera. Results are not linearly proportional to the titre.

15.2.4.7. The Multiple Of Normal Activity (MONA) method

This procedure has the advantage of stepless titration and requires a single serum dilution only. Felgner (1978) considered an approximately parabolic relationship between the concentration of antibody and the absorbance to calculate the MONA. Unfortunately, one equation given for these calculations is incomplete; here, a simple and more precise method (and example) is given for this useful MONA method.

MONA can be defined as the number of times a serum should be diluted (D_2) over that of the reference serum (D_1) to obtain the same absorbance as the reference serum ($= D_2/D_1$).

Fig. 15.8. shows a typical sigmoid response curve. When the re-

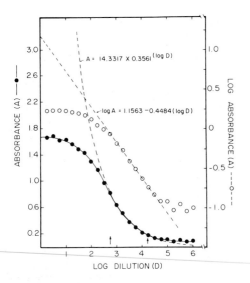

Fig. 15.8. A typical sigmoid dose–response curve and the log transformation of the lower half (between $\log_{10}$ dilutions indicated by arrows).

sponses are expressed in logarithms, a straight line is obtained over a reasonably long range (either exponentially increasing or decreasing part of the curve). The exact slope (regression coefficient m) of this straight line, which can be calculated by linear regression of log absorbance vs. log dilution, is very important to establish a precise MONA.

The absorbance of the various sera (diluted by the same factor) is determined after the EIA. A basic assumption of the MONA concept is that all dose–response curves are parallel. Each absorbance is, therefore, representative of a dose–response curve and, irrespective of the initial dilution, the factor of dilution is the same to obtain the same EIA-response for another serum (Fig. 15.9). This dilution factor (MONA = D_2/D_1) can be calculated with the slope m as shown in this Fig.:

$$\log \frac{D_2}{D_1} = \log \text{MONA} = -\frac{\log A_1/A_2}{m}$$

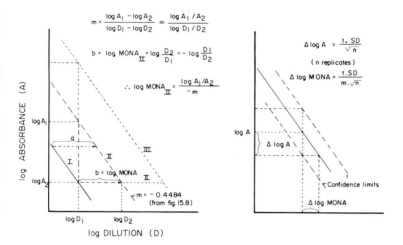

$$m = \frac{\log A_1 - \log A_2}{\log D_1 - \log D_2} = \frac{\log A_1 / A_2}{\log D_1 / D_2}$$

$$b = \log MONA_{II} = \log \frac{D_2}{D_1} = -\log \frac{D_1}{D_2}$$

$$\therefore \log MONA_{II} = \frac{\log A_1/A_2}{-m}$$

$$\Delta \log A = \frac{t \cdot SD}{\sqrt{n}}$$

(n replicates)

$$\Delta \log MONA = \frac{t \cdot SD}{m \cdot \sqrt{n}}$$

Fig. 15.9. Determination of the Multiple Of Normal Activity (MONA). It is assumed that all sera to be tested have parallel dose–response curves (I–III), the slope (m) of which with simple regression analysis is obtained from the log transformation in Fig. 15.8. The number of times a serum should be diluted over that of the reference serum (MONA) can then be calculated and is independent of the original dilution (i.e., $a = b = MONA_{II}$). However, to obtain the MONA of the various sera, their EIA-absorbance values are determined at the same dilution (e.g., D_1). The confidence interval of the mean of MONA-values, important for seroconversion tests, can similarly be established.

For example, for the slope in Fig. 15.8. $m = -0.4484$. If EIA gives for this serum an absorbance of 0.30, for a more positive serum 0.50 and for a pool of negative sera 0.08, the MONA of the positive serum ($A = 0.30$) is antilog $[-(\log 0.30/0.08)/-0.4484] = 19.06$ and for the more positive serum 59.56. The MONA of the latter is 3.12 when calculated with respect to the less positive serum. These values are related by their product ($19.06 \times 3.12 = 59.56$). This indicates that the choice of the reference serum (Normal Activity, MONA $= 1$) should be carefully made. The slope used here to calculate the MONA is related to the parabola exponent (n) used by Felgner (1978) as $m = -n^{-1}$.

To establish the significance interval of the mean of log MONA

for a serum, the t-distribution can be applied as in Section 15.1.
Fig. 15.9 shows that in addition to the standard error, the significance
limits are also determined by the slope of the response curve. The
MONA method is advantageous in several aspects: (i) it compares
the antibody activity of the test serum to that of a reference serum,
(ii) it is more linearly proportional to the titre than most absorbance
methods; (iii) the use of internal standards obviates the need for
rigorous control of assay conditions; (iv) the detectability is improved
and a single dilution of the serum suffices if properly chosen; and,
(v) despite the strong variation in absorbance of the various sera
in the different experiments, the MONA values remain relatively
stable.

There are, however, also some important disadvantages since (i)
it is assumed that dose–response curves are parallel, (ii) the determination of MONA is greatly influenced by the choice of the positive
reference serum; and, (iii) the range from which absorbance values
are taken is only about half of the normal sigmoidal dose–response
curve.

*15.2.4.8. Percentile estimate with respect to a positive reference se-
rum*   Non-parametric methods are preferable for the estimation
of the normal range because they are valid regardless of the underlying form of the statistical population from which the data are obtained. However, more data (samples) are required to obtain the
same precision than in calculations for Gaussian or log-Gaussian
distributions. Two non-parametric methods of normal range estimation are the percentile estimate (Elveback and Taylor, 1969) and
the tolerance interval (Brunden et al., 1970).

A cumulative frequency distribution is prepared from the absorbance values of sera from a large 'normal' group (> 100). This standard
curve serves then as reference to establish the percentiles or P-values
(de Savigny et al., 1979). Above a certain absorbance value the
test sample is reported as 100th percentile or $P > 1.0$. The reference
group must be carefully selected and defined which may pose several
problems. Moreover, the percentile method requires the initial testing

of a large reference group and its results are not proportional to titres.

15.2.5. Procedures to improve precision of curve fitting for antigen dose–response curves

Dose–response curves which serve to estimate the antigen concentration are usually sigmoidal or hyperbolic. Precision of the standard curve can be considerably improved with suitable plotting systems. Plotting the absorbance data linearly or logarithmically against a logarithmic x-scale often facilitates the construction of a reliable standard curve but is not always satisfactory. Dose–response curves of solid-phase EIA are difficult to describe on the basis of mass action, because neither the actual amounts of the reactants are known, nor is the influence of the solid phase on the immunoreactivity (avidity, affinity) predictable. In contrast to the homogeneous EIA, curve fitting is still little used in solid-phase EIA.

In the following examples, the data of the typical dose–response curve of Fig. 15.8 are used (Table 15.2) so that comparisons may demonstrate the relative merits of these methods. Dose–response curves are non-linear and curvilinear fitting may provide a satisfactory solution to obtain the precise function. This can be done by transforming one or both variables (from linear to square root, logarithm or inversion), by polynomial or other curvilinear regressions, or by transformations for proportions (logit, probit, or angular, inverse sine or arcsine transformation). Details on the calculation of regression lines (Snedecor and Cochran, 1967; Armitage, 1971) are omitted since simple scientific calculators are equipped with regression functions. Berkson (1944) used the logit function for the transformation of sigmoidal response curves in bioassays and coined the term 'logit' as an abbreviation of logistic function in which the measurable quantity (absorbance) should, strictly speaking, be normally distributed (Cavalli-Sforza, 1969) . It is often used in RIA, although the logit procedure does not always transform sigmoidal curves to a linear form (Ekins, 1974; Fey, 1981). The empirical

TABLE 15.2

Absorbances observed and absorbances calculated after curve-fitting[a]

$\log_{10}$ dilution	Absorbance observed	Calculated by curve-fitting					
		$\log_{10}$ transformation	logit[b]	Least square polynomial			
				Parabola[c]		Cubic	Quintic
				a	b		
5.75	0.09	0.038	0.1046	0.314	−0.086	0.150	0.079
5.25	0.09	0.063	0.1118	0.181	−0.015	0.035	0.123
4.75	0.12	0.106	0.1301	0.134	0.086	0.048	0.108
4.25	0.18	0.178	0.1750	0.173	0.217	0.164	0.151
3.75	0.30	0.298	0.2792	0.297	0.378	0.355	0.298
3.25	0.52	0.500	0.4908	0.507	0.569	0.597	0.545
2.75	0.83	0.838	0.8232	0.803	0.790	0.864	0.850
2.25	1.17	1.404	1.1813	1.184	1.040	1.130	1.158
1.75	1.44	2.353	1.4395	1.651	1.321	1.369	1.412
1.25	1.57	3.942	1.5768	2.204	1.632	1.555	1.574
0.75	1.62	6.607	1.6381	2.843	1.972	1.607	1.621
0.25	1.67	11.071	1.6634	3.569	2.343	1.668	1.662

[a] The absorbances observed in example from Fig. 15.8 were fitted by different methods, such as log transformation (Fig. 15.8), logit transformation (Fig. 15.10) or polynomials (Fig. 15.11). The absorbances expected for the same dilutions were then recalculated by the regression curves given in those figures.

[b] The expected absorbance, A, from the logit curve can be calculated since:

$$\frac{A - A_0}{A_m - A} = \exp(\text{logit } Y); \text{ hence, } A = \frac{A_0 + A_m \cdot \exp(\text{logit } Y)}{1 + \exp(\text{logit } Y)}$$

using $A_m = 1.68$ and $A_0 = 0.10$.

[c] The parabola (second degree polynomial) can only be fitted over a limited range (Fig. 15.11). For case a, the parabola is fitted between the log dilutions of 3 and 4.5 (regression formula in Fig. 15.11), whereas in case b the regression curve is fitted between the log dilutions of 1 and 5 (regression formula: $A = 0.6754 - 0.4417 (\log D) + 0.0599 (\log D)^2$). Cubic, quartic, or quintic polynomials were calculated by the methods discussed in great detail by Snedecor and Cochran (1967).

basis of logit in fitting data has been reported by Rodbard and McClean (1977) and Wellington (1980) and an example will be given below. Linearization of sigmoidal curves leads to a severe heteroscedascity (Section 15.1). A significant drawback of the proportional transformation is that symmetry of the sigmoid curve (about inflection point) is assumed.

A solution in cases where the logit function fails to linearize response curves is the non-linear least squares method (Cook and Wellington, 1978) by changing the exponent in the logistic function (below) to provide for curvature. This sophisticated method does not assume a linear response curve and is more generally applicable. In addition to the four-parameter logistic curve, Cook (cited by Wellington, 1980) suggested several models of five-parameter logistic curves for EIA.

The general form of the four-parameter logistic function is:

$$\frac{A' - A_0}{A_m - A_0} = \frac{1}{1 + (D/c)^b} \quad \text{or} \quad A' = \frac{A_m - A_0}{1 + (D/c)^b} + A_0$$

in which A' corresponds to the absorbance of the test sample divided by the maximum absorbance, i.e., that at high antigen concentration, A_m is the maximum dose absorbance, A_0 is the zero dose absorbance, D is the test calibration dose or dilution and c is a constant which corresponds to the value of D at $(A_m + A_0)/2$. This equation resembles the Hill equation (Section 9.1.3; Section 15.3), although the thermodynamic terms of the parameters may differ (De Lean et al., 1978). In this expression b determines the curvature of the dose–response curve and corresponds to the slope in the logit–log plot:

$$\pm b = \frac{d(\text{logit}\,(A' - A_0)/(A_m - A_0))}{d \ln D}$$

Iterative fitting of the standard curve can be done with a weighting function depending on the presence of a systematic non-uniform variance. This weighting function is $1/\sigma^2$, for n replicate standards giving a mean response A' at a given dose.

The logit transformation can then be computed, after replacing $(A' - A_0)/(A_m - A_0)$ by proportion p:

$$\text{logit} \frac{A' - A_0}{A_m - A_0} = \text{logit}\, p = \ln \frac{p}{1-p}$$

In the example (Table 15.2; Fig. 15.10) the maximum and background absorbances are 1.68 and 0.1, respectively and, e.g., at a value of $A = 0.40$, logit $p = \ln (0.30/1.58)/(1 - 0.30/1.58 = -1.45$. The logit p values thus calculated give a virtually straight line (d is logit p extrapolated to log $D = 0$):

$$\text{logit}\, p = d + b \log D$$

the regression of which can serve to calculate the dose or dilution:

$$D_{\text{test}} = \text{antilog} \frac{(\text{logit}\, p) - d}{b}$$

Alternatively, plotting the dose–response curve on logit–log paper is convenient for the direct estimation of D. Probits are not used

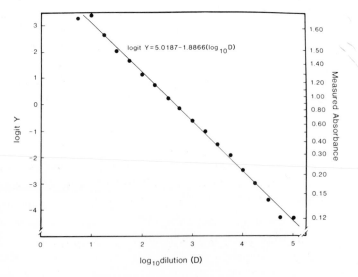

Fig. 15.10. Logit transformation of the dose–response curve of Fig. 15.8. Details on the calculation are given in Section 15.2.5.

for this purpose though they are based on the similar principle and will yield comparable results.

Fitting of data with a polynomial is very popular in bioassays. The fit can be achieved by Lagrangian interpolation or, alternatively, by the least squares (Wellington, 1980). However, these polynomials lack monotonicity of the curves and are distorted by outlying values. Nevertheless, they have been adapted with success for AA-type EIA (Platt et al., 1981).

Curvilinear fitting with polynomials may avoid the distortion of the error structure encountered with logits. In the polynomial model, successive powers of D (dose or dilution):

$$A = A_0 + c_1 \cdot D + c_2 \cdot D^2 + c_3 \cdot D^3 + ... + c_n \cdot D^n$$

are regarded as separate predictor variables. The polynomial can be fitted by applying the standard methods after defining $D = x_1$, $D^2 = x_2$, etc. Fig. 15.11 shows that the fitting by second degree polynomials is useful only for a limited range, since least square parabolas are produced. The regression line is, however, reliable over a larger range than with the log transformation. Enlarging the range for fitting outside the exponential part of the curve produces poor fitting (Fig. 15.11). The log–log transformation gives a parabola-like curve for a large range and fitting should be excellent for:

$$\log A = \log A_0 + c_1 \cdot \log D + c_2 \cdot (\log D)^2$$

The fitting by higher polynomials (cubic, quartic, quintic) is closer (Table 15.2), however, outlying observations tend to bend the curve and calculation without automation is time-consuming.

15.3. Calculation procedures for activity-modulation assays

AM-type EIA can be divided into two groups: heterogeneous (solid-

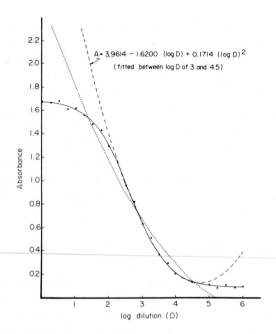

Fig. 15.11. Curve-fitting by second degree polynomials of the sigmoid curve given in Fig. 15.8. The least square parabolas will fit well if the range used for fitting is small and only that range is considered. Enlarging the range to log D of 1–5 will result in poor fitting.

phase) EIA and homogeneous EIA. The curves obtained and the calculations with AM-type EIA are quite similar to those discussed above.

Solid-phase AM-type EIA are increasingly subjected to data reduction and linearization procedures for more accurate results with the least possible testing (Signorella and Hymer, 1984). This accuracy can be similar to, or even exceed, that obtained with a large number of data processed in a less sophisticated manner.

The omnipresence of desk-top programmable calculators, such as the TI-59, or of microcomputers, in particular when interfaced with other equipment and printers, increases significantly their use for the evaluation of EIA. They decrease the risks of obtaining erroneous results and reduce thereby the necessity of plotting manually the data. Computer programs for the rapid and precise analysis of the data of solid-phase AM-type EIA have been designed by Canellas and Karu (1981) and Ritchie et al. (1981).

Homogeneous EIA lend themselves better to dose–response curve linearization than solid-phase EIA. This type of EIA is generally used for the determination of concentrations of small molecules (haptens, drugs). The major supplier of this type of EIA kits (Syva Co.) recommends the plotting of the response variable ('EMIT Units') vs the log of the concentration or the presentation of the results on special non-linear graph paper provided by them, which is, in fact, logit–log paper.

Oellerich et al. (1982) compared 5 different data processing methods for 5 EMIT kits which were adapted for the Cobas Bio Centrifugal analyzer. These methods were the 4-parameter logistic function (log–logit model), the 5-parameter logit, the 5-parameter exponential, the 5-parameter polynomial and the spline approximation. The 4-parameter logistic function gave the best results which explains its general popularity.

Rodbard and McClean (1977) applied the 4-parameter logistic model, discussed in Section 15.2.5, to a number of EMIT assays for various drugs with a fully mechanized enzyme rate analyzer. The standard curves are usually constructed to span the therapeutic range. A practical difficulty encountered with this method is to determine A_0, the absorbance at the background plateau, which is usually measured at a dose of hapten 10–50 times higher than the highest dose for the standard curve (antibody virtually completely saturated), since some of the drugs or haptens may not be soluble at the dose required. To circumvent this difficulty, Rodbard and McClean (1977) used a cross-kit, i.e., a similar kit for another more soluble drug. The validity of such an approach is questionable and depends strongly on the uniformity of the reagents and on the absence of cross-reactivity. Dietzler et al. (1983) observed a marked variation in the value of A_0 using different equipments or reaction conditions.

In an earlier study, A_0 was estimated simply by omitting the antibody from the mixture, instead of trying to saturate the available antibody with an excess of the hapten (Dietzler et al., 1980). The importance of a correct value for d to obtain linear curves is illustrated in Fig. 15.12. The graph paper provided by Syva Co. with their kits is based on an assumed uniformity in $(A_0 - A_m)$, which is designated as K_C (printed in the lower left side of the paper). Adaptation of the ordinate to the real value of the (maximum absorbance–minimum absorbance) results in a straight line (Fig. 15.12).

Dietzler et al. (1980) used an equation:

$$A = A' - A_0 = \frac{A^*}{1 + (H_{1/2}/H)^n} \quad \text{or} \quad A' = \frac{A^*}{1 + (H_{1/2}/H)^n} + A_0$$

which is analogous to the Hill equation (Atkinson, 1966; Section 9.1.3) and in which A is the net change in absorbance ($\times 1000$), A_0 is the absorbance ($\times 1000$) at zero dose, A^* is the change in absorbance from infinite dose to zero dose, H the hapten concentration and $H_{1/2}$ is the hapten concentration at $A' = A^*/2$. This procedure has the advantage that it can be applied under any reaction condition and without the use of the kinetic analyzer (Fig. 15.12).

The slope of the response curve is often quite low (about 0.5–0.8; Rodbard and McClean, 1977) which means that a wide range of concentrations (up to 4 orders of magnitude) can be tested. Changing the experimental protocol to obtain a steeper slope decreases the useful span but, at the same time, increases the precision and sensitivity of the method (Section 15.1).

Fig. 15.12. I. Representative curve for theophylline using graph paper and $A^* = 216$ milliabsorbance units provided by Syva Co.. With the ABA-100 analyzer some of the calibrator points are above the projected straight line. II. A saturation curve for theophylline with the EMIT assay, using the ABA-100 in the normal kinetic mode, showed that the A^* is significantly higher. III. The data shown in II can be fitted to a Hill equation, using the computer program of Atkins (1973), giving $A^* = 514$, $H_{1/2} = 300$ μg/ml, and $n = 0.56$. The various instrumental adaptations will result in different values of A^*, $H_{1/2}$, and n. From Dietzler et al., 1980; courtesy Dr. D. N. Dietzler and *Clinica Chimica Acta*.

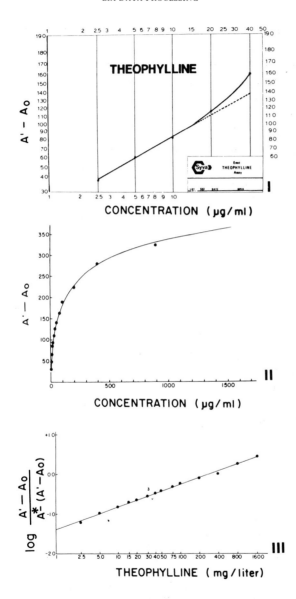

A drawback of the logit transformation is the introduction of a severe non-uniformity of the variance, which makes it highly desirable to use weighted regression. Fey (1981) designed a computer program to replace the logit–log procedure.

15.4. Standardization and optimization of assays

Optimization with the goal to maximize precision of results, to determine optimum assay conditions, and to assess the effect of changes on the assay requires a rigid statistical evaluation of the error structure of the assay. The approach of Ekins (1979) for RIA is valid for EIA as well and is based on rather simple concepts. Rodbard (1978) used a much more complex approach to analyze the error structure of EIA.

In the method of Ekins, a response–error relationship (RER) is established by plotting the error of the response variable against the response (e.g., 10 replicates for each dose; plotting the SD against the response; Fig. 15.13).

The precision profile (Ekins, 1976) gives the relation of SD of concentration (ΔC) or CV of concentration ($\Delta C/C$) as a function of the dose (Section 15.1; Fig. 15.13). This is readily obtained by dividing the SD of the response (from the RER curve) by the sensitivity (Section 15.1) of the dose-response curve for that dose. A change in the assay is reflected on the precision profile. These curves indicate which of the assay alternatives has the higher detectability or the higher precision. For example, to establish the optimal antibody concentration for an AM assay, a dose–response curve is established with different antibody concentrations in the presence and absence of competing immunoreactant (Fig. 15.14). The optimal antibody concentration is that for which the ratio of the change in response (dR) and the error at that point (SD) is maximal. This is generally not at the antibody concentration at which the difference between the two curves (with and without antigen) is maximal, where the error is minimal or where the sensitivity of the curves is maximal.

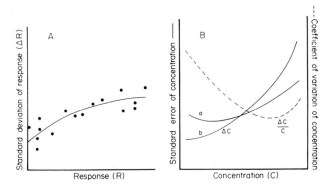

Fig. 15.13. Response error relationship (A) and precision profiles (B) to optimize (particularly AM-)EIA according to Ekins (1979). The immunoreactant concentrations which will give minimum variance, will give also minimum variance when small amounts of sample are added and allows the highest detectability. First, the *R* is measured at different responses (reliability is not high with a few replicates, Section 15.1). The error in dose (ΔC) or the relative error ($\Delta C/C$: coefficient of variation) can then be determined by the ΔR (corresponding to the *R* of that dose) and the sensitivity of the dose–response curve as shown in Fig. 15.1. A change in, e.g., the antibody concentration may change the precision profile from (a) to (b), which has a greater detectability, but less precision at high antigen concentrations.

Fig. 15.14 demonstrates some essential differences between EIA and RIA in this respect.

A large list of criteria can be made for ideal material standards (stability, homogeneity, absence of contaminants, accurate division into smaller aliquots, uniform and low moisture content, identity of properties with the test substance). Activity of standard material is quantitated in internationally accepted units (IU in immunology, U in enzymology; in enzymology IU denotes inhibitory international units).

Standardization defines the concentrations or activities of substances which cannot be characterized adequately by chemical or physical means (Rowe et al., 1970a, b, c; World Health Organization, 1972; Batty and Torrigani, 1980). Attempts have been made to standardize conjugates for EIA (Batty and Torrigani, 1980).

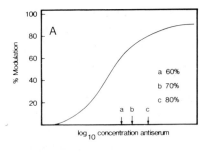 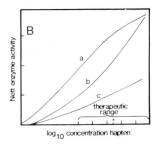

Fig. 15.14. Assay optimization of AM-type EIA such as EMIT (Kabakoff and Green-wood, 1982). In a first step, the concentration of antibody to modulate (inhibit) a given amount of enzyme conjugate is determined. Here, maximum inhibition is about 90% (inhibition should not be confounded with 'deactivation' of enzyme due to conjugation). In the next step, several ratio's antibody and enzyme conjugate are compared over the therapeutic range. Though detectability is highest for a, the highest sensitivity over the therapeutic range is obtained with b. Precision profiles (Fig. 15.13B) help then to optimize the assay. Cross- or shared reactivity is determined at the geometric mean (*) of the hapten concentration (= square root of product of highest and lowest concentration of the therapeutic range), in contrast to radioimmunoassays where 50% displacement of label is customarily measured. For example, if the geometric mean is 5 µg/ml (range 1–25 µg/ml) and the CV(%) is 15%, then cross-reactivity is expressed as the concentration of non-specific hapten needed to elevate the response to 6.5 µg/ml (i.e., 5 + 2×CV). Cross-reactivity can be selectively reduced by the addition of less-specific antibodies to block the cross-reactant or by desensitization of the assay by adding cross-reactant to the antibody reagent (in commercial assays).

15.5. Quality control and quality assessment

Quality control serves to ensure that levels of precision, accuracy, detectability, sensitivity and specificity are adequate. It has been stressed earlier that considerable confusion exists with some of these terms which have been defined in Section 1.3 and Section 15.1. These parameters are interrelated which easily leads to interpretational discrepancies.

Two types of quality assessment schemes can be distinguished: external quality assessment (between laboratories) and internal quality control (within laboratories; Hunter et al., 1980). The principal aim of internal quality control is to improve or maintain reproducibility, whereas external quality assessment considers the fundamental design of the assay, as compared to other available designs. Control and assessment procedures are usually directed against 2 different errors, imprecision for internal control and bias for external control.

Reproducibility which applies to all 5 concepts, may refer to within-assay or between-assay variation. Sometimes within-assay reproducibility is designated as repeatability (Palmer and Cavallero, 1980)

SD itself does not yield useful information, unless compared to the mean (%CV; Section 15.1). Between-assay variation is generally greater than within-assay variation, but care should be taken with the latter to reduce bias by randomly distributing the duplicates. The between-assay variation is usually of more value to estimate the accuracy of the procedure and, plotted on a quality-control chart, may indicate trends, such as deterioration of reagents (bias-type error; Section 1.3). An example of the calculation of the within-assay and between-assay variability is given in Table 15.3. In this example, the SD of between-assay results is about 5–6 times higher than for the within-assay results. For a satisfactory EIA, this factor should be less than 2–3 and the between-assay variability should be less than 10%.

A useful but not yet universally accepted parameter is the acceptable limit of error (ALE) which is generally set in each laboratory. The rule-of-thumb proposed by Tonks (cited by Palmer and Cavallero, 1980) is illustrative, although it may be too restrictive for many EIA:

$$\text{ALE} = \frac{1/4 \text{ length of normal range}}{\text{midpoint of normal range}}$$

For example, for the serum IgG levels of adult caucasian males (normal range 77–171 IU/ml), this would be 18.95%. In order to obtain information on the reliability of such EIA, the knowledge of the magnitude of the variation of measurements is essential. This can be obtained by appropriate statistical analyses of accumulated data over repeated tests. Quality control samples can then be included

TABLE 15.3

Example of calculation of within-assay and between-assay variability
(adapted from Rodbard, 1974)

Assay	Response		Mean	SD
	Test 1	Test 2		
1	74	70	72	2.38
2	93	93	93	0
3	105	110	107.5	3.54
4	102	102	102	0
5	105	95	100	7.07
6	78	82	80	2.83
7	87	88	87.5	0.71
Mean	92	91.43	91.71	2.43
SD	12.81	13.11	12.71	
SD_m [a]	4.84	4.96	4.80	

[a] SD_m = standard error of the mean = $SD/\sqrt{n}$.

SD-within assays:–for single sample: (mean of SD) = *2.43*
  –for means of duplicates: $(SD/\sqrt{n} = 2.43/\sqrt{2}) = 1.72$
  –$SD/\sqrt{r}$ responses are mean of r replicates.
-between assays: –for single sample: $(12.81 + 13.11)/2 = 12.91$
  –for means of duplicates = 12.71
  Nota bene, not $12.91/\sqrt{2}$, since the between-assay SD contains an intrinsic component of variation, SD_b, which is the lower limit and equals
  $[(SD \text{ of assay means})^2 - (\text{mean } SD)^2/r]^{1/2} = (12.71^2 - 2.43^2/2)^{1/2} = 12.59 - [\text{mean } SD]^2/r + SD^2_b]^{1/2} = (2.43^2/r + 12.59^2)^{1/2}$, if responses are means of r replicates.

CV(%): -within assays: –for single sample: $((2.43/91.71) \times 100) = 2.65$
  –for means of duplicates: $((1.72/91.71) \times 100) = 1.88$
  –for means of replicates $(2.43/91.71 \times \sqrt{r}) \times 100$
  -between assays: –for single sample: $((12.91/91.71) \times 100) = 14.08$
  –for means of duplicates: $((12.71/91.71) \times 100) = 13.86$
  –for means of replicates $(2.65^2/r + 13.73^2)^{1/2}$
t-test for difference between the 2 tests (SD of differences is 5.12 and $SD_m = 1.94$):

$$\frac{\text{average difference}}{SD_m} = \frac{(+4 + 0 - 5 + 0 + 10 - 4 - 1)/7}{1.94} = 0.3 \text{ (not significant).}$$

in the tests to monitor the measurement variations at different concentration levels and to ensure the quality of the tests.

Hunter et al. (1980) reviewed several causes of bias encountered with external quality assessment. A most important cause of bias is related to the suitability of standards, i.e., miscalculation due to incorrect dilutions and lability of standards on storage. Other causes may be related to the separation system or to over-wide working ranges. In order to recognize bias, monitoring of precision (independent of other parameters) is extremely important (Woodhead et al., 1980).

Quality assessment schemes aim to establish whether or not the test results are within accepted limits and to demonstrate the possible necessity to correct test design (Batty, 1977).

Localization and identification of electrophoretically separated antigens after their transfer from gel to membrane

Electrophoretic analysis is the most generally used method in the analysis of complex mixtures of proteins and the most widely employed supporting material is polyacrylamide gel (PAG), particularly in the presence of sodium dodecyl sulphate (SDS).

The use of SDS is popular, since this detergent solubilizes and complexes with essentially all proteins in a proportion of about 1.4 g SDS/g protein. The extreme diversity in the structure, charge and solubility of proteins is then minimized and separation of the SDS-proteins reflects differences in their molecular weights. The proteins separated on such gels are usually stained with Coomassie Brilliant Blue (CBB; detection limit ≈ 100 ng/mm^2) or with the ultra-sensitive silver stain (detection limit $0.01 - 1$ ng/mm^2) which can reveal 150 polypeptides from a single human fingerprint (Marshall, 1984)). A drawback of such procedures is that the proteins are stained without revealing the nature of each band or spot, unless they are enzymes and an enzymic stain is applied. However, enzymic revelation is often unsuccessful in the presence of the anionic detergent SDS. In recent years, the method used originally to transfer nucleic acids from agarose to membrane filters (Southern, 1975) proved to be also excellent for the transfer of proteins from PAG to membranes. Faithful replicas can be obtained from the gel and the various bands or spots can then be analyzed by the methods used in EIH (Chapter 17) with a detectability similar to the silver staining. This transfer of proteins from gels to filters ('protein blotting') is often referred to as 'Western' blotting (Gershoni and Palade, 1983), by analogy to the original 'Southern' blotting technique for the transfer of DNA to filters and the transfer of RNA which was named 'Northern' blotting by Alwine et al. (1977). This method combines the high capacity of EIA to identify antigens with the high resolving power of PAGE (Table 16.1).

16.1. Gel electrophoresis of proteins

The PAGE of proteins can be classified according to the buffer systems, continuous or discontinuous, depending on whether the same buffer or different buffers are used in the gel and electrode compartments, and according to the presence or absence of dissociating agents. Detailed reviews on the practice of PAGE of proteins have been published by Gordon (1975; volume 1 of this series)

TABLE 16.1

Advantages of transferring proteins from polyacrylamide gels to membrane filters prior to EIA

– Easy handling of filters.

– Localization of separated, specific proteins as highly concentrated bands by EIA with a detectability at least 100 times higher than by conventional, nonspecific staining of the gel. This detection limit is similar to that of autoradiography or silver staining.

– Possibility of the preparation of multiple replicas from the same gel for different EIA or auxiliary tests.

– Stability of replicas for months prior to use.

– Affinity purification of antibodies, i.e., adsorption onto and elution from a certain band, is possible. This method is useful for the identification of individual proteins or peptides ('epitope mapping').

– Small amounts of proteins recovered from slices of gels can be used for immunization of animals, producing excellent reagents for EIA on blots.

and by Hames and Rickwood (1981). Here, only the most frequently used gel systems are discussed.

16.1.1. Gel electrophoresis in the presence of SDS

SDS dissociates most proteins and reacts with them so as to equalize their charge properties. The electrophoresis protocols for SDS-proteins are, hence, not as diverse as for native proteins.

The continuous SDS-buffer of Shapiro et al. (1967) and Weber and Osborn (1969) is widely used. In this system the same phosphate buffer (100 mM, pH 7.0) is used, both for the gels and the electrode compartments. Protein separation under such conditions is consequently slow. The discontinuous system of Laemmli (1970), adapted from the system earlier described by Davis (1964) and Ornstein (1964), produces considerably faster separation than the continuous system.

The percentage of polyacrylamide to be used depends both on the proteins to be separated and on the buffer system selected. This percentage (w/v) is expressed both in terms of total polyacrylamide (acrylamide + bisacrylamide) and of percentage of bisacrylamide of the total polyacrylamide. As a general rule, a higher acrylamide concentration gives smaller pores and permits smaller proteins to pass. The relationship with bisacrylamide (cross-linker) is, however, more complicated. With increasing concentrations of bisacrylamide, the pore size first decreases, but over about 2.5% of the total polyacrylamide the pores become larger (Gordon, 1975; Tijssen and Kurstak, 1979a).

Migration in PAG also depends on the buffer system. In general, small polypeptides which migrate with the buffer front are not separated: in the continuous buffer system these limiting molecular weights are 8000 at 15% PAG, 12000 at 10% and 20000 at 5%; in the discontinuous buffer system these values are 8000, 16000 and 60000, respectively. A most useful method for the separation of proteins with a wide range of molecular weights is the use of PAG gradients which have the added advantage that they tend to sharpen the bands (Tijssen and Kurstak, 1979b).

Anomalous migration of proteins may be due to poor binding of SDS, which is the case with glycoproteins (Segrest and Jackson, 1972) or to the presence of disulfide bridges (Tijssen and Kurstak, 1981). Very basic proteins, such as histones, also tend to migrate more slowly than expected on the basis of their molecular weight (Panyis and Chalkley, 1971).

Stock solutions can be prepared for SDS (10 or 25%), the various buffers and the acrylamide–bisacrylamide mixture. The latter should be shielded from light and handled with care, since it is neurotoxic in its unpolymerized form. The catalyst, $(NH_4)_2S_2O_8$, is prepared fresh daily. The composition of the gel and the electrode buffers for the continuous system (Weber and Osborn, 1969) and for the discontinuous system (Laemmli, 1970) are presented in Tables 16.2 and 16.3. The samples are prepared for the continuous system in 10 mM sodium phosphate buffer, pH 7.0, containing 2% SDS, 2% 2-ME and 10% glycerol, and for the discontinuous system in 25 mM Tris–HCl buffer, pH 6.8 (as stacking gel buffer), containing 5% SDS, 2% 2-ME and 10% glycerol. The content for each protein present in these samples should, for CBB staining, be at least 0.3 µg/mm² slot surface for the continuous system and 0.1 µg/mm² slot surface for the discontinuous system. Bromophenol blue (0.001%) is included to indicate the buffer front. During electrophoresis the proteins migrate to the anode (+). It is good practice to operate at a constant voltage, since only this will give constant mobility during electrophoresis. For the continuous system, a potential of 3 V/cm is suitable, whereas for the discontinuous system the voltage is usually about 3–4 times higher (but the amperage is lower). After electrophoresis, the proteins may be stained, recovered from the gel for further use (e.g., immunization) or transferred to membranes for enzyme immunodetection.

16.1.2. Two-dimensional SDS-electrophoresis for simultaneous peptide mapping of proteins contained in a mixture

A simple method for peptide mapping and analysis of epitopes is

TABLE 16.2

Preparation of gels for continuous SDS-containing phosphate buffer systems[a]

Solutions	Volumes (ml) required for gels with final polyacrylamide concentration (%) of				
	15.0	12.5	10.0	7.5	5.0
Acrylamide/ bisacrylamide[b]	15.0	12.5	10.0	7.5	5.0
300 mM sodium phosphate buffer, pH 7.0	10.0	10.0	10.0	10.0	10.0
10% (w/w) SDS	0.3	0.3	0.3	0.3	0.3
Distilled water	4.5	7.0	9.5	12.0	14.5
TEMED[c]	0.015	0.015	0.015	0.015	0.015
10% (w/w) ammonium persulfate	0.2	0.2	0.2	0.2	0.2

[a] The solutions should be added in the same sequence as given in the Table and the mixture should be deaerated after adding the water. Ammonium persulfate, a strong oxidizing agent which acts as a catalyst for the polymerization, is added under mixing, just before casting. To insure flat surfaces, 0.1% SDS should be layered over the gel if cast in tubes, or a gel-comb is inserted in the top of the slab.

[b] Acrylamide (29.2 g) and bisacrylamide (0.8 g) are dissolved in 70 ml distilled water. After complete dissolution, the volume is brought to 100 ml and the container is wrapped in aluminum foil.

[c] TEMED: N,N,N',N'-tetramethylethylenediamine (1 ml = about 0.77 g).

offered by a two-dimensional SDS-electrophoresis system combined with limited proteolysis (Tijssen and Kurstak, 1983). In this method, the polypeptides are first separated by conventional discontinuous SDS-PAGE (Section 16.1.1). The strip of gel containing the unstained polypeptide bands is then embedded into a second stacking gel, perpendicularly to the direction of electrophoresis, 1–2 cm above the resolving (gradient) gel. The protease is loaded onto the stacking

TABLE 16.3

Preparation of gels for discontinuous SDS-containing Tris buffer systems[a]

Solutions	Stacking gel	Volumes (ml) required for resolving gel with final concentration polyacrylamide (%) of				
		15.0	12.5	10.0	7.5	5.0
Acrylamide/ bisacrylamide[b]	1.25	15.0	12.5	10.0	7.5	5.0
Stacking gel buffer[b]	1.25					
Resolving gel buffer[b]		3.75	3.75	3.75	3.75	3.75
Distilled water	7.3	10.75	13.25	15.75	18.25	20.75
10% (w/w) SDS	0.1	0.3	0.3	0.3	0.3	0.3
TEMED[c]	0.008	0.015	0.015	0.015	0.015	0.015
10% ammonium persulfate	0.1	0.2	0.2	0.2	0.2	0.2

[a] Prepare gels by mixing the solutions in the sequence of the table (deaerate the mixture after adding water). Persulfate is added last under mixing, just before casting the gel. The stacking gel (0.5–1 cm high) is gently layered over the resolving gel and the comb is immediately inserted into the stacking gel solution.

[b] Acrylamide-bisacrylamide solution is prepared as described in Table 16.2. Stacking gel buffer (1 M Tris–HCl, pH 6.8) is made by dissolving 12.1 g Tris in 60 ml 1.25 M HCl, adjusting the pH to 6.8 with 1.25 M HCl and bringing to 100 ml final volume with distilled water. Resolving gel buffer (3 M Tris–HCl, pH 8.8) is prepared by dissolving 36.3 g Tris in 48 ml 1 M HCl and bringing to 100 ml final volume with distilled water.

[c] TEMED: N,N,N',N'-tetramethylethylenediamine.

gel and brought into contact with the substrate by electrophoresis (e.g., for 30 min). The buffers are selected so as to bring the proteins contained in the original strip into contact with the protease in a sharp band (Fig. 16.1). At this point the electrophoresis is stopped to obtain the desired degree of digestion. The peptide fragments are subsequently separated in the resolving (gradient) gel underneath.

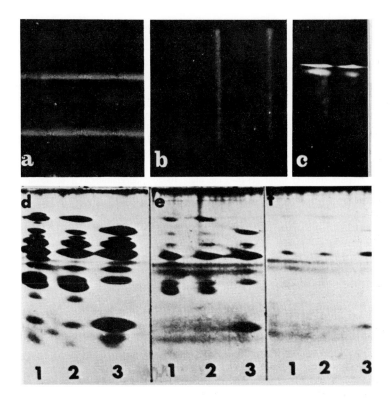

Fig. 16.1.Principle of epitope mapping using a two-dimensional electrophoresis procedure (proteins were dansylated only for visualization). The polypeptides are first
separated by conventional SDS-electrophoresis (a) and a strip containing the separated
polypeptides is embedded perpendicular to the direction of electrophoresis in a second
gel (b). The protease, loaded on top of this second gel, is concentrated with its
substrate (c) in the spacer gel through moving boundary electrophoresis. The peptides
thus generated are separated in the resolving gel (d, e, f; 1000, 100, and 10 ng
total protein, respectively) and can be stained or transferred to nitrocellulose membranes (0.1 μm pores instead of the usual 0.45 μm should be used) and epitopes
can be traced back to the various fragments of the same protein (from Tijssen
and Kurstak, 1983; courtesy of *Analytical Biochemistry*).

These fragments may then be transferred to membranes and the
epitope composition analyzed. Table 16.4 lists problems that may

TABLE 16.4

Two-dimensional simultaneous electrophoretic peptide mapping of protein mixtures

1. Separate proteins or polypeptides according to the method given in Table 16.3 (e.g., on 7.5 or 10% polyacrylamide gel).

2. Cut a gel strip (0.5–4 cm wide, depending on the protein concentration) containing the proteins of interest and incubate for 30 min in 125 mM Tris–HCl buffer, pH 6.8, supplemented with 0.1% SDS (no stirring). Drain excess liquid from the gel and place it horizontally between the glass plates, at 8 cm from the bottom so that the polypeptide bands are oriented parallel to direction of electrophoresis.

3. Prepare small gradient gel (6–7 cm high; 10–20% acrylamide, 5% bisacrylamide with respect to total polyacrylamide) of the same thickness as in step 1, using the following composition (volumes in ml; for acrylamide-bisacrylamide, see note in Table 16.2):

	Acrylamide concentration	
	10%	20%
Acrylamide-bisacrylamide (respectively 28.5 and 1.5 g/100 ml)	2.09	4.17
Resolving gel buffer	0.78	0.78
Distilled water	3.19	0.55
Glycerin		0.62
10% (w/w) SDS	0.07	0.07
10% (v/v) TEMED	0.06	0.03
10% (w/w) ammonium persulfate	0.06	0.03

Deaerate after first four solutions are mixed and add rest (persulfate last). Prepare the linear gradient with a gradient mixer equipped with chambers of equal cross-sections. The top of the gradient should be at least 1 cm below the gel strip and immediately overlayered with 1 ml of a 0.1% SDS solution.

4. After polymerization of the gradient gel, the stacking gel is prepared according to Table 16.3, with the following modifications: 1.87 ml acrylamide solution is used, the water (6.78 ml) should contain 5 μg riboflavin/ml, and ammonium sulfate is omitted (deleterious to proteases). Tilting the slab apparatus while pouring the stacking gel prevents trapping of air bubbles under the gel strip. The stacking gel solution should be about 1 cm above the gel strip and is overlayered with 0.1%

SDS. Polymerization is achieved by riboflavin, using illumination with a day-light fluorescent lamp from a distance of 2–5 cm.

5. The enzyme solution (in 62.5 mM Tris–HCl buffer, pH 6.8, containing 10% glycerol, 0.1% SDS and 0.001% bromophenol blue) is layered over the gel. Optimum enzyme concentrations are 2 ng papain or 8 ng *Staphylococcus aureus* protease V8 (Miles) per mm^2 of slot surface. It is better to dilute the enzyme solution so that the overlay produces a layer of about 3 mm high, in order to avoid possible artefacts if the gel is not perfectly horizontal.

---

arise. In practice, after the gel is prepared, electrophoresis is first carried out at 2.5 V/cm for 15 min and subsequently at 7.5 V/cm, until the bromophenol blue band moves to 2–5 mm above the resolving gel. The current is then interrupted for 30 min and resumed at a potential of 10 V/cm until the dye indicator reaches the bottom. Analysis of the fragments is carried out as in Sections 16.1.4 and 16.2.

16.1.3. Electrophoresis in non-dissociating buffer systems

Native proteins differ widely in their solubility and charge properties. Consequently, for their electrophoretic separation they require different experimental conditions (Gordon, 1975; Hames and Rickwood, 1981). A given ionic strength may be too low for some proteins resulting in aggregation, whereas a higher ionic strength may produce excessive heat.

For the discontinuous buffer systems, the three widely used protocols, i.e., for high pH (Davis, 1964; Ornstein, 1964), neutral pH (Williams and Reisfeld, 1964) and low pH (Reisfeld et al., 1962), are in Table 16.5. The neutral buffer system has a poor buffering capacity and is only useful for proteins which are unstable in the high pH system. The low pH system is used for basic proteins (histones, several of the POase isozymes). It is imperative to check carefully the pH of all solutions.

The discontinuous buffer systems are designed in such a way

TABLE 16.5

Non-dissociating, discontinuous electrophoresis systems[a]

Solutions	Stacking gel	Volumes (ml) required for resolving gel with polyacrylamide concentration (%) of				
		15.0	12.5	10.0	7.5	5.0
Acrylamide/ bisacrylamide	1.25	15.0	12.5	10.0	7.5	5.0
Stacking gel buffer[b]	1.25					
Resolving gel buffer[b]		3.75	3.75	3.75	3.75	3.75
Distilled water	6.50	8.75	11.25	13.75	16.25	18.75
TEMED[c]	0.015	0.015	0.015	0.015	0.015	0.015
Riboflavin[c] (40 μg/ml)	1.0	2.5	2.5	2.5	2.5	2.5
10% ammonium persulfate[c]		2.5	2.5	2.5	2.5	2.5

[a] Mix solutions in the sequence given in the table. Deaerate after adding water. Stock solution for acrylamide-bisacrylamide is the same as in Table 16.2.

[b] *Buffer solutions:*

High pH (for neutral and acidic proteins; Davis, 1964):

    The stacking gel and resolving gel buffers are the same as in the Laemmli system (Table 16.3).

    The reservoir buffer contains 25 mM Tris and 19.2 mM glycine.

Neutral pH (Williams and Reisfeld, 1964):

    Stacking gel buffer: dissolve 4.95 g Tris in 40 ml distilled water and titrate to pH 5.5 with 1 M orthophosphoric acid. Complete to 100 ml with distilled water.

    Resolving gel buffer: dissolve 6.85 g Tris in 40 ml distilled water and titrate to pH 7.5 with 1 M HCl. Complete to 100 ml with distilled water.

    Reservoir buffer contains 55.2 g diethylbarbituric acid and 10.0 g Tris in 1 l distilled water.

Low pH (for basic proteins; Reisfeld et al., 1962)

    Stacking gel buffer: add 48 ml 1 M KOH and 2.9 ml glacial acetic acid to distilled water, check the pH (should be 6.8) and complete to 100 ml with distilled water.

that a moving boundary is generated between the relatively rapidly migrating charged species (leading ions) and the somewhat more slowly migrating species (trailing ions). The National Technical Information Service lists the principal properties of more than 4000 buffer systems ('Jovin' output) capable of generating moving boundaries (Public Board Numbers 268309 to 259312, catalogue no. 196090) (Jovin, 1973; Chrambach and Rodbard, 1981) which are available at a nominal cost.

For the continuous buffer systems, the buffer concentrations are usually between 10 and 100 mM. Above pH 7.0, the most often used buffers are 20–50 mM Tris buffers (Tris-glycine or Tris-borate for pH 8.3–9.3; Tris-acetate for pH 7.2–8.5; Tris-citrate for pH 7.0–8.5). For basic proteins the buffer β-analine (10–50 mM)-acetate (pH 4–5) can be used (Hames, 1981). Table 16.6 summarizes the preparation of continuous gel systems.

The samples should be dissolved in a two-fold diluted stacking gel buffer for the discontinuous systems or in a 5–10 times diluted gel buffer for the continuous systems and should always contain 10% glycerol (or sucrose). A tracking dye (0.001%, bromophenol blue for alkaline and neutral gels and methyl green or pyronin for acidic gels) may also be included. Some recurrent problems and their correction are listed in Table 16.7.

Resolving gel buffer: add 48 ml 1 M KOH and 17.2 ml glacial acetic acid to distilled water, check pH (should be 4.3) and complete to 100 ml with distilled water.

Reservoir buffer: dissolve 31.2 g β-alanine in 80 ml distilled water and add 8 ml glacial acetic acid, check pH (should be 4.3) and complete to 100 ml with distilled water.

[c] Riboflavin should be used as catalyst (instead of ammonium persulfate) if enzymes or other macromolecules sensitive to persulfate are to be separated. Riboflavin is also more effective at lower pH than persulfate. The amount of TEMED (N,N,N',N'-tetramethylethylenediamine) should be increased 10-fold for the low pH, discontinuous gel preparations.

TABLE 16.6
Continuous, non-dissociating gel systems[a]

Solutions	Volumes (ml) required for gel with final polyacrylamide concentration (%) of				
	15.0	12.5	10.0	7.5	5.0
Acrylamide/bisacrylamide	15.0	12.5	10.0	7.5	5.0
Buffer (5 × concentrated)	6.0	6.0	6.0	6.0	6.0
Distilled water	7.5	10.0	12.5	15.0	17.5
TEMED[b]	0.015	0.015	0.015	0.015	0.015
Ammonium persulfate (1%) or Riboflavin (40 μg/ml)	2.5	2.5	2.5	2.5	2.5

[a] Acrylamide/bisacrylamide stock solution is prepared as given in Table 16.2. The most widely used buffer solutions are mentioned in Section 16.1.3. Riboflavin should be used instead of ammonium persulfate if persulfate-sensitive proteins (such as enzymes) are present or for acidic gels. The concentration of TEMED should be increased 10-fold for acidic gels. The reservoir buffer is the same as for the gel.

[b] TEMED: N,N,N',N'-tetramethylethylenediamine.

16.1.4. Staining of proteins after electrophoresis

CBB R250 or G250 (0.1%) in methanol-water-glacial acetic acid (5:5:2), filtered before use, is the most frequently used stain. The gel is incubated in this solution for 1 h; for SDS-containing gels the volume of the stain should be at least 10 times larger than that of the gel and destained by electrophoresis or by simple diffusion in 7.5% glacial acetic acid and 5% methanol in water (renewed from time to time to discard the unfixed stain).

The various silver stains are more tedious but have a much higher detectability, particularly in the methods of Morissey (1981) and Marshall (1984) for 'black-and-white' staining and of Sammons et

TABLE 16.7
Possible problems in electrophoresis and their remedies

1. Too fast or too slow polymerization. Incorrect catalyst concentration (TEMED, ammonium persulfate, riboflavin) or incorrect temperature of stock solutions. Polymerization may be slowed down, (e.g., for the preparation of gradients) by using cold solutions (with Tris buffers [deaerate!] but not with SDS-containing phosphate buffers). Omission of deaeration (oxygen in mixture may inhibit polymerization, as may high concentrations of thiols). In general, polymerization should be ready 10–30 min after casting; otherwise the polymers formed may be uneven.

2. Protein bands across the gel point to contamination. The presence of 2-ME may give two artificial bands corresponding to apparent molecular weights of 68000 and 54000 (Tasheva and Dessev, 1983; the role of 2-ME has been both confirmed and disputed by others).

3. Protein streaking from top of the gel points to overloading or to protein precipitation (too little SDS, wrong ionic strength or pH). Streaking in the gel as may be apparent after silver-staining points to (bacterial) contamination of the solutions mixed.

4. Precipitation in SDS systems is often due to the presence of K^+. A small amount of K^+ will precipitate SDS, as will several other metal ions.

5. Formation of air bubbles between gel and glass. Excessive heat (usually at high polyacrylamide gel concentrations) which can be prevented by more efficient cooling or lower voltage.

6. Collapse of the top of the gels. Probably presence of nucleic acid (highly charged).

al. (1981) for color staining (Tijssen and Kurstak, 1983). However, the latter produces a significantly higher background staining. These methods are presented in Table 16.8. In these ultrasensitive techniques utmost care should be taken to avoid contamination of the gels (fingerprints) or of the solutions used in the electrophoresis.

16.1.5. Use of stained protein bands for immunization

A very useful method to produce antibodies against proteins separated by electrophoresis and stained with CBB has been reported by Boulard and Lecroisey (1982). In this method (Section 5.2.1)

TABLE 16.8
Silver-stain methods[a]

A. *Black and white staining* (Morissey, 1981)
  1. Prefix gel in 50% methanol and 10% glacial acetic acid for 30 min.

  2. Fix gel another 30 min with 5% methanol and 7% glacial acetic acid.

  3. Fix gel for 30 min with 10% GA.

  4. Rinse or incubate gel in large bath with distilled water for at least 2 h. Rinse gel another 30 min with distilled water.

  5. Soak gel for 30 min in distilled water containing dithiothreitol (5 μg/ml).

  6. Pour off solution and without rinsing add 0.1% $AgNO_3$ and incubate for 30 min.

  7. Rinse gel rapidly with about 20 ml of water and twice with about 20 ml of developer (50 μl of 37% formaldehyde in 100 ml 3% Na_2CO_3).

  8. Soak gel in developer and stop the reaction once the desired staining intensity is obtained (usually 10–15 min) by the addition of 5 ml 2.3 M citric acid and agitate for 10 min.

  9. Wash several times with water and store in 0.03% Na_2CO_3.

B. *Polychromatic silver stain* (Sammons et al., 1981)
  1. Fix gel in 50% ethanol and 10% glacial acetic acid for 2 h or overnight.

  2. Wash in the following sequence:
     a. 2 h with 50% ethanol and 10% glacial acetic acid.
     b. Twice for 1 h with 25% ethanol and 10% glacial acetic acid.
     c. Twice for 1 h with 10% ethanol and 0.5% glacial acetic acid (can be stored in this solution for later staining).

  3. Equilibrate the gel with $AgNO_3$ (1.9 g/l) for 2 h, using a 3-fold excess of solution.

  4. Rinse 10–20 sec with deaerated distilled water.

  5. Reduce Ag^+ by incubation in a solution containing 87.5 mg $NaBH_4$ and 7.5 ml formaldehyde (17%) per 1 l of 0.75 M NaOH. Silver-staining will appear after 5–6 min: do not exceed 10 min of incubation.

  6. Incubate twice for 1 h in Na_2CO_3 (7.5 g/l) solution. The colors are optimal after about 6 h.

[a] Unless stated otherwise, the volume of the solutions should be in 6-fold excess to the gel volume.

the bands are cut from the gel (after destaining) and equilibrated with water for 30 min, and used immediately or stored frozen until needed. Although incomplete Freund's adjuvant was added to the homogenate and the animals were injected frequently (twice a week), it is also possible to use the gel fragments directly and to decrease the number of injections. In this case, however, a slower response is obtained (3–6 weeks vs. 2–4 weeks). Frequently, the immunization scheme of Section 5.2.1 is sufficient. The immune response is not influenced by the acrylamide gel, the nature of the gel (pH, SDS) or the dye. The gel should be destained by diffusion since with electrophoretic destaining minute amounts of other proteins, contained in the rest of the gel or in the solution, may contaminate the separated proteins. The antibodies are produced against the proteins in the same state (denatured, native) as later present on membrane blots.

16.2. Transfer of proteins from gel to membrane

Blotting of proteins can be viewed as the result of two operations (Gershoni and Palade, 1983): (i) their elution from the gel; and, (ii) the immobilization of the eluted proteins on the membrane with the smallest possible loss in resolution.

16.2.1. Elution of polypeptides from the gel

Proteins may be eluted from gels by diffusion, solvent convection or electro-elution.

Diffusion is simple but rather slow and resolution may be poor compared to the other methods. The gel is placed between two sheets of nitrocellulose membranes, which are in turn inserted between two filter papers covered with foam pads and rigid screens (Bowen et al., 1980; Aubertin et al., 1983; Table 16.9). High-molecular weight polypeptides are transferred less efficiently in the presence of SDS. Nevertheless, in the presence of SDS more faithful replicas

TABLE 16.9
Techniques for the diffusion-driven transfer of proteins

A. *Diffusion-driven transfer in the absence of SDS* (Bowen et al., 1980)
   1. Immerse the gel after electrophoresis in 10 mM Tris-HCl buffer, pH 7.0, containing 2 mM EDTA and 50 mM NaCl (transfer buffer) for 3 h.

   2. Place the gel between 2 sheets of wetted nitrocellulose membrane (pore size 0.45 μm or, preferably, 0.2 μm), avoiding any air bubbles. Cover each membrane with filter paper, foam pad and rigid screen, all previously wetted and attach with rubber bands.

   3. Submerge for prolonged periods (up to 48 h) in transfer buffer.

B. *Diffusion-driven transfer in the presence of SDS* (Aubertin et al., 1983)
   1. Complete the transfer buffer of step A.1 with 0.1% SDS.

   2. Proceed as in step A.2.

   3. Incubate for 2 h at 37°C or overnight at room temperature. In the latter case, 1 mM NaN$_3$ may be added to the buffer if it does not interfere with the enzyme activity.

---

can be obtained, particularly with DNA-binding proteins and proteins which have a limited solubility in the absence of SDS (Aubertin et al., 1983). Inclusion of urea in the transfer buffer enlarges the gel pores and facilitates the diffusion of proteins. When possible, PAG with lower solid content should be used for the transfer of proteins. The efficiency of this method, for the two replicas together, may be up to 75% (Bowen et al., 1980).

Convection or mass flow of solvent across the gel can be achieved, as in the original method of Southern (1975), by placing absorbing pads or paper towels above the gel which causes the buffer to flow through the gel and transport the proteins to the membrane between the gel and the pads. This method can also be adapted for bidirectional transfer (Reinhart and Malamud, 1982) but the two replicas will not be identical. This method is, except for SDS-containing systems, more efficient, less time-consuming and yields better resolution than the diffusion method. The methods based on convection are given in Table 16.10.

TABLE 16.10

Convection transfer of proteins from gel to membrane

Macromolecules are eluted from the gel by a buffer flow from the reservoir through gel and membrane to an absorbant stack (Fig. 16.2) according to the method of Southern (1975). In this method the macromolecules are bound by the membrane more efficiently and in less time than with diffusion blotting, but this method is less well-suited to dense gels.

1. Place in a container sponge pads covered with wetted filter paper.

2. Apply gel and cover carefully with wetted membrane.

3. Cover with dry filter paper and absorbant stack of dry towels and a weight.

4. Add buffer to container (less than height of sponge pads) and allow extraction to take place, e.g., overnight. The application of a vacuum can accelerate the mass flow and reduce considerably the elution time required (Peferaen et al., 1982).

Electro-elution is widely used (Table 16.11). A potential is applied across the gel to provide a homogeneous field over the entire area of the gel. Specifically designed equipment is commercially available (Bio-Rad), but destainers often work reasonably well. Though slabs as electrodes generate homogeneous fields, they also produce excessively high currents. A simple apparatus built by Bittner et al. (1980) has multiple bent platinum electrodes and represents a reasonable compromise. A much higher current is obtained than common power supplies provide, nevertheless, the latter may be adequate if set at a high current mode (200 mA; Gershoni and Palade, 1982). Alternatively, 12-V battery chargers also work well (Gibsen, 1981; Adair, 1982) as does the very simple and cheap but possibly hazardous, 'power supply' system devised by Kadokami et al. (1984).

As in the other methods, the proteins are transferred to a nitrocellulose membrane (0.1 μm pores) and it is imperative to hold the gel and the membrane tightly together to prevent a loss in resolution. In addition to the buffers listed in Table 16.11, 7.5 mM Tris-1.2 mM borate, pH 8.9 (McLellan and Ramshaw, 1981), 25 mM phos-

TABLE 16.11
Electro-transfer of proteins from gels to membrane filters

A. *Method for SDS gels* (Towbin et al., 1979, as modified by Burnette, 1981)
  1. Separate proteins by electrophoresis on 12.5% polyacrylamide gel, according to the method of Laemmli (1970). See also Table 16.3.

  2. Remove stacking gel and place resolving gel between the following layers (avoid air bubbles):
     a. porous polyethylene layer ('Scotch Brite' scouring pads)
     b. three layers of wetted filter paper (Whatman No. 3)
     c. resolving gel
     d. wetted nitrocellulose sheet (0.2 μm pores)
     e. three layers of wetted filter paper
     f. porous polyethylene pad

  3. Fasten together with rubber bands.

  4. Place in the electrophoresis chamber with the transfer buffer, with the nitrocellulose membrane towards the anode. A common transfer buffer is composed of 20 mM Tris, 150 mM glycine and 20% methanol; other formulations may be necessary depending on proteins (Section 16.2.1).

  5. Apply a potential of 6–8 V/cm for 16–22 h. The potential should not exceed 10 V/cm to avoid excessive heat. The time needed is considerably longer than in the original method of Towbin et al.

B. *Method I for proteins separated in non-dissociating conditions* (Towbin et al., 1979)
  As method A with the following modifications:
     a. transfer buffer is 0.7% acetic acid
     b. nitrocellulose membrane is placed on the cathodic side of the gel.

C. *Method II for proteins separated in non-dissociating conditions* (according to Kakita et al., 1982)
This method also resembles method A; however, the buffer differs and an extra step is introduced to link the small protein transferred (in their case insulin) covalently to the membrane. This adaptation could be advantageous for other methods as well (e.g., for elution of antibodies). The electrophoresis system used to resolve the proteins was the one of Davis (1964; Table 16.5).

  1. Proceed as in method A steps 1–4 but the buffer should contain 25 mM Tris and 192 mM glycine (pH 8.3).

  2. Apply a potential of 4–5 V for 4 h at room temperature.

  3. Soak the blot with 4% BSA in 10 mM phosphate buffer, pH 7.4, for 1 h at 40 °C.

4. Prepare an *N*-hydroxysuccinimidyl-*p*-azobenzoate (HSAB; Pierce Chem. Co.) solution by dissolving 1.7 mg in 250 μl DMSO and dilute 50 times with the phosphate buffer.

5. Perform photolinkage by adding 10 ml of the HSAB solution to the blot for 2 min in a darkened room at 4 °C and subsequent photolysis for 10 min with long wave UV (about 365 nm) held 15 cm from the membrane.

6. Terminate the reaction by adding 1/50 volume 1 M Tris–HCl buffer, pH 7.5.

7. Wash twice at room temperature for 5 min with 10 ml of the phosphate buffer.

---

phate buffer, pH 6.5 (Bittner et al., 1980) and 15.6 mM Tris-120 mM glycine, pH 8.3 (Gershoni and Palade, 1982) can also be used. Towbin et al. (1979) included 20% methanol in the buffer which seemed to increase the binding capacity of nitrocellulose, although it reduced the elution efficiency for SDS-proteins. Buffers of low ionic strength without methanol tend to swell the gels and enlarge the pores. However, the ionic strength should not be too low to avoid the precipitation of proteins. Swelling is complete after 1 h of incubation. Omitting this step before the transfer distorts the bands. The pH of the transfer buffer and the charge of the proteins determine which electrode is at the membrane side of the gel.

Protein transfer by electro-elution has been achieved from various gels, such as agarose (McMichael et al., 1981), urea-polyacrylamide (Towbin et al., 1979), SDS-polyacrylamide (Table 16.11A; Gershoni and Palade, 1982; Erickson et al., 1982); lithium dodecyl sulfate-polyacrylamide (Gershoni et al., 1982), two-dimensional polyacrylamide systems (Symington et al., 1981; Anderson et al., 1982) and polyacrylamide prepared with non-dissociating buffers (Kakita et al., 1982).

Sometimes the elution of proteins of low molecular weight is unsuccessful (Legocki and Verma, 1981). This may be due to the charge of the protein and may be improved with another buffer. Also, a large fraction of the proteins may pass through the membrane due to the size of the pores (Anderson et al., 1982), particularly in the absence of methanol.

Multiple replicas of the gels may be obtained by two methods, both of which fail to yield identical replicas: (i) layering as many as 10 nitrocellulose membranes on top of each other (Gershoni and Palade, 1982) and performing the electro-transfer in the absence of methanol (fraction of each protein band passes through the membrane, resulting in a progressive decrease of concentrations and less representative replicas); and, (ii) the use of one membrane at the time, with short blotting periods (Legocki and Verma, 1981; McLellan and Ramshaw, 1981). Theoretically, the latter method can be optimized to obtain better-resembling replicas by varying the blotting period.

Membrane blots may be stored for at least 1 year in dry and cool conditions.

16.2.2. Membranes used for the immobilization of proteins

Immobilization of proteins from solutions has been discussed in Section 13.3. Several matrices can be used for the transfer of proteins from gels, the most widely used being nitrocellulose. Other alternatives are diazobenzyloxymethyl-cellulose (DBM filters; Alwine et al., 1979), diazophenylthioether-cellulose (DPT filters; Reiser and Wardale, 1981), cellulose-acetate or paper activated with CNBr (Clarke et al., 1979), commercially available nylon-based membranes such as Gene screen (New England Nuclear), Zetabind (available from Bio-Rad as Zeta Probe). Nitrocellulose is better for EIA than Zeta Probe (considerably less background).

The structure of nitrocellulose membranes has been discussed by Gershoni and Palade (1983). The nitric acid-esterified cellulose is solubilized either with acetic acid-acetone or ether-alcohol. The latter solvent mixture seems to produce better membranes for blotting (Towbin et al., 1979). The films of these solutions are allowed to gel by meticulous control of the evaporation of the solvent. The drying conditions determine the ultimate pore size of the membranes. About 500 million pores are present per cm^2 of membrane, accounting for about 80% of its volume. For protein blotting, the 0.45 μm pore size is traditionally used but there is a tendency towards the 0.2 μm type (Burnette, 1981). Proteins are not captured primarily by a sieving process but by an as yet poorly understood non-covalent interaction (Wallis et al., 1979; Presswood, 1981). In many of the experimental conditions, the net charge of both the proteins and the membrane is negative, pointing to the importance of hydrophobicity. This may be responsible for the non-uniform and non-quantitative recovery of components from the various protein bands, for the adverse effects of non-ionic detergents on protein blotting (Farrah et al., 1981; Section 13.3), and for the prevention of adsorption of proteins to membranes by Tween 20, e.g., during immunostaining (Batteiger et al., 1982). Another problem, rarely mentioned, is the change of the adsorptive affinity of the membrane during prolonged storage. Schneider (1980) regenerated aged nitrocellulose sheets by immersion in a 1% solution of 3-methyl-1-butanol at 60°C for 15 min, washing 5 times with distilled water and subsequent bathing in 8% glycerol. The membranes were then pressed gently against filter paper to remove excess of glycerol.

DBM filters offer the irreversible covalent attachment of the proteins via the azo linkage to the membrane (Fig. 13.4; Alwine et al., 1979). Glycine should then be avoided in the transfer buffer. The proteins transferred are probably first bound by electrostatic interactions which are then slowly converted to covalent links. The diazonium groups are rather unstable so that a slow transfer of proteins results in a low efficiency of binding (Stellwag and Dahlberg, 1980). Resolution in this system is often poor due to the coarseness of the filters.

DPT filters have similar problems but seem to be more stable than the DBM filters (Gershoni and Palade, 1983).

The nylon-based membranes have several advantages over the derivatized cellulose membranes. They are thin, much more durable and have a much higher capacity (up to about 0.5 mg/cm^2; Gershoni and Palade, 1982), probably due to its numerous positive charges. These membranes are particularly efficient with SDS-proteins. A disadvantage of nylon-based membranes is that anionic dyes cannot be used for staining. Covalent interaction is not achieved with these membranes, and their high capacity results in high background staining in EIH.

16.2.3. Staining of proteins on membranes

Nitrocellulose-bound proteins can be stained with amido black 10B (Towbin et al., 1979), CBB (Burnette, 1981), and several other dyes (aniline black, Ponceau S, fast green, toluidine blue; Gershoni and Palade, 1983). The recently developed immunostain for proteins on nitrocellulose filters (Wojtkowiak et al., 1983) is very sensitive (Section 16.3.1).

Nitrocellulose membranes are not very stable in acidic methanol and prolonged use of such solvents should be avoided. Staining with CBB is carried out in 40% methanol, 10% acetic acid and 0.2% dye for 5 min. Destaining is performed rapidly (2 min) in 90% methanol. Alternatively, 0.1% amido black 10B in 45% methanol and 10% acetic acid can be used for 5 min, followed by a 2–3 min destaining with 90% methanol and 2% acetic acid.

16.3. Enzyme immunoassays and related techniques with protein blots

Protein blots can be used: (i) to identify various constituents of a mixture and to establish their relationship(s) by EIH (epitope mapping); (ii) to localize these constituents by the sensitive immunostain after their haptenation and subsequent reaction with labeled anti-hapten antibodies; and, (iii) to elute antibodies immobilized to a certain protein band ('poor man's monoclonals').

16.3.1. General immunostain of blotted proteins

Wojtkowiak et al. (1983) devised a simple, universal and very sensitive, but time-consuming method for the detection of proteins on blots.

After blotting of the proteins, they are dinitrophenylated (Section 12.5). This hapten is then detected with anti-DNP antibodies (Miles, Inc.) by one of the methods discussed below. Detectability by this method is at least equal to that of autoradiography (<1 ng). The intensity of the staining, however, is not representative of the stoichiometry of the protein in the blot. Kittler et al. (1984) haptenated the amino groups of the blotted proteins with pyridoxal-5′-phosphate. This method requires no organic solvents and can also be used with Zetabind membranes.

16.3.2. Specific detection of particular antigens or haptens

Before antigens are reacted with their corresponding antibodies, it is necessary to quench all sites on the membrane which bind proteins non-specifically. The filters can be saturated with a non-interfering protein added to the antisera or enzymes. Triton X-100 or Tween 80 may elute the specific antigens from the blot (Section 16.2.2). However, incubation of the blots for 2 h in 0.05% Tween 20 (used throughout the procedure) gives very good results (Batteiger et al., 1982).

The protein used for quenching is mostly BSA (3%) in 10 mM Tris–HCl buffer, pH 7.4, containing 0.9% NaCl, for 1 h at 40°C (Towbin et al., 1979) or 0.5% for 24 h at room temperature (Erickson et al., 1982), but ovalbumin, hemoglobin or gelatin can also be used (White et al., 1981; Gershoni and Palade, 1982; Lee et al., 1982). After quenching, the membranes are rinsed with Tris-buffered saline.

The numerous procedures for the detection of specific antigens are similar to those used in EIH at the light microscope level, and details can be found in Section 17.3. A typical procedure is given in Table 16.12. Though lectins generally have a lower affinity for glycoproteins than antibodies for antigens, enzyme–lectin conjugates may also be used (Section 17.3.2.4). For the detection of POase on blots (Section 17.3.3) diaminobenzidine is not as suitable as in EIH (high background) and is usually replaced by 4-chloro-1-naph-

TABLE 16.12
Detection of antigens on nitrocellulose (adapted from Batteiger et al., 1982; Hawkes et al., 1982)

1. Wash membrane for 5 min in 50 mM Tris–HCl buffer, pH 7.4, containing 200 M NaCl (TBS).

2. Block remaining active sites with 3% BSA and 1% normal serum in TBS and leave for 15 min at room temperature (or 2 h with 1% BSA). Instead of this blocking step, 0.05% Tween 20 may be included in the various solutions containing the immunoreactants. Zetabind or Zeta-Probe membranes require very rigorous blocking conditions due to their high adsorptive capacity (12 h at 50°C with 10% BSA), but are then still less useful for this purpose.

3. Incubate with primary antibodies (3 h at room temperature, overnight for high dilutions). Antiserum dilutions are made in blocking solutions.

4. Wash for 30 min with several changes of TBS and repeat step 2.

5. Incubate with the conjugate in blocking solution (2 h; about 2 μg conjugate per ml).

6. Repeat step 4 (but not step 2).

7. Reveal enzyme. Prepare for POase detection a stock solution of 4-chloro-1-naphthol (3 mg/ml in methanol), which can be stored in the dark for about 10 days (until yellowing occurs). Dilute before use with 5 volumes TBS and 0.003% H_2O_2. Time required is usually 5–15 min.

thol (Section 17.3.3). Towbin et al. (1979) used ODA at 25 μg/ml and 0.01% H_2O_2 in 10 mM Tris–HCl buffer, pH 7.4. The blots are washed for 30 min with water and immediately dried to prevent background staining. APase may be stained as in Section 17.3.3.2.

Non-specific staining may be due to several causes (Section 17.3.4.1 and Section 17.3.4.2) which can be corrected by appropriate measures (Section 17.3.4.3).

An elegant variant has been described by Muilerman et al. (1982). They were faced with the problem to identify a particular enzyme after it had been denatured and separated from other proteins by SDS–PAGE. After transferring the denatured proteins to nitrocellulose membranes and quenching of the blot, the membrane was overlayered with anti-enzyme antibodies in excess, so that only one of the two combining sites reacted with the denatured antigen. A crude enzyme preparation was added in the next step which combined with the antibody reacted with the inactivated enzyme on the blot. Enzyme activity on the blot revealed the position of the denatured enzyme in the gel.

Zwitterionic detergents (0.1–0.4%) in the electrotransfer buffer may restore the antibody-binding capacity of conformational epitopes of antigens denatured by SDS (Mandrell and Zollinger, 1984).

16.3.3. Purification of antibodies on protein blots

Affinity purification of antibodies on protein blots has been described by Olmsted (1981). In this study DPT filters were used, but CNBr-activated paper or nitrocellulose works equally well (Gershoni and Palade, 1983).

The blotted proteins are reacted with their corresponding antibodies (Section 16.3.2). The bands are excised and eluted with 3 ml 200 mM glycine–HCl buffer, pH 2.8, during 2 min at 0°C. The solution is then neutralized with NaOH and concentrated to 0.1–0.2 ml. The monospecific antibodies obtained can then be used for other EIA (blots, titration, EIH). Though the blot can be used several times to extract monospecific antibodies from the serum, the amounts obtained are not excessive. It can be advantageous to link the antigen to the blot by the method given in Table 16.11C.

Enzyme immunohistochemistry (EIH) in light and electron microscopy

17.1. Overview

One of the classical procedures employed in immunodiagnosis for the identification and localization of antigens and the titration of antisera has been the immunofluorescence method (Nairn et al., 1960; Coons, 1961). Fluorescent antibodies to trace antigens in tissues are increasingly replaced by enzyme-conjugated antibodies which proved very powerful for studying the function, development and processing of antigens in their natural environment, i.e., in cells. The relative advantages of these two labels are compared in Table 17.1.

The ideal enzyme label for EIH should convert a soluble substrate to an insoluble product so that an identifiable precipitate forms immediately at the site of enzyme action, whereas the substrate should not contribute to background staining. The precipitate in the cell can then be seen with a light microscope and may be rendered, in some systems, electron opaque for studies by electron microscopy. In particular POase (Avrameas and Uriel, 1966; Nakane and Pierce, 1966) and GOase are useful for this purpose. In EIH an amplification of the signal is possible to a degree seldom attained in enzyme cytochemistry and often much less tedious. Recent developments in EIH made routine applications of these techniques possible (reviews: Bullock and Petrusz, 1982; Van Noorden and Polak, 1983).

The low penetration rate of antibodies through cell membranes

TABLE 17.1

Advantages and disadvantages of methods using enzyme-labeled antibodies compared to fluorescent antibodies

---

Advantages

– Normal light microscope can be used.

– Cellular structure can be easily appreciated.

– Can be used at the ultrastructural level.

– Preparations are often permanent.

– Detectability with certain procedures is significantly higher (> 100 ×).

– Less background staining.

– Long shelf-life of reagents.

– Highly sensitive unlabeled-antibody procedures possible.

Disadvantages

– More laborious to prepare conjugates.

– May be more expensive.

– Health hazard for laboratory personnel, i.e., products for some of the methods may be carcinogenic.

– Assay more laborious since enzyme labels are revealed histochemically at the end of the antibody–antigen reaction.

---

may constitute a main obstacle in demonstrating intracellular antigens, particularly in electron microscopy. On the other hand, increased permeabilization by any of the techniques available should not: (i) interfere with the immunoreactivity of the epitopes; (ii) solubilize the antigen or allow diffusible antigens to redistribute; and, (iii) change the morphological features of the tissue preparation. The optimal fixation conditions for the last 2 requirements involve rapid and complete fixation, whereas preservation of immunoreactivity usually requires the lowest degree of fixation. Therefore, a compromise between the opposing criteria of fixation and permeabilization should be established in every case.

Original strategies consisted in simple direct and indirect methods, which differ from the immunofluorescence procedures mainly in the nature of the label. However, the particular properties of enzymes made much more sophisticated designs possible. Popular among these designs is the POase–anti-POase (PAP) method (Sternberger, 1979), in which the immunogenicity of the enzyme is exploited (Section 11.3). The use of avidin–biotin–POase complexes (ABC), based on a similar bridge principle, potentially has a higher detectability and lower background staining. For ultrastructural studies, however, these large complexes are not always satisfactory since they do not penetrate easily into cells as do smaller probes. PAP-complexes usually are employed on thin sections for the localization of antigens ('post-embedding staining'), but recent advances made pre-embedding staining also practical.

Another development in EIH is the double immunoenzymatic staining in which two different antigens are detected in the same tissue preparation. In the initial technique two different substrates were used: the first antigen was localized by the usual methods, the enzyme revealed and the antibodies subsequently selectively eluted without removing the colored product, followed by incubation with antisera and conjugate against the second antigen, but using another substrate giving a product of different color (Vandesande and Dierickx, 1975). In subsequent studies, Sternberger and Joseph (1979) found that antibody removal may not be necessary if certain conditions are met. The use of two unrelated enzymes on two different antibodies offers many advantages, e.g., they may be applied simultaneously rather than sequentially. Consequently, the only additional manipulation is the revelation of the second enzyme (about 5 min).

Mason and Sammons (1979) introduced an elegant method to lower background staining, caused by non-specific adsorption of IgG to tissue sections, by coupling the enzyme to purified antigen. An excess of the primary antibody is incubated with the tissue preparation, but among the IgG adsorbed only the antibodies reacting with the antigens in the section are capable of binding subsequently added enzyme-labeled antigen. This method is also very rapid, i.e., it takes about 30 min, but it is limited to systems where the tissue antigen is available in pure form.

Enzyme-lectin histochemistry has many features in common with EIH. Lectins are of non-immune origin but recognize fine differences in complex saccharide structures. Usually lectin specificity is expressed as reactivity to a given monosaccharide, but it has been demonstrated repeatedly (e.g., Debray et al., 1981) that this is an oversimplification (Section 3.4). It is becoming increasingly clear that cellular differentiation, maturation and neoplastic transformation are associated with changes of carbohydrate composition of the cell membrane (Ponder, 1983).

Methods used in EIH may be extended to other techniques where identification and localization of antigens are important: the protein and nucleic acid transfer blots (Chapter 16) may be subjected to these methods. As with EIA, epitopes rather than antigens or molecules are recognized by EIH methods. Shared reactivity and cross-reactivity (Section 8.6) may, therefore, interfere as in the AA-type assays (Section 2.3).

17.2. Enzymes suitable for the localization of antigens

POase (Section 10.1.1) in EIH is so universal that the techniques described here have been widely known as immunoperoxidase. The popularity of POase is due to the fact that several H-donors fulfill the requirements of suitable substrates, the enzyme is stable, of moderate size, and affordable.

Some effort has been devoted to obtain even smaller probes, i.e., smaller enzymes conjugated to Fab. An early candidate was cytochrome *c* (Singer, 1974) which has only 1/3 of the molecular weight of POase, though its diameter is only 30% smaller, but it has the disadvantage of low enzymatic activity. Digestion of cytochrome *c* (Section 10.3.1) yields the active site (microperoxidase, MPOase) with a much higher activity than the original cytochrome c (Section 10.3.1.2), but a somewhat lower activity than POase and is used only in electron microscopy.

APase has also been used for the probes to localize antigens in cells (Mason and Sammons, 1978), in the form of immune complexes of this enzyme (APAAP; Section 11.3.2). Naphthol AS phosphate in combination with Fast Red TR gives an intense red reaction product which counterstains well with hematoxylin, whereas in combination with Fast Blue BBN it produces a blue color.

GOase is becoming more popular due to the low background staining. It can also be used in combination with POase for sequential double staining (Campbell and Bhatnager, 1976).

17.3. Enzyme immunohistochemistry procedures in light microscopy

17.3.1. Permeabilization and fixation of tissues and cells

The material to be investigated may be: (i) large pieces of tissues, directly from the organism or maintained as explants, usually fixed and/or frozen before sectioning and incubation of the free floating or mounted sections with antibodies; and, (ii) small pieces of tissue, cell suspensions or cells grown in vitro, which do not require sectioning, if rendered permeable to facilitate the access of the antibodies to the antigen.

From large pieces of tissue, paraffin sections of fixed tissue or cryostat sections of fresh or fixed tissues are prepared. Many laboratories prefer cryostat sections since antigen preservation is superior and paraffin cannot be used for lipid-soluble antigens. Paraffin is removed from the sections with toluene or xylene and hydration through a graded series of alcohol baths. Further details can be found in textbooks of histochemistry or specialized literature (Culling, 1974; Nairn, 1976; and, Pearse, 1980).

Cells in small pieces of tissue can be permeabilized either by chemical agents (most frequent) or by freezing and should be accompanied by a fixation to prevent both a loss of internal structure and a loss, or diffusion, of antigen. Optimal procedures vary for every system and should be determined empirically. The fixation procedure which causes minimal denaturation of the antigen depends on the antigen. Table 17.2 lists some of the common procedures used for permeabilization and fixation. The goal of fixation is to avoid structural decomposition, to hinder diffusion of soluble compo-

TABLE 17.2

Common procedures to obtain permeabilization and fixation of cells in enzyme immunohistochemistry by light microscopy (adapted from Jessen, 1983)[a]

	Procedure				
	1	2	3	4	5
Detergent extraction with Triton X-100 or NP40	−	−	−	+	+
Cross-linking with formaldehyde or *p*-benzoquinone	−	+	+	+	+
Precipitation/extraction with acid–alcohol, methanol, or acetone	+	−	+	−	+

[a] In all procedures, the last step is followed by washing with physiological saline. Diffusible proteins can also be removed prior to fixation by washing the tissue pieces extensively in PBS at 4°C.

Non-ionic detergents are often used prior to fixation to demonstrate cytoskeletal proteins. Detergents or pH treatments, or a combination (e.g., acid urea) can also be used after fixation to expose hidden antigens.

Cross-linkers denature particularly large proteins but are the method of choice for the immobilization of small antigens. Treatment with sucrose may partially restore antigenicity. A local high protein concentration will lead to more cross-linking and to a more pronounced denaturation. This uneven antigen masking subsequently causes artefacts in the distribution of staining. In contrast, methanol will yield better immobilization without antigen masking when protein concentrations are high.

Methanol or ethanol are relatively mild precipitants and proteins may be redissolved in a fairly native state, particularly after ethanol precipitation. Though often satisfactory, the absence of diffusion artefacts is far from guaranteed. Shrinkage due to dehydration may cause less morphological preservation.

nents and to fortify the tissue. Preservation of antigenicity is probably the most important factor for success in EIH.

Fixation with organic solvents, such as methanol or acetone, is often used for light microscopy, though some antigens may be extracted by these solvents. Lipids are removed from tissues, particularly from the membranes, and proteins are precipitated. The most frequently used 'precipitant fixatives' are 100% methanol, 100% acetone, or 5% acetic acid in absolute ethanol. Slides or coverslips carrying the tissue or cell preparations are submerged in these solvents for about 15 min (often at $-20°C$) and washed with physiological saline or buffer until the pH is neutral. Small antigens are best preserved with fixatives based on cross-linking (FA, GA, PBQ).

Freshly prepared FA is a better fixative in EIH than GA since it cross-links proteins less than GA, permeabilizes cell membranes and provides an improved penetration of the immunoreactants due to the limited cross-linking. Fixation with FA is highly pH dependent (Berod et al., 1981) and is extremely slow at pH 6.5. This phenomenon can be used to advantage, particularly for large tissue fragments, by first distributing the fixative uniformly throughout the tissue at low pH and then cross-linking the preparation evenly by raising the pH to about 10–11 (with sodium borate). Depolymerized paraformaldehyde should be used since commercially available FA solutions (37%) contain stabilizers and methanol, which may be deleterious for EIH techniques (Farr and Nakane, 1981). The fixative is prepared by dissolving 10 g of paraformaldehyde in 50 ml distilled water at 60°C under continuous stirring. The addition of 2–6 drops of 100 mM NaOH clears the solution, which is then diluted to 500 ml with 110 mM sodium phosphate buffer, pH 7.5 (or other pH) and 1 g NaCl is added (final concentrations: 2% FA, 100 mM sodium phosphate buffer and 0.2% NaCl). Tissues are usually fixed at room temperature. Sometimes, the addition of picric acid, a precipitant fixative, may be advantageous (Stefanini et al., 1967). Bouin's fixative (75 ml saturated aqueous picric acid, 25 ml formalin and 5 ml glacial acetic acid) is another common fixative for the PAP method.

Over-fixation with FA-based solutions may sometimes conceal the antigens. This may often be corrected by treatment with a protease (Huang, 1975; Radaszkiewicz et al., 1979; Stein et al., 1980), probably by releasing some of the fixative and thus making more epitopes accessible. Trypsin is used as a 0.1% solution in 50 mM Tris–HCl buffer, pH 7.8. or in a 0.1% CaCl₂ solution adjusted to pH 7.8 at the working temperature (37°C) due to the variation of pH with temperature. Incubation of the sections should not exceed 30 min and they should be well rinsed before immunostaining. Alternatively, pronase is also used at 0.1% but at most for 15 min. PBS containing 2 mg/ml glycine is an effective inhibitor of pronase. The balance between over- and underdigestion is delicate and treatment may not always improve localization, particularly after acidic FA fixation (e.g., with Bouin's; Brandtzaeg, 1982). Proteolytic digestion may also eliminate xylene-induced antigen impairment (Matthews, 1981). Sections mounted on slides may become detached during protease treatment. Therefore, such sections should be mounted on slides coated with poly-L-lysine (MW > 150000; Farr and Nakane, 1981). This film is applied by placing a drop of a 0.01% solution on the end of the slide and spreading with another slide under an angle of about 30° to the other end. The film dries quickly, becomes invisible (mark the coated side), and will keep its stickiness up to one week. Stock poly-L-lysine solutions should be stored frozen.

PBQ is a bifunctional cross-linking agent (Section 11.2.3.1.2) for tissue constituents and is, therefore, used at lower concentrations (0.4–0.5% in PBS). Fixation for 30 min at room temperature has been particularly successful for the visualization of neuropeptides and other small molecules (Jessen et al., 1980; Jessen, 1983). PBQ reacts not only with proteins but also with sugars.

The non-ionic detergents Triton X-100 and NP40 are frequently used in studies of the cytoskeleton. They are applied either prior to fixation with a cross-linker in the presence or absence of precipitant fixatives or after fixation to remove remaining lipids. Generally, 0.3% of detergent in PIPES buffer containing 0.1 mM EGTA is used for 1 to 3 min.

Permeabilization by repeated freeze-thaw cycles may be a method of choice in cases where it is important to avoid modifications in the avidity of antibody–antigen reactions. Coverslips with the cell preparation upwards are placed on a metal plate cooled with dry ice. The cells freeze in a few seconds as indicated by the white color of the frozen film of culture medium. The coverslip is then removed for a few minutes to thaw and the cycle is repeated several times. Diffusion of antigens, due to the lack of anchorage, can be reduced by layering the sample with primary antibodies before and after the freeze-thaw procedure.

To distinguish diffusible from bound antigens, cryostat sections are often preferred. Pre-fixation diffusion artefacts (e.g., passive uptake of non-specific antigens by cells, particularly of the lymphoid system; Mason et al., 1980), which occur quite often, may be revealed by double EIH staining (e.g., κ and λ chains should normally not be present in the same cell) and counteracted by rapid fixation or removal of diffusible antigens by washing with cold saline. Post-fixation diffusion artefacts are also frequently noticeable, e.g. after ethanol fixation (Brandtzaeg, 1982).

Some antigens or epitopes may be hidden, e.g. J-chain in IgA or IgM in ethanol-fixed tissues, which may be exposed after treatment for 1 h at 4°C with 100 mM glycine-HCl buffer, pH 3.2, containing 6 M urea (Brandtzaeg, 1976).

17.3.2. Detection of antigens in cells by light microscopy

A frequent source of poor results in EIH techniques is the failure to rinse the preparations after fixation to neutrality.

Etching the area around each section and drying the slide around this etch after each washing minimizes running of the solutions applied. Sera can be diluted with almost any neutral isotonic buffer. The slides should be incubated in humid chambers (a closed Petri dish with wet cotton) to prevent the drying of the immunoreactants; this non-specifically adsorbed material is very difficult to remove by washing. Slides incubated with different immunoreactants should not be washed in the same jar. Coverslips can be inverted on a large drop on Parafilm.

17.3.2.1. Immune reactions with enzyme-conjugated antibodies
The principles of these techniques are illustrated in Fig. 17.1. and
resemble the corresponding immunofluorescence methods, though
they have somewhat better detectabilities. For example, the nuclear
antigen of Epstein Barr virus (EBNA) is detected with the indirect
immunoperoxidase technique (Fig.17.2; Kurstak et al., 1978), whereas
with immunofluorescence it can be detected only with the more
sensitive anti-complement procedure (Reedman and Klein, 1973;
Kurstak et al., 1978).

17.3.2.1.1. Direct method   The direct method is simple and,
consequently, requires few controls (Fig. 17.1a). Its main drawbacks
are that for each antigen the corresponding specific antibodies should
be purified and conjugated and that its potential detectability is
not as good as with most other techniques. The direct method is
a reasonable choice when the same antigen–antibody reaction is
frequently used (e.g., autoimmune diseases) or when the detection
limit is not the main concern.

The enzyme-labeled antibodies at a convenient concentration

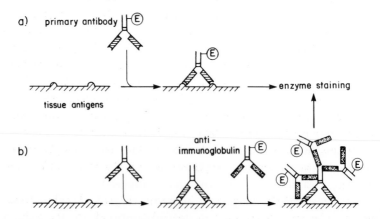

Fig. 17.1. Direct (a) and indirect (b) EIA-detection methods, in which the primary
antibody and an Ig are enzyme-labeled, respectively. The different shading of the
Fab parts of the antibodies indicates the different species in which antibodies are
raised.

(mostly 20–100 µg/ml) are applied to the coverslips or slides carrying the fixed cell preparations, which are then incubated for 1–2 h in a humid chamber, often at 37°C. It may be advantageous to incubate at room temperature, e.g. for 'cold antibodies' (Section 8.2).

17.3.2.1.2. Indirect method   In this method labeled anti-IgG antibodies are used to reveal the presence of primary antibodies complexed to antigens in situ (Fig. 17.1b). Since several anti-IgG antibodies may react with each primary antibody, an increase in detectability of the order of about 5 to 10-fold can be expected. A single conjugate may be used to reveal an unlimited number of different antigens, provided the primary antibodies (which need not to be purified) are from the same species. Disadvantages are the increased number of incubation steps, and the greater number of controls required.

Cell or tissue preparations are first incubated with the primary antibody (1–25 µg/ml) in a humid chamber for at least 1 h at room temperature. The preparations are washed three times with PBS for 5 min and enzyme-labeled anti-IgG antibodies (5–100 µg/ml) are subsequently reacted with the primary antibody for 90 min at room temperature. Tween 20 at 0.05% in PBS is often beneficial.

A convenient alternative in the indirect method is the use of SpA-enzyme. SpA, which reacts with primary antibodies from the majority of mammalian species (Section 7.1.9.1), can thus be employed virtually as a universal probe and may be readily conjugated to POase (Section 11.2.2). In many cases SpA-POase has a greater specificity than anti-IgG (Dubois-Dalcq et al., 1977), particularly for tissues which contain Fc receptors. Background staining is generally considerably less and SpA-POase penetrates better than anti-IgG-POase. In this incubation step, anti-IgG is simply replaced by SpA-POase (2–10 µg/ml).

Falini et al. (1980) compared the indirect enzyme-labeled antibody method, the SpA-POase method, the PAP method and the indirect enzyme-labeled antigen method. The big difference of the SpA-POase method with the other methods was the almost complete absence of background staining, though the detectability was lower than

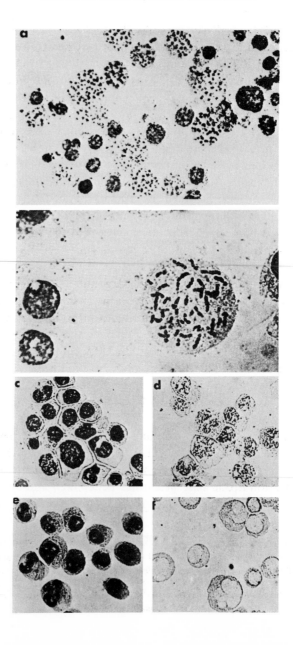

with the PAP method. The cost of SpA may be considerably reduced by producing and purifying it in the laboratory (Section 3.3.1).

17.3.2.1.3. Anti-complement method   A powerful variant of the indirect method is the anti-complement method. Complement is fixed by antigen–antibody complexes containing IgM or certain subclasses of IgG. Since complement is antigenic, these complexes can then be revealed by enzyme-labeled anti-complement antibodies. Experimental details are similar to those in the indirect methods, the only difference being the addition of fresh complement (e.g. 1:50; if serum is not fresh) to the primary antibody sample.

17.3.2.2. Unlabeled antibody–enzyme methods   Covalent labeling often diminishes the efficiency of detection of antigens in EIH due to inactivation of a fraction of the enzyme molecules. Antibody labeled with an inactive enzyme competes with the antibody labeled with the active enzyme for the available epitopes. (Inactivation of a fraction of the antibody molecules merely necessitates a higher concentration of the conjugate but does not decrease the maximum staining.)

Mason et al. (1969) and Sternberger (1969) developed simultaneously the unlabeled antibody–enzyme method in which the enzyme/antigen ratio is increased, thus improving the detection limit. Drawbacks of this method (Section 11.3.1) led to the development of the PAP method (Sternberger et al., 1970) and of the ABC (avidin–biotin–peroxidase complex) method and its variants (Guesdon et al., 1979; Hsu et al., 1981), further increasing in detectability and decreasing background staining. Principles of these various procedures are illustrated in Fig. 17.3.

Fig. 17.2. Detection of Epstein Barr virus nuclear antigen (EBNA) in B lymphocytes with the indirect anticomplement method (a–d, f). Cells arrested in metaphase (a,b) revealed that EBNA is linked to chromosomes. The indirect (anti-Ig) method (e) has higher background levels due to Ig or receptors on the membrane. In (f) antiserum was omitted. Dilutions used: 1:600 (a, b, c), 1:5000 (d), and 1:200 (e). From Kurstak et al., 1978; courtesy *Journal of Medical Virology*.

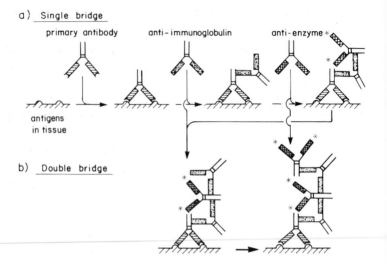

Fig. 17.3. Anti-enzyme antibodies linked by a bridge (anti-Ig) to the primary antibody can immobilize enzyme molecules (at *), which can be revealed subsequently. This can be repeated by several layers (double bridge, etc.) until the avidity of the antibodies used becomes the limiting factor. Instead of anti-enzyme, avidin can be used if enzyme and primary antibodies are biotinylated. The last step (addition of enzyme) is not illustrated. In the PAP-method, POase-anti-POase complexes are preformed.

17.3.2.2.1. Original unlabeled antibody–enzyme method   The original unlabeled antibody–enzyme method obviated problems encountered in conjugation, but required purified anti-POase antibodies. Fig.17.3a shows the four sequential steps in this technique. The anti-POase antibodies should be pure, to prevent the bridging antibody to capture Ig other than anti-POase antibody. Anti-POase antibodies can be purified with specific immunosorbents (Section 7.1.9.2), but mainly antibodies with lower affinities are recovered which are easily lost during washing (Section 8.5).

The method is performed at room temperature with incubation periods of 1 h each, though longer periods are sometimes used for the primary antibody and shorter for the subsequent steps. After each incubation, 3 washings of 5 min with PBS should be carried out. Primary antibodies should be used at high dilutions (i.e. 400–10000, mostly 1000) and the incubation period can be increased up to 48 h with primary antibodies of lower affinity. In contrast, the bridging antibody is diluted only about 20 times to obtain the necessary excess of anti-Ig antibodies. The preparations are then incubated with anti-POase antibodies (50 µg/ml), followed by POase (5 µg/ml) in 0.1% ovalbumin and the histochemical revelation of the enzyme.

Detectability with this technique can be increased through the use of a double bridge. After the anti-POase step, another incubation with bridging antibody can be introduced, followed by incubations with anti-POase and POase, at the same concentrations as above (Fig.17.3).

17.3.2.2.2. Improved unlabeled antibody–enzyme methods   In these methods soluble enzyme anti-enzyme complexes (Section 11.3.2) are used instead of separate incubations with anti-POase and POase. The PAP method avoids the problem of the original method of non-antibody Ig in the anti-POase serum. With the increase in detectability, the fixation method can be chosen more in favor of the preservation of morphology than of antigen.

The first two steps of the PAP method are similar to those of the original unlabeled antibody–enzyme method. In the following step, PAP (40 µg/ml; in buffer containing 1% normal serum from the same species as the bridging antibody) is applied to the preparation, followed by the revelation of POase. Detectability can be increased by a double bridge procedure: after the last incubation step, another incubation with bridging antibody (anti-Ig) and with soluble PAP is carried out at the same concentrations as above.

A weak staining in the PAP method may sometimes be corrected by further incubation with POase (5 µg/ml) in 0.1% ovalbumin. A cause of false negative results might be the binding of primary antibodies at a too high density. This causes both combining sites of the bridging antibody to react with the primary antibody (Bigbee et al., 1977; Vandesande, 1979). Density of the binding of antibodies may be influenced by: (i) the concentration, cellular distribution and accessibility of tissue antigen after fixation; (ii) the titer and dilution of the primary antiserum; and, (iii) the temperature and length of incubation.

SpA is also convenient for the PAP procedures. SpA reacts with IgG of many mammalian species, particularly if IgG is complexed with the specific antigen (Section 3.3). Moreover, SpA has two reactive sites which enables this protein to link two Ig, like the bridging antibody, with the additional advantage that it can act between IgG of two different species. The requirement that the antibodies in the PAP complex should be produced in the same species as the primary antibody is, therefore, eliminated. Among the PAP complexes prepared with anti-POase raised in the rabbit, guinea pig, rat or goat, only those from the rabbit and guinea pig gave excellent results with SpA (Notani et al., 1979; Table 7.1). SpA is used at the dose of 25–400 µg/ml for 30 min or, if enhanced sensitivity is desired, between the anti-IgG antibodies and the PAP probe in double-bridge experiments. Methods employing SpA can attain detection limits not unlike those of commonly used EIA (i.e., dilutions of 1:25000 of the primary antiserum). If the primary antibody is not reactive with SpA, an incubation with an anti-Ig from a convenient (reactive) species can be inserted. For example, if the primary antibodies were chicken IgY, rabbit anti-IgY antibodies could render the complex reactive towards SpA. SpA can be used as crude extract for this bridging step. However, SpA cannot be used on tissues which have abundant Igs in their interstitium or numerous IgG-containing plasma cells (Hsu and Raine, 1981).

17.3.2.2.3. Avidin–biotin complex methods   Avidin acts as a universal bridging molecule between biotinylated molecules. Biotinylation is possible without impairing immunological activity of antibodies or catalytic activity of some enzymes (POase, GOase); BGase is only slightly affected and APase activity is severely reduced (Section 3.2.4.4). If the enzyme is affected by biotinylation, avidin can be linked to the enzyme directly.

Avidin and biotin can be used in different EIH systems. In the direct method, either biotinylated antibody is reacted with avidin-labeled enzyme or biotinylated enzyme is linked to biotinylated anti-body by avidin (Guesdon et al., 1979). The indirect method may be modified similarly. Alternatively, the avidin–biotin–POase complex (ABC) can be preformed by incubating avidin with biotin–POase (optimum ratio, w/w, 4:1) for at least 20 min (Hsu et al., 1981), making the procedure less time consuming and more sensitive than the unlabeled antibody–enzyme or PAP methods. Concentrations of the ABC should be about 10 µg/ml, at 40 µg/ml background staining is increased which cannot be abolished by treating the tissues with hypertonic salt solutions, alkaline buffers or heat-denatured avidin. An alternative for the preparation of ABC with increased detectability and economy, is presented in Section 11.4.

The high detectability of these techniques may be due to the presence of multiple biotin molecules on the proteins. Non-specific staining can be considerable at high concentrations of ABC which may be related to the fact that biotin is an important coenzyme for transcarbamylation and may be present in some tissues to bind ABC. Pretreatment with avidin and biotin, respectively, prior to the serological detection, could remedy this problem in some cases.

Incubation conditions are as in the other techniques, i.e. 1 h at room temperature in a humid chamber. Primary antibodies (dilution of serum 200–4000 times) are first complexed to the antigen in the tissue. After washings, biotin-labeled anti-Ig (dilution 1:200) is added, followed by incubation with ABC (8 µg/ml avidin and 2 µg/ml biotin–POase).

17.3.2.3. Detection of different epitopes in the same preparation
Multiple staining methods to distinguish different epitopes offer important advantages. In particular, the availability of monoclonal antibodies is likely to result in the use of this method on an increasing scale.

Multiple staining can be achieved by two, fundamentally different approaches: (i) the same enzyme is used for both epitopes but with different substrates, yielding distinctly colored reaction products; and, (ii) two unrelated enzymes are used to detect the two epitopes.

Other possibilities are the radioactive labeling in vitro of one of the monoclonal antibodies and enzyme-labeling of the other and their detection in cells by autoradiography (Tijssen and Kurstak, 1977) or the complexing of heavy metals to one of the immunoreactants (e.g., colloidal gold to SpA; Roth, 1982).

The choice for the multiple immunoenzymatic staining method is determined by several parameters: (i) whether or not the same enzyme should be used for both staining procedures; (ii) if unrelated enzymes are used, the selection of the second enzyme, in addition to the generally used POase; (iii) the design of the two systems (direct conjugation, unlabeled method, bridge method, etc.) to avoid interference between them; and, (iv) the species origin of the various antibodies.

17.3.2.3.1. Sequential localization of multiple antigens with conjugates of the same enzyme   Two distinct epitopes can be detected sequentially with the same enzyme using substrates which yield products of contrasting colors. Two approaches can be taken with this method: (i) after one epitope is localized by the production of an insoluble, colored product, the conjugates are removed (leaving behind the colored product identifying the antigen) and the second antigen is revealed with the second system; or, (ii) a pair of substrates is selected in which the first yields a product with a dominant staining over the other so that the elution step may be omitted. Nakane (1968) used this technique to localize three different antigens. Only about a decade later were further investigations reported using this technique (Vandesande and Dierickx, 1975; Erlandsen et al., 1976; Martin-Comin and Robyn, 1976; Tramu et al., 1978; Sternberger and Joseph, 1979) when problems due to spurious labeling after elution of the conjugate with acidic buffer, particularly in the case of high-affinity antibodies, were overcome. Vandesande and Dierickx (1975) and Vandesande (1979) suggested successive washings with: (i) 200 mM glycine buffer, pH 2.3, containing 500 mM NaCl; (ii) 10% DMF in 50 mM Tris–HCl buffer, pH 7.6; and, if necessary, followed by electrophoresis at 20 V/cm in 50 mM glycine buffer, pH 2.2, containing 30% DMF for 60 min. Even under these conditions, some high-affinity primary antibodies are not completely removed (Sternberger, 1979). Tramu et al. (1978) recommended oxidation with $KMnO_4$ as a simple alternative and more efficient procedure for the destruction of residual enzyme activity. Sternberger and Joseph (1979) avoided the elution of antibody altogether, since the reaction product of DAB apparently masked both the antigen and the catalytic sites of the first system and thus prevented interaction with reagents of the second system. A weak reaction in the first step produces a mixing of colors for the first antigen. Almost without exception all these methods use DAB as the first substrate and, very frequently, 4-chloro-1-naphthol (CN) as the second, which yield brown and blue colored products, respectively. A slightly modified version of the method of Sternberger and Joseph (1979) in which the same bridging antibody and PAP preparation are used for both reaction sequences, is presented in Table 17.3.

Non-specific reactions can be attributed to: (i) reaction of the bridging antibody in the second system with the primary antibody or PAP belonging to the first system; (ii) reaction of the primary antibody of the second system with the bridging antibody of the first system; and, (iii) reaction of the substrate of the second system with the PAP of the first system. Mixing of colors occurs if the two epitopes of the two systems are in close proximity (Joseph and Sternberger, 1979). The necessity to elute antibodies from the first system depends on the strength of the DAB reaction. In Nakane's original work the enzyme-labeled antibodies were less reactive which may have resulted in a less well-covered complex.

17.3.2.3.2. Simultaneous localization of multiple antigens with conjugates of unrelated enzymes   In addition to POase, the most popular enzymes for double-labeling are APase (Mason and Sammons, 1978) and GOase (Mason et al., 1983). If care is taken that the two antibody preparations labeled with two different enzymes do not interfere, the only additional procedure compared to the single immunoenzymatic technique is the histochemical step for the second enzyme.

GOase has the theoretical advantage that no endogenous enzyme

TABLE 17.3

Sequential localization of two antigens in the same specimen by peroxidase–anti-peroxidase (PAP) complexes without intermittent antibody removal

---

1. Pretreat sections or smears: dewaxing (if necessary, Section 17.3.1); inactivation of endogenous POase (if necessary, Section 17.3.4.3.2.1); application of normal serum to lower background staining (Section 17.3.4.3.2.2).

2. Apply primary antiserum (100–1000 times diluted with isotonic buffer) to one of the antigens; incubation for 1 h at room temperature.

3. Wash 4 times, 5 min each, with isotonic buffer; dry around sections or etch.

4. Apply anti-Ig antibodies (antiserum dilution 1/25); incubation as in step 2.

5. Wash as in step 3.

6. Apply PAP prepared with antibodies from the same species as the primary antibody, at a concentration of about 40 μg/ml.

7. Reveal the enzyme after washing as in step 3, with DAB (Section 17.3.3.1) until a strong staining is obtained (usually 2–5 min), followed by 3 washings as in step 3.

8. Apply primary antiserum to the second antigen as in step 2.

9. Same as steps 3, 4, 5, and 6.

10. Reveal the second reaction with 1-chloro-4-naphthol (Section 17.3.3.1).

N.B. Some modifications reported may be useful for particular situations:

step 1, (and/or steps 3 and 5), the use of hypertonic buffers (e.g., 50 mM Tris–HCl, pH 7.6, in 3% NaCl; Pickel et al., 1976; Sternberger and Joseph, 1979).

step 2, the inclusion of Triton X-100 at 0.4% with the primary antibodies and 0.025% with all other solutions (Grzanna et al., 1978). Alternatively, Tween 20 at 0.05–0.10% in all buffers improved often considerably the staining.

step 3, increased washing after the application of the primary antibodies, e.g. 5 × 15 min.

step 9, for an intensified second reaction, according to a procedure originally suggested by Vacca et al., 1975, repeat steps 3, 8, 3, 4, 5, and 6.

activity is found in mammalian tissues, in contrast to POase (or POase-like) activity (e.g., peroxisomes) and APase (Rathlev and Franks, 1982). In practice, this advantage is often not important, since these endogenous activities, if present, can be blocked (Section 17.3.4.3.2.1).

The techniques employed may be any of the direct or indirect methods. To avoid color mixing, it is necessary to prevent the interaction of the Ig of the two systems. For the more complex and sensitive indirect methods, this may necessitate the use of antibodies from several species. Due to the extensive structural homologies of Ig of different species (Section 6.1.2), it is not surprising that cross-reactions among Ig of various species are considerable. This is exemplified by several studies in EIH which took advantage of this phenomenon (Erlandsen et al., 1975; Parsons et al., 1976; Grzanna et al., 1978). For example, antigens can be revealed with a primary antiserum from the guinea pig or monkey followed by goat or sheep anti-rabbit Ig and rabbit PAP (Sternberger and Joseph, 1979). Though good results are reported in a number of instances with the conventional methods, the use of haptenated antibodies and of anti-hapten antibodies (or biotin–avidin) instead of the less specific anti-IgG antibodies may be advantageous.

The simultaneous localization of antigens may be complicated if monoclonal primary antibodies are used for both epitopes. Monoclonal antibodies are often of the IgG1 subclass, which cannot be distinguished by secondary antibodies. Hapten-labeling or biotin–avidin bridging could be of considerable value to circumvent this problem.

Mixing of colors is less easily detected with enzyme methods than with double immunofluorescent labeling where filter systems in the microscope are more effective in segregating the staining intensities of the two labels. The use of fluorescent antibodies and enzyme-labeled antibodies for the different epitopes may lend itself particularly well to assess co-distribution of epitopes.

Fig. 17.4 illustrates several systems used for simultaneous localization of two epitopes and Table 17.4 gives the details for double immunoenzymatic analysis of cellular constituents by the PAP and APAAP methods (modified from Mason and Sammons, 1978).

Intestinal APase is the most used second enzyme for antigen local-

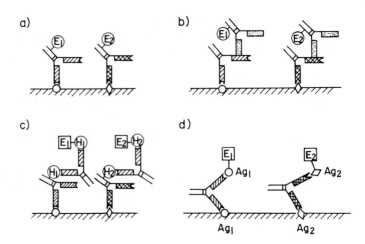

Fig. 17.4. Different approaches to simultaneous, differential staining of unlike antigens. In (a) two different antigens in the same preparation are detected simultaneously using different enzymes conjugated to separately prepared antibodies. In (b) different antigens are detected sequentially. This can be done in the direct or indirect mode with different enzymes, or the same enzyme if the first stain is dominant. In (c) antibodies with different specificities are labeled with different haptens (one of which may be biotin) so that they can be detected separately. In (d) antigen-labeled enzymes are used after excess of the bridging antibody is allowed to react with the solid-phase antigen permitting the other antigen-binding site of the Ig to bind the corresponding enzyme conjugate.

ization. However, *E. coli* APase may be better suited for localization purposes since its pH optimum is considerably lower than that of intestinal APase (Section 10.1.3.1). An alkaline buffer in the enzyme revelation may dissociate complexes and produce a diffuse staining in the preparation.

17.3.2.4. Enzyme-lectin histochemistry   Carbohydrate components in cells and, in particular, on the cell membrane seem to be associated with cell differentiation and transformation (Burridge, 1976; Salik and Cook, 1976; Ponder, 1983). The finding of affinity between a particular lectin (Section 3.4), among the many hundreds known, and certain glycoproteins of a particular phenotype is virtually always empirical.

TABLE 17.4
Simultaneous detection of two antigens by peroxidase–anti-peroxidase antibody (PAP)
and alkaline phosphatase–anti-alkaline phosphatase (APAAP) complexes

1. Pretreat sections as in Table 17.3.

2. Apply primary antibodies (100–1000 times diluted in isotonic buffer) to both antigens. Incubation for 1 h at room temperature in a humid chamber.

3. Wash as in step 3 (Table 17.3), apply both anti-IgG as in step 4 (Table 17.3), wash again.

4. Apply enzyme–antibody complexes (PAP and APAAP at a concentration of about 40 μg/ml). Alternatively, instead of APAAP, anti-APase antiserum (1:400) plus APase (5.0 U/ml of intestinal enzyme) may be applied.

5. Washing as in step 3.

6. Enzymatic revelation. First POase is revealed with DAB (brown color) and then APase with naphthol AS phosphate plus Fast Blue BBN, according to Section 17.3.3.2.

For preliminary experiments commercial kits of conjugates of representative lectins may be very useful. Conjugated lectins are also useful at the ultrastructural level (Ponder, 1983). Appropriate sugars provide adequate controls for the specificity of lectin-based histochemical stains. If a particular lectin is found to be of value after a first screening, it may be worth purifying the lectin from raw material (Colowick and Kaplan, 1972) and preparing the appropriate conjugates. Details of the histochemical application of lectins, according to Ponder (1983), are given in Table 17.5. Specificity of binding is controlled with 100 mM of the appropriate sugar. This may not be sufficient, even at higher concentrations, for Con A and for lectins from *Ricinus communis*, *Alrus precatorius*, and *Phaseolus limensis* (Ponder, 1983). Beside the currently used direct method (Table 17.5), indirect and even more complex systems to enhance sensitivity are possible through the use of anti-lectin antibodies.

17.3.2.5. Enzyme-labeled antigen methods   Non-specific adsorp-

TABLE 17.5
Peroxidase–lectin histochemical staining of cellular markers

1. Wash specimen with PBS, containing 0.5% BSA.

2. Blot excess moisture away.

3. Dilute lectin-conjugate with PBS–BSA to a concentration of 10 μg (check for particular lectin), applied and incubated according to standard conditions (Section 17.3.2.2). For control slides 100 mM of the appropriate monosaccharide is added to the lectin-conjugate during incubation.

4. Wash 3 times by flooding with PBS, or in 3 baths of PBS.

5. Stain and counterstain as in Section 17.3.3.

tion of non-antibody IgG from the primary antiserum is a common cause for background staining. Primary antisera often have less than 10% specific antibodies and most of the non-specifically adsorbed IgG is irrelevant. This background staining can often be minimized with enzyme-labeled antigen, which reacts only with its corresponding antibody–antigen complex (one binding site of antibody free) and not with non-specifically adsorbed Ig or antibodies bound to minor, but strongly immunogenic, contaminants.

The essential feature of this technique is that specificity depends on the purity and nature of the labeled antigen. Only antibodies having affinity for this antigen are revealed. This technique is conceptually similar to that described for immunofluorescence (Beutner et al., 1965). Mason and Sammons (1979) noted two important characteristics in this method. The high concentrations of the primary antiserum (up to undiluted), needed to prevent binding of the antibody by both sites, does not increase background staining, nor weakens the specific staining (prozone effect), in contrast to conventional two-stage methods. Moreover, the length of the washing after incubation with the primary antiserum has no effect on the reaction: just rinsing for a few seconds produces as good results as repeated washings for 5 min. These features make it possible to reduce the overall time needed for the detection of a specific antigen: from paraffin section to counterstained, mounted slide in about 30 min. Table 17.6 summarizes this method.

17.3.2.6. Localization of specific nucleic acid sequences in situ
Biotinylated nucleic acids, particularly with B-cap-NHS (Section 3.2.4.3), are very useful for in situ hybridization (as for molecular cloning and blotting) since such probes have a much longer half-life (at least a few years) than radioactively labeled probes and have at least similar detectabilities. This approach was successful for the localization of specific DNA sequences in *Drosophila* polytene chromosomes (Langer- Safer et al., 1982), in the mapping of satellite DNA (Manuelidis et al., 1982) and the localization of MVM (a parvovirus) sequences in infected cells (Brigati et al., 1983).

In the method of Brigati et al., culture cells or dewaxed formalin-fixed sections are hydrated briefly in PBS and treated for 10 min with 0.02 N HCl. The samples are then washed twice with PBS (3 min), once with 0.01% Triton X-100 in PBS (1.5 min) and twice 3 min in PBS. The preparations are then treated with pronase (Section 17.3.1). This is the most critical step of this procedure. The pronase concentration which causes cells to begin to round after 10 min is determined and half of this concentration is used for 10 min. An RNase treatment can be included if DNA is to be detected. Haase et al. (1982) observed that a paraformaldehyde postfixation

TABLE 17.6
Two-stage enzyme-labeled antigen method

1. Pretreat sections as in step 1 of Table 17.3.

2. Incubate in a humid chamber with primary antiserum in isotonic buffer (dilution 1:50, 30 min; dilution 1:5, 10 min) at room temperature.

3. Rinse by dipping preparation for a few seconds in isotonic buffer.

4. Apply enzyme-labeled antigen (concentration depending on size of antigen about 5–100 μg/ml). Incubation for 10–30 min at room temperature.

5. Stain and counterstain, according to Section 17.3.3.

at this stage reduces markedly the loss of cellular DNA during hybridization (5 min with 4% paraformaldehyde in PBS and two washes of 3 min with PBS). The samples are then dehydrated. The hybridization mixture contains 50% (v/v) deionized formamide, 10% (w/v) dextran sulfate, 300 mM NaCl and 30 mM sodium citrate ('2 × SSC'; pH 7.0), 250 µg/ml sonicated carrier DNA (herring sperm) and 2 µg/ml of probe DNA. The cells are overlayered with this solution, the temperature rapidly increased to 80°C, left for 2 min at 80°C, and lowered rapidly to 40°C or less. After hybridization for 16 h at 37°C, the samples are washed in 50% formamide and 2 × SSC and twice with 2 × SSC with decreasing temperatures. The immobilized probe is detected as in Section 17.3.2.2.3. The use of streptavidin instead of the currently used avidin is recommended.

17.3.3. Chromogens for enzyme immunohistochemistry

17.3.3.1. Detection of peroxidase   The substrate universally used for POase is H_2O_2 which has a rather narrow optimum concentration range (Tijssen et al., 1982). The lack of taking this into consideration is one of the most common and unrealized causes of poor results. At low concentrations the activity is considerably decreased, whereas at concentrations higher than optimum, substrate inhibition can be substantial, e.g. doubling the concentration may cause 50% inhibition. The POase used in EIH, isozyme C, has the highest activity in solution at a H_2O_2 concentration of 0.003%. As noted in Section 9.2.2, solid phase in EIA may considerably aggravate or lessen this inhibition or the different effects may cancel each other. This should be established for each new batch of solid-phase material (glass or plastic plus cells plus fixation method). The substrate concentration is often used at 0.01% though this is frequently not optimal. The most useful concentration is easily established by doubling concentrations of substrate on a small series of samples. In many cases it may be preferable to incubate the tissue preparation first in a solution of the H-donor to saturate the specimen (pre-reaction soak) before adding the substrate. H_2O_2 is not stable during storage and the actual concentration should be measured by the simple method given in Section 10.1.1.5. Among the H-donors, 3,3'-diaminobenzidine (DAB) is the most generally used for the detection of antigens in cells, whereas CN is the most frequently used for immunoblots (on nitrocellulose). The chemical relationship of DAB to benzidine, an established carcinogen, suggests that DAB might be carcinogenic, though definite proof is still lacking (Tubbs and Shebani, 1981). Until final proof, DAB should be handled as a carcinogen. Instead of weighing small samples every time, a stock solution of DAB may be stored frozen in sealed vials until use. The DAB solution is prepared by dissolving 50 mg of DAB·4HCl, its most soluble form, in 100 ml of 50 mM Tris–HCl buffer, pH 7.6 and filtered just before use. H_2O_2 is added to the desired concentration (0.01–0.003%, see above). Staining is performed as in Table 17.7. Spills should be 'neutralized' with bleach (NaOCl).

Intensification of the DAB staining is a simple way to enhance detectability. A simple method of post-intensification is the deposition of metallic silver on the end-product of the DAB reaction, increasing detectability by about 100-fold (Gallyas et al., 1982). To avoid strong background staining it is recommended to incubate the preparation with the substrate solution just for the minimum period necessary to obtain good contrast. The procedure is based on the capacity of the DAB end-product to catalyze the deposition of metallic silver from silver ions in the presence of a reducing agent. The catalytic capacity of the tissue is suppressed by treatment with mercaptoacetic acid, which does not affect catalysis by the polymerized DAB. The tissue section is treated with a solution containing 20 ml concentrated mercaptoacetic acid, 5 ml concentrated HCl and 75 ml distilled water for 4 h at room temperature. The preparation is then washed three times for 5 min with distilled water, transferred to the developer solution until the desired degree of intensification is obtained, washed with three changes of 10% acetic acid, 10 min each, dehydrated and mounted with Canada balsam. The developer is prepared by slowly adding (in the sequence stated) an equal volume of a 5% Na_2CO_3 solution to a solution containing

TABLE 17.7

Staining procedure for peroxidase in light microscopy

The complete staining procedure takes place at room temperature.

1. Wash with isotonic buffer (3 × 5 min).

2. Equilibrate (1 × 5 min) with buffer used for substrate (Section 17.3.3.1) (optional: prereaction soak with hydrogen donor, 2 min).

3. Stain with DAB for 1–5 min or with HY[a], CN[a], or AEC[a] for about 5–10 min while stirring gently. Development of stain can be checked from time to time under microscope. DAB development can be prolonged considerably if Tween 20 was used. The substrate solutions are prepared according to Section 17.3.3.1.

4. Wash with buffer used for substrate (1 × 5 min).

5. Counterstain if desired: DAB lightly with hematoxylin or 0.1% methyl green (chloroform washed) in veronal–acetate buffer, pH 4.0; HY with neutral red or carmalum; AEC with hematoxylin (lightly) since product is alcohol-soluble and differentiation of the hematoxylin with acid–alcohol should be avoided.

6. Mount: DAB can easily be mounted with usual methods; HY will also withstand alcohols and solvent-based mounting media but deteriorates upon storage; AEC and CN are soluble in alcohol or other current mounting media with the exception of water-bound mountants such as glycerin jelly; CN products are probably most stable if mounted in acid-buffered glycerin, pH 2.2. It is advisable to examine and photograph immediately if a hydrogen donor other than DAB is used.

[a] HY, Hanker-Yates reagent; CN, 4-chloro-1-naphthol; AEC, 3-amino-9-ethylcarbazole.

0.2% NH_4NO_3, 0.2% $AgNO_3$, 1% silicotungstic acid and 0.5% FA.

Another simple method for intensification of the DAB-based product with heavy metal was reported by Adams (1981). In this procedure, 100 mg DAB are dissolved in 33 ml water and 66 ml 300 mM phosphate buffer (pH 7.3) are added. While stirring, 5 ml 1% $CoCl_2$ and 4 ml 1% nickel ammonium sulfate are added dropwise in this sequence. The tissue is incubated about 15 min in this mixture, followed by the addition of 0.66 ml 3% H_2O_2. After another 15 min incubation, the sections are rinsed and mounted. This method is also applicable for the detection of proteins transferred to membranes.

As alternatives to DAB or for double immunoenzymatic staining, Hanker-Yates (HY) reagent, composed of p-phenylenediamine-HCl and two parts of pyrocatechol, 3-amino-9-ethylcarbazole (AEC), 3,3'-5,5'-tetramethylbenzidine (TMB), CN and α-naphthol/pyronin have received the most attention (Tubbs and Shebani, 1981; Sofroniew and Schrell, 1982). HY yields a purple-brown, almost black product, AEC a reddish product and TMB, CN a dark-blue product and naphthol/pyronin a red/purple product.

The capricious HY-chromogen (Polyscience), is prepared according to Tubbs and Shebani (1981) by preweighing just before use and adding 75 mg of the mixture to each of six chemically clean and dry Coplin jars. The buffer, 200 mM Tris–HCl, pH 7.6, is added just prior to immersing the slides. H_2O_2 (20 μl, 30%) is added immediately after and the solution is agitated during color development. The incubation time is longer than for DAB and slides should be transferred from one jar to another containing fresh HY when the chromogen turns brown. Background staining is very low, since this reagent seems to be specific for plant POase and does not react with endogenous POase.

AEC stock solutions (0.4% in DMF) are stable at room temperature. The incubation solution is prepared by adding 0.5 ml AEC stock solution to 9.5 ml 50 mM acetate buffer, pH 5.0, followed by 1–10 μl 30% H_2O_2. The solution is filtered onto the sections and left for 3–10 min at room temperature. This reaction is generally weak.

The conversion of TMB is highly pH dependent and is most effective at lower pH (2.5–4.0) and weak at pH 5.0 (Mesulam, 1978). Since the recommended procedure involves a pre-reaction soak for 20 min at pH 3.3, this method is less suitable for EIH than for cytochemistry (unless immune complexes are fixed as in ultrastructural studies, Section 17.4.2.1).

CN is prepared by dissolving 40 mg in 0.2–0.5 ml of absolute ethanol. While stirring, 100 ml of 50 mM Tris–HCl buffer, pH 7.6, and 10–100 μl of 30% peroxide are added. Usually a white precipitate forms which is removed by filtration. Heating the incubation medium to 50°C before use produces a stronger stain (Buffa, cited by Van Noorden and Polak, 1983). This hot solution is filtered on a coarse filter paper and used immediately. CN staining is weaker than with DAB, but yields much less background staining in immunoblots.

17.3.3.2. Alkaline phosphatase staining   An early method for APase staining is Gomori's method which yields a black deposit of CoS (Burstone, 1962) and is compatible with dehydration and mounting. In EIH, the methods of Mason and Sammons (1978) are preferred since they stain more evenly.

A stock solution (10 mg/ml) of naphthol AS-MX, or naphthol AS phosphate, or naphthol AS-BI phosphoric acid sodium salt (Sigma) in DMF is prepared and diluted 50 times with 100 mM Tris–HCl buffer, pH 8.2. The solution is stable at 4°C for several weeks (in their original work, Mason and Sammons used naphthol AS phosphate and a buffer of pH 9.0). The substrate solution is prepared by dissolving Fast Blue BBN or Fast Red TR (1 mg/ml) in the naphthol stock solution.

Fast Red gives the most intense (red) reaction product which contrasts well with hematoxylin. For double immunostaining (in combination with POase/DAB) Fast Blue is preferred due to its contrast with oxidized DAB. Naphthol AS-MX (Stage and Avrameas, 1976) gives comparable results to naphthol AS phosphate.

The slides are first washed, shaken to drain all excess buffer and the substrate solution is pipetted directly onto the slides. If the substrate solution is cloudy, it is preferable to filter it directly onto the slide. Staining is complete after 10–15 min and can be followed under the microscope. The reaction is stopped by washing in a jar with isotonic buffer and extensive rinsing under tap water. The slides should be mounted in aqueous material, such as Apathy's mountant.

Endogenous enzyme activity is suppressed as discussed in Section 17.3.4.3.2.1.

17.3.3.3. Glucose oxidase staining   Rathlev and Franks (1982) obtained very good results with glucose, *t*-nitroblue tetrazolium chloride (*t*-NBT) and *m*-phenazine methosulfate (*m*-PMS) for the revelation of GOase conjugates.

The two chromogenic reagents (Sigma) are dissolved at 2.5 mM (*t*-NBT) and 0.6 mM (*m*-PMS) in 100 mM phosphate buffer, pH 6.6, containing 41.7 mM glucose, about 1 h before staining (to allow mutarotation of glucose to occur).

Tissue sections are covered with 50 μl of the staining reagent and the slides are placed in an opaque plastic box. The box is closed and placed for 30 min in a water bath at 50°C. After the incubation, the slides are rinsed twice with PBS, pH 7.2, mounted and examined by light microscopy. Background stain usually is completely absent. Staining produces an insoluble stable formazan due to an electron transfer between *m*-PMS and *t*-NBT, which appears as a finely granular purple-colored deposit at the site of the immune complex. The reagents are not carcinogenic (Rathlev and Franks, 1982; but see also Table 18.1).

17.3.4. Nature, recognition and prevention of non-specific staining

17.3.4.1. Nature of non-specific staining   Two sources of non-specificity can be distinguished in EIH: (i) immunological non-specificity (e.g., antibodies against contaminants); and, (ii) methodological non-specificity resulting in background staining. The latter may originate from: (i) endogenous enzyme activity; (ii) non-immunological adsorption of antiserum, conjugated antibodies or conjugated antigen: and, (iii) methodological errors such as insufficient washing, incorrect buffer, pH, substrate concentration, etc. These two types of non-specific reactions have different characteristics: immunological non-specificity is often localized in some specific pattern and is quite difficult to eliminate, whereas methodological non-specificity tends to give a diffuse staining distributed evenly over the preparation (except for endogenous enzyme activity) and is mostly quite easy to correct.

Immunological non-specificity is due to the presence of the same (shared reactivity) or similar (cross-reactivity) epitopes on different antigen molecules. As discussed earlier (Section 8.6), antibodies recognize epitopes, not the antigens, implying that immunization with a pure antigen does not reduce non-specificity if different antigens share the same epitope(s). However, polyclonal antisera often have a 'specificity bonus' (Section 8.6), absent for monoclonal antibodies. For example, if two antigens have 10 epitopes each, one of which is the same (epitope 'X'), the relative staining intensity with a polyclonal antiserum against the specific antigen (if all affinities are the same) is about 10 times stronger than against the non-specific antigen. In contrast, with monoclonal anti-'X' antibodies both specific and non-specific antigens have equal staining, whereas with monoclonal antibodies against an epitope other than 'X' staining is completely specific for the antigen. This situation may arise in double immunoenzyme staining procedures where the secondary antibodies (anti-Ig) are not absolutely specific for antibodies from one species only but are often reactive with those of many other species. This phenomenon is not necessarily harmful and has been, in fact, exploited in various situations. Thus, Marucci and Dougherty (1975) used PAP complexes made with baboon antibodies in conjunction with human primary antibodies and guinea pig antibodies to human Ig. An alternative sequence which theoretically should have been more successful, i.e., (human primary antibody)–(rabbit anti-human IgG)–(guinea pig anti-rabbit Ig)–(rabbit PAP), yielded strong background staining. In this sequence, selective omission of individual components revealed that the rabbit anti-human IgG was adsorbed non-specifically to the tissue and was revealed with the PAP probe. However, using a heterologous sequence by omitting the rabbit anti-human IgG, PAP complexes reacted only with the guinea pig anti-rabbit Ig antibodies which had reacted with the primary antibody. This effect is a major contribution to the specificity of the PAP method.

Endogenous enzyme activity is readily recognizable in some cases (e.g. staining of peroxisomes with POase substrates) and can be inhibited specifically (Section 17.3.4.3.2.1).

Examples of non-immunological adsorption of various reagents to the tissue preparation abound. Virus receptors on cell membranes may remain intact during manipulation and can adsorb viral antigens. Similarly, Fc receptors may adsorb antibodies, particularly in the form of PAP complexes. Another main cause of non-immunological adsorption is denaturation of proteins during or after conjugation. The stickiness of the tissue preparation after fixation or of the conjugate due to cross-linkers (e.g., Molin et al., 1978) may occasionally cause important non-immunological adsorption. An often difficult cause to eliminate in non-specific reactions is the electrostatic binding to tissue components. Early studies with immunofluorescence showed that a change of the pI of the Ig due to a high fluorescein/protein ratio enhances non-specific staining (Grossi and Mayersbach, 1964; Hebert et al., 1967). PAP was also observed to adsorb non-specifically to all neurophysin-containing structures of the pig hypothalamus in paraffin sections (Watkins, 1977). Non-specific adsorption may also occur on the embedding material in post-embedding techniques.

A common problem with the indirect covalently labeled enzyme methods is that anti-Ig antibodies often adsorb non-specifically to the tissue, resulting in background staining: (i) when long incubation or staining periods are used; and, (ii) when the ratio of specifically bound and non-specifically adsorbed antibodies becomes smaller (sparsity of antigens or primary antibodies; large excess of anti-Ig antibodies).

17.3.4.2. Recognition of non-specific staining   Methodological non-specific reactions can be recognized: (i) by staining of tissue preparations not containing the specific antigen; (ii) by staining with conjugated normal, non-immune serum; and, (iii) when staining is not prevented by the blocking or neutralization test (Fig.17.5). The controls can, therefore, be divided into three groups: controls for antigen, antibody and methodology, with each of which difficulties may arise.

Staining of control slides without the application of the immune serum reveals endogenous enzyme activity: cells devoid of the specific

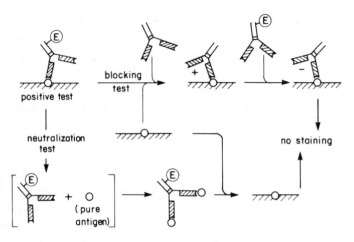

Fig. 17.5. Blocking and neutralization tests. In the blocking test, positive staining can be prevented by pre-incubation of the tissue with the specific antibody, whereas in the neutralization test staining is prevented by adding pure antigen to the immunoreactants prior to incubation with the tissue.

antigen should remain unstained after the application of the substrate. However, the specimen may be unique or of pathological origin and appropriate control tissue may not be available. In such situations the blocking test is a good alternative if the affinity of the antibodies is high (otherwise antibody may be released from the blocked sites and replaced by conjugate). Blocking tests in indirect methods or of more complex designs require that the blocking antibody does not react with the other antibodies used in the test. If pure specific antigen is available, neutralization can be used to recognize non-specific staining. This method may be extended to the use of purified antigen fragments (containing one or several epitopes).

Non-specific adsorption of the immunoreactants can be recognized by a simple method. Serial sections of the tissue preparation are incubated with the reagent of the last step, of the last two steps, etc., e.g., one section with PAP, the second with bridging antibody plus PAP, etc.

Immunological specificity is best inferred from neutralization or blocking tests. It is fallacious to deduct degrees of cross-reactivity or shared reactivity of a given antiserum in EIH from the results of EIA. Sensitivity and specificity are determined to a high degree by the design of the test as shown in Chapter 2 for the AA and the AM tests, and may, therefore, be very different in EIH and EIA.

17.3.4.3. Prevention of non-specific staining

17.3.4.3.1. Prevention of immunological non-specificity   Any method which renders an antibody population more specific for a given antigen, i.e., the elimination of antibodies directed against epitopes not found on the specific antigen but on contaminants, by neutralization or immunosorption (Section 7.1.9.2), can be used to reduce or eliminate non-specific staining. Instead of polyclonal antisera, monoclonal antibodies may be used to detect a given epitope.

Another approach to exclude immunological reactions of the primary antiserum with epitopes not found on the specific antigen is the labeling of pure antigen. Subsequent to the reaction of the primary antiserum, pure antigen is bound only to the specific antibodies complexed to the antigen in the tissue preparation.

Immunological non-specificity is not restricted to primary antibodies, as sometimes stated (Vandesande, 1979; Sternberger, 1979). The simultaneous detection of two or more antigens in the same sample requires that the immunological reagents in the consecutive steps do not interreact. Such non-specificity is, nevertheless, quite common (Section 17.3.4.1) and can be eliminated by replacing the linking anti-Ig antibodies by anti-hapten antibodies and using appropriately haptenated antibodies (primary antibodies, enzyme-conjugated antibodies, etc.) (Farr and Nakane, 1981). For the different layers of the reaction different haptens can be used (Section 12.5). This method is also convenient when the antibodies against two epitopes come from the same species (e.g., mouse hybridomas). In the preparation of haptenated proteins utmost care should be taken to avoid sensitization (delayed-type hypersensitivity) with reactive compounds. The avidin–biotin system may also be used to circumvent immunological non-specificity of secondary antibodies.

Another potential cause of immunological non-specificity involves allo- or auto-antibodies. Anti-IgG antibodies cannot discriminate between endogenous Ig and the primary antibodies from the same species or, frequently, from other species. This problem may also be overcome by the use of haptenated or biotinylated primary antibodies.

17.3.4.3.2. Prevention of methodological non-specificity

17.3.4.3.2.1. Inhibition of endogenous enzyme activities. In mammals APase is found in two forms: one is confined to the intestine, the other is distributed in a variety of tissues but not in the intestines. Tetrahydrophenylimidazothiazole (levamisole, Sigma) inhibits the non-intestinal form of the enzyme, but has no effect on the intestinal enzyme which is used as a label (Van Belle, 1972; Borgers, 1973). Ponder and Wilkinson (1981) suppressed the endogenous enzyme activity by the inclusion of 1 mM levamisole in the substrate used for revelation of conjugated APase and found this method very efficient. Endogenous APase may also be inhibited by treatment with 20% acetic acid in water or ethanol for 15 sec at 4°C (both types of enzymes). Heat stability of different APases is also different (Ponder and Wilkinson, 1981) but this property is difficult to exploit for EIH. Another approach for the selective inhibition of endogenous enzyme(s) which is worth further exploration is the differential sensitivity of APases to a variety of anions (Freiman et al., 1962). Bulman and Heyderman (1981) inactivated endogenous APase by oxidation with $NaIO_4$.

POase activity in tissue or cell preparations is usually eliminated prior to the test. In some cases, endogenous POase is confined to peroxisomes and does not interfere with the test. Fixation in methanol is often accompanied by a decrease in peroxidatic activity. The method of Straus (1971) using 1% sodium nitroferricyanide and 1% acetic acid in methanol, is effective to abolish endogenous POase, but also weakens the immunohistochemical reaction. Streefkerk (1972) used H_2O_2 at high concentrations, e.g. 0.5% H_2O_2 in methanol for about 30 min, as an effective inhibitor of POase. Zehr (1978) coated the sections for about 15 min with 3% H_2O_2 in 10% ovalbumin. Acidified methanol (0.075% HCl in methanol) may also be used for inactivation of endogenous POase for light microscopy. Weir et al. (1974) destroyed endogenous POase activity by treatment with 10 mM HIO_4 for 10 min followed by a treatment with $NaBH_4$ (0.1 mg/ml in water) for 10 min prior to the test. All these methods are performed before the primary antiserum is applied. Another method useful for both light and electron microscopy inactivates endogenous enzyme by the addition of 5 mM NaN_3 to the substrate solution (Farr and Nakane, 1981).

   17.3.4.3.2.2. Prevention of non-immunological adsorption of immuno-reactants to tissue preparations. The frequent use of cross-linkers both in the preparation of conjugates and fixation of the samples may result in a 'stickiness' of the preparations. Most of these cross-linkers react via amino groups. Molin et al. (1978) reduced background staining by the inclusion of 20 mM lysine, with or without 1% BSA, in the incubation steps.

   In cases where Fc receptors in the tissue are a problem (cells of the lymphoid system, central nervous system and some epithelia) the use of Fab may offer a solution. Pretreatment of the samples with 2% normal serum may also obviate this problem.

   One of the most effective means to reduce background staining is to improve the detection limit of the test, so that antisera may be used at higher dilution. Several suitable procedures are listed in Table 17.8.

   The classical method for the prevention of non-specific adsorption of antibodies to the sample, particularly in the PAP method, is the pretreatment of the tissue preparation with normal serum from the species which produced the antiserum (3% normal serum in the pretreatment, 1% normal serum included in the next steps; Sternberger and Joseph, 1979). Grube and Weber (1980), however, reported that IgG or F(ab')$_2$ from non-immune serum was bound non-specifically to gastrin cells (to unidentified anionic constituents) and

TABLE 17.8
Some methods to improve detectability

1. The use of high-titered antisera with high affinity.

2. Microscopy with differential interference optics (e.g., Zeiss–Nomarski amplitude-contrast optics; Webster et al., 1974).

3. Increasing incubation time with primary antibodies, but at higher dilutions; This, in turn, reduces background staining (Petrusz et al., 1975).

4. Repetition of layers to increase enzyme/epitope ratio. This may be achieved by the use of additional layers of anti-Ig or by extra bridges (e.g., double PAP method, Vacca et al., 1975; double bridge, Ordronneau and Petrusz, 1980).

5. Reduction of background staining due to nonspecific adsorption by pretreatment with normal serum: by hypertonic buffers; by addition of detergents (Triton X-100; Tween 20) to buffers; by inhibition of endogenous enzyme activity (may be particularly prominent in cryostat sections).

6. The composition of the buffer or its pH may also influence background staining; Tris usually produces lower background staining than phosphate. A buffer- or pH-induced lowering of the activation energy required for substrate product transformation would increase spontaneous product formation and cause a decrease in the signal/noise ratio.

interfered with the EIH procedure. Pickel et al. (1976) used hypertonic instead of isotonic buffers (3% instead of the 0.9% NaCl in 50 mM Tris–HCl buffer of Table 17.3) and reduced background staining.

Neutralization tests (Fig.17.4) are not reliable controls under these conditions. Meaningful results from neutralization tests are obtained only if high-titered antisera (dilution at least 1:500) and hypertonic buffers are used (Grube, 1980). Isotonic buffers often favor non-specific staining (Grube and Weber, 1980), whereas hypertonic buffers (with 3% NaCl) and a pH closer to the pI of the Ig strongly decrease non-specific reactions (Grube, 1980). The latter also varies with the batch of antiserum. Among the additives used for the gastrin cell-system, Triton X-100 and BSA were without any effect for the majority of the sera, whereas a pre-incubation with normal serum prior to the antiserum reduced background staining remarkably. Hypertonic buffers are efficient not only in the incubation step but also in the rinsing to reduce non-specificity. However, rinsing even up to 20 h with isotonic buffers has no effect.

17.4. Enzyme-immunohistochemistry procedures in electron microscopy

17.4.1. Overview

The essential difference between light and electron microscopy is the degree of resolution. To obtain this higher resolution in electron microscopy, it is essential to have a better preservation of the ultrastructure. This requirement creates at the same time an obstacle for the demonstration of intracellular antigens by EIH, since the penetration of antibodies or of antibody–enzyme conjugates through membranes decreases considerably upon improved preservation.

Several approaches have been tried to circumvent these difficulties. One general way is to improve permeability of membranes and to detect the antigens prior to embedding ('pre-embedding staining methods'), the other is the detection of antigens on ultrathin sections after embedding and sectioning ('post-embedding staining'). Pre-embedding staining methods were considered to be futile, since immunoreactants penetrate too sluggishly (Sternberger, 1979). However, this misgiving was dispelled by other studies (Pickel et al., 1976; Bohn, 1978). Moreover, it was shown that under certain conditions pre-embedding might yield considerably higher resolution. For example, in the triple-layer PAP method (post-embedding), the product is deposited on the thin section at a maximum distance of 40 nm from the antigenic site and staining is, therefore, found within an area with a diameter of 80 nm. Sternberger et al. (1977) observed about 20 times higher resolution with pre-embedding staining methods, probably due to the restricted antibody orientation in the tissue, and were, thus, able to localize myelin basic protein to the intraperiod line of 6–9 nm (not to the major dense line as surmised from earlier studies).

Only those methods will be discussed which are pertinent to ultrastructural EIH and supplement the usual techniques employed in electron microscopy. Many of the concepts discussed above also apply in electron microscopy.

17.4.2. Ultrastructural EIH by pre-embedding staining

Almost all pre-embedding staining procedures consist in the following steps: (i) prefixation to obtain maximum permeabilization of the tissue with the best acceptable structural preservation and minimal loss of antigens; (ii) immunohistochemical incubations; (iii) further fixation; (iv) revelation of the enzyme; (v) postfixation (e.g., with osmic acid to render the DAB product electron dense); and, (vi) dehydration and embedding. Extensive washings are included between the various steps. The enzyme-generated product should be insoluble, both in water and alcohol.

To improve permeability after fixation or to unmask antigenic sites (Curran and Gregory, 1977), proteolytic enzymes (Section 17.3.1; Kuhlmann et al., 1974; Mepham et al., 1979)., freezing and thawing (Leduc et al., 1969) or treatments with digitonin (Dales et al., 1965) or saponin can be used. Saponin (Graham et al., 1967; Seeman, 1967; Speth et al., 1972; Bohn, 1978; Willingham et al., 1978) gives quite satisfactory results.

In the method developed by Pickel et al. (1976), organs or animals are perfused with fixative, followed by the preparation of sections (about 20 μm) which are then treated with detergent (Triton X-100) to increase permeability. Subseqent EIH staining, as in light microscopy (Section 17.3.3), gives suitable results for the outer 2–3 μm layer of thick sections.

Instead of further increasing permeabilization of the tissues, it is possible to decrease the size of the tracer, by conjugating Fab with MPOase (Section 10.4.1).

17.4.2.1 Fixatives for prefixation of tissue prior to immunocytochemical staining The best fixative for the preservation of cellular morphology is GA (Sabatini et al., 1964; Hayat, 1970). Unfortunately, GA has several drawbacks in EIH: extensive cross-linking reduces permeability, denatures proteins or changes their immunological properties (Habeeb and Hiramoto, 1968) and introduces reactive groups which may enhance background staining. Reactive groups may be blocked by treatment with 50 mM NH_4Cl before the application of the immunohistochemical reagents. Because of its superiority, it is useful to test GA first for a new antigen. Satisfactory fixation can often be obtained with as little as 0.125% GA in 5% sucrose at room temperature for 3 h. GA can also be used in conjunction with other cross-linkers, such as EDC (Section 7.1.9.2.3; Willingham et al., 1978).

FA does not cross-link as extensively as GA. Though structure preservation with FA is inferior to that obtained with GA, it has the advantages of improved penetration of the immunoreactants, generally good retention of antigenicity and its compatibility with other fixatives. A combination which can be used with reasonably good results is FA and picric acid (Stefanini et al., 1967). Singer (1974) investigated several combinations of GA and FA for the detection of H-1 virus antigens. Fixative concentrations which are sub-optimal separately, were adequate in combination and 4% FA and 0.25% GA gave acceptable results for H-1 virus.

McLean and Nakane (1974) developed another fixative based on FA and containing $NaIO_4$ and lysine (PLP: periodate-lysine-paraformaldehyde). $NaIO_4$ oxidizes carbohydrates to create aldehyde groups which are then interconnected by the lysine through Schiff's bases. PLP offers the advantage that it also cross-links carbohydrates, reducing thus the need for extensive cross-linking of proteins.

OsO_4 sharply decreases antigenicity and is not considered suitable as prefixative, though Baskin et al. (1979) employed it successfully for some hormones.

The preparation of the most frequently used fixatives for ultrastructural EIH are given in Table 17.9.

TABLE 17.9

Fixatives used in ultrastructural enzyme immunohistochemistry

A. *Glutaraldehyde*
–   Biological grade GA (25–50%) or 'pure' GA (8%) is diluted to the desired concentration just before use. Storage at room temperature or at neutral or alkaline pH should be avoided. The important properties of this reagent are discussed in Section 11.2.3.1.1.

B. *Formaldehyde–picric acid* (Stefanini et al., 1967)
–   Paraformaldehyde (20 g) is added to 150 ml double-filtered saturated aqueous picric acid solution.

–   Paraformaldehyde is depolymerized by heating this solution to 60 °C and the subsequent addition of a few drops of 200 mM NaOH until clearing of the solution.

–   After cooling and filtration, the solution is diluted to 1 l and the pH brought to 7.3 by the addition of 100 mM phosphate buffer (final osmolarity; 900 mosM). This fixative is stable for 1 year at room temperature.

C. *Periodate–lysine–paraformaldehyde*
Two stock solutions are prepared, one with lysine (solution A) and one with formaldehyde (solution B).

Solution A (stable for 1 week at 4 °C):
        L-Lysine is added to distilled water (1.83 g/50 ml) and the pH adjusted to 7.4 with 100 mM Na_2HPO_4. This solution is diluted to 100 ml with 100 mM sodium phosphate buffer.

Solution B:
        8% formaldehyde is prepared from paraformaldehyde in distilled water.

PLP fixative:
        Three parts of solution A are mixed with one part of solution B just before use and 214 mg $NaIO_4$ are added to 100 ml of fixative. (The final composition of the fixative is 75 mM lysine, 2% FA, 100 mM $NaIO_4$ in 37.5 mM sodium phosphate, pH 6.2, with an osmolarity of about 700 mosM). At this pH, FA reacts slowly (Section 17.3.1).

D. *Saponin–glutaraldehyde–formaldehyde* (Bohn, 1980)
–   1.   GA and FA solutions are prepared separately at a concentration of 8% and 4%, respectively.

–   2.   Sodium phosphate buffer, 300 mM, pH 7.3, is prepared.

– 3. Same phosphate buffer with 75 mg saponin (Merck 7695, Darmstadt, F.R.G.) per 100 ml is prepared.

Preparation of fixatives:

Fixative I is prepared with 10 ml of a solution 3 and with 0.2 ml of the GA and 3.75 ml of the FA solutions, completed with 1.05 ml distilled water.

Fixative II is prepared by adding the same amounts of GA, FA and water to 10 ml of buffer 2. The final concentration of GA can be changed from 0.0125% to 0.05%.

17.4.2.2. Methods of prefixation   Different approaches are used for tissue fragments, cell monolayers (cell culture) or cell suspensions. For the latter, the cells may be kept in suspension throughout and centrifuged after each step. The last pellet is then embedded directly for ultramicrotomy. In another method the suspended cells are fixed, adsorbed on a solid phase (slide, filter) and then treated as a cell monolayer. For this purpose, clean glass microscope slides are immersed and rinsed for several minutes in 70% ethanol containing 1% HCl. The slides are then dipped in acetone and air-dried.

Cells are often adsorbed on slides coated with ovalbumine or poly-L-lysine (Farr and Nakane, 1981). The ovalbumine solution is prepared by mixing one egg white with 1 ml of concentrated NH_4OH and 500 ml distilled water, stirring for 10 min and filtering through several layers of gauze. The clean slides are placed for 1 min in this solution, excess is drained off and the slides are air-dried at room temperature (if relative humidity is low) or at higher temperatures (up to 60°C) for 2–18 h. These slides can be stored indefinitely.

A cytocentrifuge is used to deposit poly-L-lysine (Sigma; 50 μl of a 0.1% solution in water) on the slide, followed by 10^5 fixed cells (10^6 cells/ml in PBS containing 10% sucrose) with a brief (10–15 sec) high-speed centrifugation. The slides are then quickly transferred to a PBS- sucrose bath. Lysine imparts a positive charge to the slide, so that negatively charged cells (or tissues) are attracted.

Fixed tissue fragments are usually chopped with a semi-automatic tissue sectioning system (e.g., the vibratome) or with a razor blade into sections of about 20–50 μm. The sections are stained and washed in clean test tubes in the same way as sections adsorbed to slides. After dehydration, the sections are oriented on a clean slide and embedded.

The following method (Bohn, 1978, 1980) is particularly suitable for monolayer cells. Fixation with FA (1%) and 0.0125% GA gives poor penetration of sera, even after 18 h of incubation. Saponin enhances penetration, and thus the detection of intracellular antigens whereas pretreatment with saponin is unsatisfactory for the preservation of morphology. Several combinations of GA and saponin were investigated at constant FA concentrations. Best results were obtained with the mixture given in Table 17.9D and Table 17.10.

TABLE 17.10

Some methods of prefixation

Selected methods are presented for different tissues. However, it is possible to interchange these procedures.

A. *Saponin–glutaraldehyde–formaldehyde* (for cell monolayers)
Intracellular antigens:
    Monolayers are briefly rinsed with 200 mM phosphate buffer, pH 7.3, pretreated with fixative I (Table 17.9D) for 5 min at 4°C and briefly rinsed with buffer. The cells are then fixed with fixative II (Table 17.9D) for 45 min at 4°C, rinsed for 30 min at 4°C and incubated with albumin or normal serum in phosphate buffer for 1 h at 4°C.

Membrane-associated antigens:
    Monolayers are rinsed with phosphate buffer, fixed with fixative II (Table 17.9D) for 45 min at 4°C, rinsed with buffer and incubated with albumin or normal serum as for intracellular antigens.

B. *PLP method* (for small tissue fragments)
    Small pieces of tissues are fixed in PLP for 4 h at 4°C on a rotatory shaker, washed overnight at 4°C in 100 mM phosphate buffer, pH 7.4, containing 10% sucrose, followed by several washings: 15% sucrose in buffer (overnight at 4°C), 20% sucrose in buffer (4 h at 4°C), 20% sucrose plus 20% glycerol (1 h at 4°C). The pieces are embedded in OCT medium (Miles), in a small cup of heavy aluminum foil, by snap-freezing in ethanol–dry ice bath while avoiding contact between ethanol and OCT. Frozen sections are cut, 6–12 μm thick, mounted on albuminized slides and washed 3 times 10 min with PBS–10% sucrose.

C. *Glutaraldehyde–paraformaldehyde perfusion* (for large tissue fragments)
Method described by Pickel et al. (1976) to obtain fixed tissues from rodents for light and electron microscopy.

1. Anesthesize animal with pentobarbital (50 mg/kg).

2. Perfuse the animal for 15 min through the ascending aorta with either 4% paraformaldehyde (*p*-FA) in 100 mM phosphate buffer, pH 7.2 (for light microscopy) or with 1% GA and 1% *p*-FA in 100 mM sodium cacodylate buffer, pH 7.15 (for electron microscopy). Heat fixative to 40 °C before use.

3. For light microscopy: remove tissue to be investigated and post-fix for 6 h in picric acid-formalin, prepared as described in Table 17.9B. The post-fixed tissue is washed overnight with 10 mM phosphate buffer, pH 7.1 and embedded in paraffin or polyethylene glycol (Mazurkiewicz and Nakane, 1972). The tissue is sectioned on a microtome.

4. For electron microscopy: prepare sections (thickness 20 μm) on a vibration microtome while fragments are immersed in cacodylate buffer. At this stage Pickel et al. incubated the sections with 0.2% Triton X-100 for 30 min to improve specific detection.

D. *Glutaraldehyde–borohydride–saponin* (procedure of Willingham (1983) for cells)
1. Wash cells in PBS.

2. Fix cells for 15 min in 0.4% GA in 80% PBS at room temperature.

3. Wash again with PBS.

4. Treat the cells for 5 min with freshly prepared (0.5 mg/ml) $NaBH_4$ in PBS at room temperature.

5. Wash 5 times with PBS.

6. Incubate the cells in 0.1% saponin – 4 mg/ml normal goat globulin – 1 mM EGTA/PBS for at least 30 min at room temperature.

7. Wash the cells in 0.1% saponin–PBS.

8. Proceed with steps for immunohistochemistry (dilutions made in the solution of step 6).

The PLP method (McLean and Nakane, 1974; Farr and Nakane, 1981) is suitable for tissue fragments (Table 17.10B). PLP in the first step may be replaced by other fixatives, depending on the nature of the antigen.

The method of Pickel et al. (1976) is simple for large tissue fragments if the antigen withstands fixation. Organs or animals are perfused with a warm mixture of 1% GA and 1% paraformaldehyde in 100 mM sodium cacodylate buffer, pH 7.15. Microtome sections are pretreated with Triton X-100, normal serum and hypertonic buffer prior to immunostaining.

17.4.2.3. Immunocytochemical incubations, postfixation and embedding
        Prefixed cells are thoroughly washed; all incubation and washing steps are similar to those used for the detection of antigens by light microscopy (Section 17.3.2). However, the lengths of the incubation periods depend on the site of the target, the penetrability of the cells and the size of the conjugates. Doubling or tripling these periods is reasonable in preliminary experiments with large complexes, such as PAP, or for cells prefixed with GA-containing fixatives. Shortening of the incubation time and better penetration can be achieved with Fab-MPOase conjugate (Section 10.3.1).

POase or MPOase in combination with DAB as the H-donor is used almost universally for ultrastructural EIH. POase activity is hardly affected by GA. After completion of the immune reactions in the tissue and sufficient washing (sluggishly entering Ig also leaves sluggishly), but prior to the enzyme revelation, sections are incubated in a solution of 2% GA in PBS–10% sucrose for 30 min at 4°C to prevent further deterioration of the morphology and to stabilize immune complexes. The latter is particularly important if the pH of the substrate solution is far from neutrality (e.g., for MPOase: pH 10.5) which otherwise dissociates immune complexes. FA fixation is reversible to a certain limit (Section 17.3.1) and may act as a temporary stabilizer during immunocytochemical incubations, whereas fixation with GA is permanent. It is possible to improve preservation of morphology by an incubation, after fixation with 2% GA and washing, with 1% gelatin in 100 mM phosphate buffer, pH 7.4, for 15 min at room temperature. The section is then rapidly air-dried, again fixed with 2% GA in PBS–10% sucrose for 10 min and washed three times in PBS–10% sucrose, 10 min each.

For the revelation of POase activity, sections are first soaked for 30 min with DAB (0.05% in 50 mM Tris–HCl buffer, pH 7.6, containing 0.9% NaCl and 10% sucrose), followed by H_2O_2 (0.003–0.01%, see Section 17.3.3.1) in the same medium for 2–10 min at room temperature. The reaction is stopped by three washings for 10 min with PBS–10% sucrose.

The oxidized product of DAB is not visible by electron microscopy unless rendered electron dense with OsO_4 (the reaction product is very osmiophilic). This postfixation is carried out with 2% OsO_4 for 30 min or with 1% (Millonig's solution) for 1 h. The preparation is washed again with three baths of PBS–10% sucrose (10 min each) prior to embedding.

The specimen is dehydrated through a graded series of ethanol to 100% (10 min per bath), infiltrated by the resin, covered with a capsule of embedding resin and polymerized. Resins most frequently used are Araldite (Glauert and Glauert, 1958; Luft, 1961), Epon-Araldite (Abelson et al., 1969; Hayat, 1970), and Epon 812 (Bohn, 1980). Glycol methacrylate, which is extensively used in routine histopathology, has so far been unsatisfactory for pre-embedding immunostaining (Van Noorden and Polak, 1983).

The block with the tissue section is trimmed and ultrathin sections are cut with an ultramicrotome. The enzyme product may be hazardous for diamond knives, so that normal glass knives should be used.

17.4.3. Ultrastructural enzyme immunohistochemistry by post-embedding staining

In these methods antigens are exposed by cutting through organelles and membranes, and are detected on ultrathin sections mounted on grids. However, several problems may arise: (i) initial fixation, dehydration and embedding may all be detrimental for antigenicity; (ii) plastic embedding materials adsorb non-specifically proteins; (iii) epitopes are covered by plastic, which should then be etched or partially removed; and, (iv) staining products spread out more on the surface than intracellularly, giving relatively poor resolution. Nevertheless, many of these problems have been (partially) circumvented and post-embedding methods remain popular.

Samples may be fixed, processed and immunostained by a standard procedure (Table 17.11), but, in case of unsatisfactory results, loss of antigenicity must be suspected. The temperature (heat-cured resin sections) and the composition of the fixative, the dehydration of the sample and the polymerization of the embedding resin may all be the cause.

TABLE 17.11
Immunohistochemical procedures for post-embedding staining

I. *General method*
(All solutions should be filtered; avoid drying of sections)

1. Fix as given in Table 17.10 and embed according to standard method.

2. Cut sections to about 80–60 nm (light gold to silver) and pick up from water on 300 mesh bare gold or nickel grids (copper grids are not suitable since they react with osmium).

3. Etch Araldite- or Epon-embedded sections to expose the antigenic sites. Kuhlmann and Peschke (1982) found a treatment of 1% NaOH in 50% ethanol for 10 min easier to handle or more beneficial than sodium ethoxide or peroxide treatments. The sections are then 'jet washed' by a spray of PBS from a plastic spray bottle and blotted by holding the grid edgewise on filter paper.

4. Incubate section with normal serum, diluted 1:30 with isotonic Tris–HCl buffer, pH 7.6, for 5 min (on drops on a wax or Parafilm strip). Drain and blot excess but do not wash. Tween 20 in subsequent solutions (p. 461, 476, 486) is sometimes beneficial.

5. Incubate with diluted ($>1000\times$) antiserum for 48 h at 4°C in a humid chamber (wet sponge on bottom and covered) and re-equilibrate for 2 h to room temperature (rest of procedure at room temperature). Wash for 10 min in PBS and for 5 min in 1:30 normal serum.

6. Follow one of the procedures of Table 17.11, II.

7. For staining, place the grids in a Hiraoka supporting plate (Polysciences), which is suspended with a paper clamp in the stirred substrate solution.
   Substrate (DAB or CN; both in 50 mM Tris–HCl, pH 7.6):
   DAB: 0.0125% DAB and 0.0025% H_2O_2 for 3–5 min. Solution is freshly prepared and filtered (0.2 μm pore size) before use.
   CN: 16 mg/ml is dissolved in 0.25 ml 95% ethanol and added to 100 ml of buffer. Reaction is initiated by adding 0.02% H_2O_2 while stirring for 1 min.

8. Rinse grids first in Tris buffer and then in 2 baths of PBS (30 sec each) and dip in water.

9. Float grids on a 2% solution of aqueous OsO_4 for 10–15 min, wash again in water and allow to dry. Examine with microscope.

II. *Unlabeled variants of immunocytochemical steps* (for step 6 of section I)

A. Single-bridge method (Mason et al., 1969)

   1. Incubate with anti-Ig antiserum (1:100 in PBS plus 1% normal serum) for 10 min and rinse by dipping in three baths of PBS

   2. Float grids on 2% normal serum for 5 min.

   3. Incubate sections with anti-POase antibodies (1:100 in PBS plus 1% normal serum) for 10 min, and wash three times with PBS.

   4. Incubate with POase (5 μg/ml in a 0.1% ovalbumin solution) for 10 min and rinse thoroughly in PBS.

B. Double-bridge method (Ordronneau and Petrusz, 1980)

   1. Proceed as in steps 1–3 of the single-bridge method and incubate with 2% normal serum in PBS (5 min).

   2. Repeat steps 1–3 of the single-bridge method.

   3. Incubate with POase as in step 4 of the single-bridge method.

C. Single-PAP method (Sternberger et al., 1970)

   1. Incubate as in steps 1–2 of the single-bridge method.

   2. Incubate with PAP, diluted with PBS to about 65 μg anti-POase/ml, for 5 min and rinse thoroughly with PBS. If PAP preparations are less active, an incubation with POase as in the single-bridge method can be included.

D. Double-PAP method (Vacca et al., 1975)

    1. Proceed as in the single-PAP method step 1 and 2, and place grids for 5 min on 1:30 diluted normal serum.

    2. Repeat steps 1 and 2 of the single-PAP method.

Similarly to pre-embedding methods, relatively mild fixatives are necessary to preserve antigenicity. Some antigens (e.g. Ig) could not be localized with the PAP method by post-embedding staining (Sternberger, 1979). In most post-embedding methods, samples are fixed by the conventional aldehyde method followed by dehydration and embedding in Araldite or Epon, according to standard procedures. Rodning et al. (1978) and Coulter and Terracio (1977) obtained much better preservation of antigenicity by freeze-drying of the tissue and fixation in water-free medium. Thin slices of tissue are quickly frozen through direct contact with a polished copper bar at the temperature of liquid nitrogen. The sample is then transferred to a Cooper specimen block, removal of water monitored with a partial pressure analyzer and the temperature raised at a rate of 10°C/h. Tissue devoid of water is apparently more resistant to further denaturation than hydrated tissue (Sternberger, 1979). The dried tissue is then fixed with FA vapor and embedded directly into Spurr's low-viscosity Epon by infiltration in vacuo. The blocks can be used for thick (2 μm) or semi-thick (0.1–1 μm) sectioning for light microscopy or for thin sectioning (<0.1 μm) for electron microscopy. The possibility to investigate the same tissue by both light and electron microscopy is particularly convenient if antigens are sparsely distributed. However, embedded tissue should be freed from plastic after the sectioning to allow detection of antigens by light microscopy. The sections are mounted on slides, e.g. by heat (90°C for 30 min) and the resin is removed with sodium methoxide (Mayor et al., 1961). This section is then investigated by light microscopy, whereas the adjacent section is stained for electron microscopy (Table 17.11).

Early experiments with post-embedding revealed that plastic adsorbs immunoreactants giving rise to high background staining. Hydrophobic embedding media, such as Araldite, Epon 812 and Spurr's low-viscosity Epon, seem to have a somewhat lesser, but still significant capacity to adsorb proteins than glycol methacrylate. Incubation with protein prevents the adsorption of subsequently applied PAP complexes, indicating a saturation of the non-specific adsorption sites. Therefore, post-embedding EIH should be preceded by incubation with normal serum from the same species (if possible pre-immunization sera). Hypertonic buffers with detergents may also reduce or eliminate non-specific staining (Pickel et al., 1979; Grube, 1980).

Glycol methacrylate (Leduc and Bernhard, 1967), which may be used with the modifications suggested by Spaur and Moriarty (1977), has the advantage that etching is not always necessary. H_2O_2 can be used for etching and seems also to swell the plastic, thus increasing accessibility (suitable for Epon and Araldite; Moriarty and Halmi, 1972). Kuhlman and Peschke (1982) obtained superior results with 1% NaOH in 50% ethanol (10 min) for Epon 812 over peroxide or ethoxide treatments.

Ultrathin sections are picked up on bare nickel or gold grids (copper reacts with OsO_4) and incubated, section down, on a drop of antiserum (e.g., on Parafilm or in a microtitre plate) and washed in multiple grid holders. Dilutions of antisera and incubations are as for light microscopy. The primary antibodies, however, are usually incubated for prolonged periods (up to 48 h) at higher dilutions.

Potential toxic hazards associated with enzyme immunoassays

Comparisons of RIA and EIA generally stress the radiological hazards of RIA without mentioning possible health hazards of EIA. Stochastic and non-stochastic effects on health can be distinguished (Gosling, 1980). Non-stochastic effects are of short-term, giving irritation, dizziness, aches, etc., whereas stochastic effects are often long-term, e.g. contact dermatitis, delayed hypersensitivity, induction of malignancies. Stochastic effects may also induce short-term effects, though this is rare. Laboratory workers are generally not sufficiently aware of stochastic effects due to EIA and tend to have a more superficial attitude towards safety than those using RIA.

18.1. Hazards associated with the preparation of reagents

The potential hazards associated with conjugation of proteins are important, even though labeling is performed infrequently due to the long shelf-lives of conjugates. Because of the cross-linking ability of many of the reagents involved, direct contact with these reagents should be carefully avoided and they should always be pipetted with safety bulbs. The preparation of stock solutions is particularly hazardous. Many of the reagents may constitute serious ecological risks, therefore, incineration is often the best method to dispose of hazardous organic compounds. An annual edition of the *Registry of Toxic Effects of Chemical Substances* is available from the Superintendent of Documents, US Government Printing Office, Washington D.C. 20402. The studies involved are accessible via the USA National Institute for Occupational Safety and Health Registry of Toxic Effects of Chemical Substances. All chemicals may be hazardous in particular circumstances, but are not necessarily so in laboratory conditions.

Borohydrides, frequently used in the conjugation of enzymes to stabilize Schiff's bases, should be handled only by those familiar with the properties and potential dangers of these chemicals. Borohydrides should be stored dry at room temperature in a well-ventilated area, since in contact with moist air or water they produce flammable hydrogen gas which may cause vigorous reactions with strong acids or salt solutions of transition metals. Personnel handling borohydrides should wear rubber gloves with sleeves inside the gloves and lab coats should not be made of nylon. Moreover, eyes should be protected with safety glasses. Spills should be immediately covered with anhydrous CaO or dry sand. For obvious reasons this should not be disposed of in an incinerator, but should be placed in a metal bucket and air-hydrolyzed at a safe location outdoors.

18.2. Hazards associated with the performance of enzyme immunoassays

In most EIA chromogens are used which produce signals measurable with a spectrophotometer or special colorimeter. Many of these chromogens have stochastic or non-stochastic effects. Table 18.1 compares several of the substrates most often employed in EIA and their resulting products. Many of these substrates are quite fluffy and easily produce a solid aerosol. o-NP is less toxic than p-NP and may be used at lower concentrations (Exley and Abuknesha, 1978).

Many of the H-donors for POase may also be dangerous, e.g., ODA and DAB. The use of the latter has even been prohibited in some countries. ABTS is a fluffy product the safety of which

TABLE 18.1
Toxicity of frequently used substrates for enzyme immunoassays

Chemical	Role	Enzyme	Known toxic effects
p-Nitrophenyl phosphate	substrate	APase	none
p-Nitrophenyl-β-D--galactose	substrate	BGase	none
p-Nitrophenol	product	APase, BGase	irritant
o-Nitrophenyl-β-D--galactose	substrate	BGase	none
o-Nitrophenol	product	BGase	irritant
H_2O_2	substrate	POase	irritant
o-Dianisidine	H-donor	GOase, POase	irritant, carcinogen
m-Phenylenediamine	H-donor	GOase, POase	carcinogen
ABTS	H-donor	GOase, POase	mutagen
5-AS	H-donor	POase	none
OPD	H-donor	POase	irritant (eyes) mutagenic
DAB	H-donor	POase	irritant, carcinogen(?)
DMAB/MBTH	H-donor	POase	none
Phenazine methosulfate	H-donor	MDase	irritant, carcinogen

is regularly claimed in the literature, but it can induce both base-pair substitutions and frame-shift mutations (Voogd et al., 1980). However, ABTS has about 100 times lower mutagenic activity on *Klebsiella pneumoniae*, at about 100 times higher concentrations than needed in EIA, than on *Salmonella typhimurium* TA 98.

OPD appears less toxic than *m*-phenylenediamine. Most of these compounds are able to induce contact dermatitis and become, like the cross-linking agents, attached to skin proteins, producing extensive immune reactions (delayed-type hypersensitivity), sometimes all over the body. OPD also exerts a mutagenic action at very low concentrations (200 times less than used in EIA; Voogd et al., 1980), confirming earlier reports by Ames et al. (1975a) and Venitt and Searle (1976). *p*- and *m*-phenylenediamine are positive in the Ames screening test for carcinogens (Hanlon, 1978), but surprisingly, they are still used in hair dyes in some countries (Gosling, 1980).

The widely used 5-AS has apparently no serious toxic effects though it has been listed as a toxin in the above-mentioned Registry (Section 18.1).

Voogd et al. (1980) observed an increase in the mutation rate with umbelliferone but not with methylumbelliferone.

References

Abelson, H.T., Smith, G.H., Hoffman, H.A. and Rowe, W.P. (1969) J. Natl. Cancer Inst. *42*, 497.

Abaturov, L.V., Nezlin, R.S., Vengerova, T.I. and Varshavsky, Ja. M. (1969) Biochim. Biophys. Acta *194*, 386.

Abraham, G.E., Swerdloff, R., Tulchinksky, D. and Odell, W.D. (1971) J. Clin. Endocrin. Metab. *32*, 619.

Ackerman, S.B. and Kelley, E.A. (1983) J. Clin. Microbiol. *17*, 410.

Adachi, H., Fukuda, T., Funahashi, S., Kurahori, T. and Ishikawa, E. (1978) Vox Sang. *35*, 219.

Adair, S.W. (1982) Anal. Biochem. *125*, 299.

Adams, R.P.L. (1980) Cell culture for biochemists. In: Laboratory Techniques in Biochemistry and Molecular Biology (T.S. Work and E. Work, eds.), vol. 9, Elsevier/North-Holland Biomedical Press, Amsterdam.

Adams, J.C. (1981) J. Histochem. Cytochem. *29*, 775.

Adams, T.H. and Wisdom, G.B. (1979) Biochem. Soc. Trans. *7*, 55.

Adams, E.C., Jr., Mast, R.L. and Free, A.H. (1960) Arch. Biochem. Biophys. *91*, 230.

Africa, B. and Haber, E. (1971) Immunochemistry *8*, 479.

Agrawal, B.B.L. and Goldstein, I.J. (1967) Biochim. Biophys. Acta *147*, 262.

Al-Bassam, M.N., O'Sullivan, M.J., Gnemmi, E., Bridges, J.W. and Marks, V. (1978) Clin. Chem. *24*, 1590.

Albert, W.H.W., Kleinhammer, G., Linke, R., Transwell, P. and Staehler, F. (1978) In: Enzyme-linked Immunoassay of Hormones and Drugs (S.B. Pal, ed.) p. 153. Walter de Gruyter Berlin.

Alberty, R.A. (1953) J. Am. Chem. Soc. *75*, 1928.

Alderton, G. and Fevold, H.L. (1946) J. Biol. Chem. *164*, 1.

Al-Kaissi, E. and Mostratos, A. (1983) J. Immunol. Methods *58*, 127.

Altschuh, D. and Van Regenmortel, M.H.V. (1982) J. Immunol. Methods *50*, 99.

Alwine, J.C., Kemp, D.J. and Stark, G.R. (1977) Proc. Natl. Acad. Sci. USA *74*, 5350.

Alwine, J.C., Kemp, D.J., Parker, B.A., Reiser, J., Renart, J., Stark, G.R. and Wahl, G.M. (1979) Methods Enzymol. *68*, 220.

Amerding, D. and Katz, D.H. (1974) J. Exptl. Med. *140*, 19.

Ames, B.N., Kammen, H.O. and Yamasaki, E. (1975) Proc. Natl. Acad. Sci. USA *72*, 2423.

Amzel, L.M., Poljak, R.J., Saul, F., Varga, J.M. and Richards, F.F. (1974) Proc. Natl. Acad. Sci. USA *71*, 1427.

Anderer, F.A. and Schlumberger, H.D. (1966) Biochim. Biophys. Acta *115*, 222.

Anderson, M.J. (1978) Med. Lab. Sci. *35*, 173.

Anderson, W.L. and Wetlaufer, D.B. (1975) Anal. Biochem. *67*, 493.

Anderson, N.L., Nance, S.L., Pearson, T.W. and Anderson, N.G. (1982) Electrophoresis *3*, 135.

Andersson, J. and Melchers, F. (1978) Curr. Top. Microbiol. Immunol. *81*, 130.

Andersson, J., Coutinho, A., Lenhardt, W. and Melchers, F. (1977) Cell *10*, 27.

Andersson, K.K., Benyamin, Y., Douzou, P. and Balny, C. (1979) J. Immunol. Methods *25*, 375.

Archer, P.G. (1976) Biometrics *32*, 369.

Arends, J. (1981) Methods Enzymol. *73*, 166.

Armitage P. (1971) Statistical Methods in Medical Research. 504 pp.. John Wiley and Sons, Inc., New York.

Arvidson, S., Holme, T. and Wadström, T. (1970) J. Bacteriol. *104*, 227.

Arvidson, S., Holme, T. and Wadström, T. (1971) Acta Pathol. Microbiol. Scand. Section B *79*, 399.

Atkins, G.L. and Nimmo, I.A. (1980) Anal. Biochem. *104*, 1.

Atkinson, D.E. (1966) Ann. Rev. Biochem. *35*, 85.

Aubertin, A.M., Tandre, L., Lopez, C., Obert, G. and Kirn, A. (1983) Anal. Biochem. *131*, 127.

Avrameas, S. (1969) Immunochemistry *6*, 43.

Avrameas, S. and Lespinats, G. (1967) Compt. Rend. Acad. Sci., Paris *265*, 1149.

Avrameas, S. and Ternynck, T. (1969) Immunochemistry *6*, 53.

Avrameas, S. and Ternynck, T. (1971) Immunochemistry *8*, 1175.

Avrameas, S. and Uriel, J. (1966) Compt. Rend. Acad. Sci., Paris *262*, 2543.

Avrameas, S., Ternynck, T. and Guesdon, J.-L. (1978) Scand. J. Immunol. *8* (suppl. 7), 7.

Axén, R., Porath, J. and Ernback, S. (1967) Nature *214*, 1302.

Bach, F.H., Bach, M.L. and Sondel, P.M. (1976) Nature *259*, 273.

Bacquet, C. and Twumasi, D. (1984) Anal. Biochem. *136*, 487.

Bailey, J.M. and Butler, J. (1967) In: The Reticuloendothelial System and Artherosclerosis (N.R. Diluzio and R. Paoletti, eds.) p. 433. Plenum, New York.

Baker, R.M., Brunette, B.M., Mankowitz, R., Thompson, L.H., Whitmore, G.F., Siminovitch, L. and Till, J.E. (1974) Cell *1*, 9.

Bale, J.R., Huang, C.Y. and Chock, P.B. (1980) J. Biol. Chem. *255*, 8431.

Banaszak, L.J. and Bradshaw, R.A. (1975) In: The Enzymes (P.D. Boyer, ed.) vol. 11. p. 369. Academic Press, New York.

Barbara, D.J. and Clark, M.F. (1982) J. Gen. Virol. *58*, 315.

Bar-Joseph, M. and Malkinson, M. (1980) J. Virol. Methods *1*, 179.

Barlough, J.E., Jacobson, R.H., Downing, D.R., Marcella, K.L., Lynch, T.J. and

Scott, F.W. (1983) J. Clin. Microbiol. *17*, 202.

Barnstable, C.J., Bodmer, W.F., Brown, G., Galfre, G., Milstein, C., Williams, A.F. and Ziegler, A. (1978) Cell *14*, 9.

Barrett, M.J. (1977) US patent 4,001,583.

Bartos, F., Dolney, A.M., Grettie, D.P. and Campbell, R.A. (1978) Res. Commun. Chem. Pathol. Pharmacol. *19*, 295.

Baskin, D.G., Erlandsen, S.L. and Parsons, J.A. (1979) J. Histochem. Cytochem. *27*, 867.

Bastiani, R.J., Phillips, R.C., Schneider, R.S. and Ullman, E.F. (1973) Am. J. Med. Techn. *39*, 211.

Batteiger, B., Newhall V, W.J. and Jones, R.B. (1982) J. Immunol. Methods *55*, 297.

Batty, I. (1977) In: Techniques in Clinical Immunology (R.A. Thompson, ed.) ch. 11. Blackwell Scientific Publications, Oxford.

Batty, I. and Torrigani, G. (1980) In: Manual of Clinical Immunology (N.R. Rose and H. Friedman, eds.) p. 1083. American Society of Microbiology. Washington DC.

Baumstark, J.S., Laffin, R.J. and Bardawil, W.A. (1964) Arch. Biochem. Biophys. *108*, 514.

Bayer, E. and Wilchek, M. (1974) Methods Enzymol. *34*, 265.

Bayer, E.A. and Wilchek, M. (1980) Methods Biochem. Anal. *26*, 1.

Bazin, H., Beckers, A. and Querinjean, P. (1974) Eur. J. Immunol. *4*, 44.

Beards, G.M., Campbell, A.D., Cottrell, N.R., Peiris J.S.M., Rees, N., Sanders, R.C., Shirley, J.A., Wood, H.C. and Flewett, T.H. (1984) J. Clin. Microbiol. *19*, 248.

Becker, V.E. and Evans, H.J. (1969) Biochim. Biophys. Acta *191*, 95.

Becker, J.W., Reeke, G.N., Jr. and Edelman, G.M. (1971) J. Biol. Chem. *246*, 6123.

Beckett, G.J., Hunter, W.M. and Percy-Robb, I.W. (1978) Clin. Chim. Acta *88*, 257.

Belanger, L., Hamel, D., Dufour, D. and Pouliot, M. (1976) Clin. Chem. *22*, 198.

Benacerraf, B. and Unanue, R. (1981) Textbook of Immunology. 292 pp. Williams and Wilkins, London.

Benacerraf, B. and Germain, R.N. (1978) Immunol. Rev. *38*, 70.

Benedict, A.A. and Yamaga, K. (1976) In: Comparative Immunology (J.J. Marchalonis, ed.) p. 335. John Wiley and Sons, Inc., New York.

Bentley, R. (1963) In: The Enzymes (P.D. Boyer, H.L. Lardy and H. Myrbäck, eds.) vol. 7, p. 567. Academic Press, New York.

Bergmeyer, H.-U. (1955) Biochem. Z. *327*, 255.

Bergmeyer, H.-U. (ed.) (1974) Methods of Enzymatic Analysis. Vol. 1–4. Academic Press, New York.

Bergmeyer, H.-U., Gawehn, K. and Grassl, M. (1974) In: Methods of Enzymatic Analysis (H.U. Bergmeyer, ed.) p. 457. Academic Press, New York.

Berkowitz, D.B. and Webert, D.W. (1981) J. Immunol. Methods *47*, 121.

Berkson, J. (1944) J. Amer. Statist. Ass. *41*, 70.

Berlin, B.S. and McKinney, R.W. (1958) J. Lab. Clin. Med. *52*, 657.

Berod, A., Hartman, B.K. and Pujol, J.F. (1981) J. Histochem. Cytochem. *29*, 844.

Berzofsky, J.A. and Schechter, A.N. (1981) Mol. Immunol. *18*, 751.

Beutner, E.H., Holborow, E.J. and Johnson, G.D. (1965) Nature *208*, 353.

Bigbee, J.W., Kosek, J.C. and Eng, L.F. (1977) J. Histochem. Cytochem. *25*, 443.

Billingham, R.E., Brent, L. and Medawar, P.B. (1953) Nature *172*, 603.

Biocca, S., Calissano, P., Barra, D. and Fasella, P.M. (1978) Anal. Biochem. *87*, 334.

Birkmeyer, R.C.,, Keyes, L.L. and Tan-Wilson, A.L. (1981) J. Immunol. Methods *44*, 271.

Birkmeyer, R.C., Dewey, T.K. and Tan-Wilson, A.L. (1982) J. Immunol. Methods *49*, 141.

Bittiger, H. and Schnebli, H.P. (1976) Concanavalin A as a Tool. 639 pp. John Wiley and Sons, Chichester, New York.

Bittner, M., Kupferer, P. and Morris, C.F. (1980) Anal. Biochem. *102*, 459.

Björk, I., Petersson, B.-A. and Sjöquist, J. (1972) Eur. J. Biochem. *29*, 579.

Blaedel, W.J. and Olson, C. (1964) Anal. Chem. *36*, 343.

Blake, C.C.F., Johnson, L.N., Mair, G.A., North, A.C.T., Phillips, D.C., and Sarma, V.R. (1967) Proc. Roy. Soc. B *167*, 378.

Blakeley, R.L., Webb, E.C. and Zerner, B. (1969) Biochemistry *8*, 1984.

Blattner, F.R. and Tucker, P.W. (1984) Nature *307*, 417.

Bleile, D.M., Schulz, R.A., Harrison, J.H. and Gregory, E.M. (1977) J. Biol. Chem. *252*, 755.

Blomberg, F., Cohen, R.S. and Siekewitz, P. (1977) J. Cell Biol. *74*, 204.

Blonde, D.J., Kresack, E.J. and Kosicki, G.W. (1967) Can. J. Biochem. *45*, 641.

Bodanszky, M. and Fagan, D.T. (1977) J. Amer. Chem. Soc. *99*, 235.

Böhme, H.-J., Kopperschläger, G., Schulz, J. and Hofmann, E. (1972) J. Chrom. *69*, 209.

Bohn, W. (1978) J. Histochem. Cytochem. *26*, 293.

Bohn, W. (1980) J. Gen. Virol. *46*, 439.

Boiteux, J.L., Lemay, C., Desmet, G. and Thomas, D. (1981) Clin. Chim. Acta *113*, 175.

Boorsma, D.M. and Kalsbeek, G.L. (1975) J. Histochem. Cytochem. *23*, 200.

Boorsma, D.M. and Streefkerk, J.G. (1976) J. Histochem. Cytochem. *24*, 481.

Borek, F. (1977) In: The Antigens (M. Sela, ed.). vol. 4. p. 369. Academic Press, New York.

Borgers, M. (1973) J. Histochem. Cytochem. *21*, 812.

Borrebaeck, C., Mattiasson, B. and Svensson, K. (1978) In: Enzyme-immunoassay of Hormones and Drugs (S.B. Pal, ed.). p. 15. Walter de Gruyter, Berlin.

Bosman, F.T., Cramer-Knynenburg, G. and van Bergen Henegouw, J. (1980) Histochemistry *67*, 243.

Boulard, C. and Lecroisey, A. (1982) J. Immunol. Methods *50*, 221.

Bowen, B., Steinberg, J., Laemmli, U.K. and Weintraub, H. (1980) Nucl. Acids Res. *8*, 1.

Bowes, J.H. and Cater, C.W. (1966) J. Roy. Microsc. Soc. *85*, 193.

Bradwell, A.R., Burnett, D., Ramsden, D.B., Burr, W.A., Prince, H.P., and Hoffenberg, R. (1976) Clin. Chim. Acta *71*, 501.

Brandt, J., Anderson, L.-O., Porath, J. (1975) Biochim. Biophys. Acta *386*, 196.

Brandtzaeg, P. (1976) Clin. Exp. Immunol. *25*, 50.

Brandtzaeg, P. (1982) In: Techniques in Immunochemistry (G.R. Bullock, and P. Petrusz, eds.) vol. 1, p. 1. Academic Press, London.

Braun, D.G., Hild, K. and Ziegler, A. (1979) In: Immunological Methods (I. Lefkovits and B. Pernis, eds.) vol. 1, p. 107. Academic Press, New York.

Brauner, P. and Fridlender, B. (1981) J. Immunol. Methods *42*, 375.

Bretscher, P. and Cohn, M. (1970) Science *169*, 1042.

Brewer, M.E. and Moses, V. (1967) Nature *214*, 272.

Brigati, D., Myerson, D., Leary, J.J., Spalholz, B., Travis, S.Z., Fong, C.K.Y., Hsiung, G.D. and Ward, D.C. (1983) Virology *126*, 32.

Briggs, G.E. and Haldane, J.B.S. (1925) Biochem. J. *19*, 338.

Bright, H.J. and Appleby, M. (1969) J. Biol. Chem. *244*, 3625.

Bright, H.J. and Porter, D.J.T. (1975) In: The Enzymes (P.D. Boyer, ed.) vol. 12. p. 421. Academic Press, New York.

Briles, D.E. and Davie, J.M. (1980) J. Exptl. Med. *152*, 151.

Brodsky, F.M., Parham, P., Barnstable, C.J., Crumpton, M.J. and Bodmer, W.F. (1979) Immunol. Rev. *47*, 3.

Brooks, K.H. and Feldbush, T.L. (1981) J. Immunol. *127*, 963.

Brown, S., Teplitz, M. and Revel, J.-P. (1974) Proc. Natl. Acad. Sci. USA *71*, 464.

Bruck, C., Portetelle, D., Glineur, C. and Bollen, A. (1982) J. Immunol. Methods *53*, 313.

Brunk, S.D., Hadjiioannou, T.P., Hadjiioannou, S.I. and Malmstadt, H.V. (1976) Clin. Chem. *22*, 905.

Bullock, G.R. and Petrusz, P. (eds.) (1982) Techniques in Immunochemistry. Vol. 1, 306 pp.. Academic Press, New York.

Bullock, S.L., and Walls, K.W. (1977) J. Infect. Dis. *136* (Suppl.), S279.

Bulman, A.S. and Heyderman, E. (1981) J. Clin. Pathol. *34*, 1349.

Bundesen, P.G., Drake, R.G., Kelly, K., Worsley, I.G., Friesen, H.G., and Sehon, A.H. (1980) J. Clin. Endocrinol. Metab. *51*, 1472.

Burd, J.F., Carrico, R.J., Fetter, M.C., Buckler, R.T., Johnson, R.D., Boguslaski, R.C. and Christner, J.E. (1977) Anal. Biochem. *77*, 56.

Burnette, W.N. (1981) Anal. Biochem. *112*, 195.

Burridge, K. (1976) Proc. Natl. Acad. Sci. USA *73*, 4457.

Burstone, M.S. (1962) In: Enzyme Histochemistry. p. 267. Academic Press, London.

Burt, S.M., Carter, T.J.N. and Kricka, L.J. (1979) J. Immunol. Methods *31*, 231.

Butler, J.E. (1981) Methods Enzymol. *73*, 482.

Butler, V.P. and Chen, J.P. (1967) Proc. Natl. Acad. Sci. USA *57*, 71.

Butler, V.P., Feldbush, T.L., McGivern, P.L. and Stewart, N. (1978) Immunochemistry *15*, 131.

Butler, J.E., Cantarero, L.A., Swanson, P. and McGivern, P.L. (1980) In: Enzyme-Immunoassay (E.G. Maggio, ed.) p. 197. CRC Press, Boca Raton, FA, USA.

Calcott, M.A. and Müller-Eberhard, H.J. (1972) Biochemistry *11*, 3443.

Calvert, P.D., Nichol, L.W., Sawyer, W.H. (1979) J. Theor. Biol. *80*, 233.

Campbell, G.T. and Bhatnager, A.S. (1976) J. Histochem. Cytochem. *24*, 448.

Canellas, P.F. and Karu, A.E. (1981) J. Immunol. Methods 47, 375.

Canfield, R.E. (1963) J. Biol. Chem. 238, 2691.

Canfield, R.E. and Liu, A.K. (1965) J. Biol. Chem. 240, 1997.

Canfield, R.E., Collins, J.C. and Sobel. J.H. (1974) In: Lysozyme (E.F. Osserman, R.E. Canfield and S. Beychock, eds.) p.63. Academic Press, New York.

Cann, G.M., Zaritsky, A. and Koshland, M.E. (1982) Proc. Natl. Acad. Sci. USA 79, 6656.

Cantarero, L.A., Butler, J.E. and Osborne, J.W. (1980) Anal. Biochem. 105, 375.

Cantor, H. and Boyse, E.A. (1977) Immunol. Rev. 33, 105.

Capra, J.D., Tung, A.S. and Nisonoff, A. (1975) J. Immunol. 114, 1548.

Carlier, Y., Bout, D. and Capron, A. (1979) J. Immunol. Methods 31, 237.

Carr, S., Outch, K. and Russell, J. (1978) Data Pathol. 10, 391.

Carrico, R.J., Christner, J.E., Boguslaski, R.C. and Yeung, K.K., (1976) Anal. Biochem. 72, 271.

Carroll, S.F. and Martinez, R.J. (1979) Infect. Immun. 24, 460.

Carter, R.J. and Boyd, N.D. (1979) J. Immunol. Methods 26, 213.

Caswell, M. and Caplow, M. (1980) Biochemistry 19, 2907.

Cavalli-Sforza, L. (1969) Grundzüge biologisch-medizinischer Statistik. Gustav Fischer, Stuttgart (FGR).

Ceska, M. and Lundkvist, U. (1972) Immunochemistry 9, 1021.

Chance, B. (1949) Arch. Biochem. 22, 224; 24, 11.

Chance, B. (1952) Arch. Biochem. Biophys. 41, 404.

Chance, B. and Maehly, A.C. (1955) Methods Enzymol. 2, 763.

Chandler, H.M. and Hurrell, J.G.R. (1982) Clin. Chim. Acta 121, 225.

Chandler, H.M., Cox, J.C., Healey, K., MacGregor, A., Premier, R.R. and Hurrell, J.G.R. (1982) J. Immunol. Methods 53, 187.

Chang, K.Y. and Carr, C.W. (1971) Biochim. Biophys. Acta 229, 496.

Chang, J.J., Crowl, C.P. and Schneider, R.S. (1975) Clin. Chem. 21, 967.

Chan-Shu, S.A. and Blair, O. (1979) Transfusion 19, 182.

Chen, T.R. (1976) Tissue Cult. Assoc. Man. 3, 229.

Cheng, Y.-C. and Prusoff, W.H. (1973) Biochem. Pharmacol. 22, 3099.

Cheng, W.C. and Talmage, D.W. (1969) J. Immunol. 103, 1385.

Chessum, B.S. and Denmark, J.R. (1978) Lancet (i), 161.

Chrambach, A. and Rodbard, D. (1981) In: Gel Electrophoresis of Proteins: A Practical Approach (B.D. Hames and D. Rickwood, eds.) p.93. IRL Press Ltd., London and Washington DC.

Christensen, P., Johansson, A. and Nielsen, V. (1978) J. Immunol. Methods 23, 33.

Citri, N. (1971) In: The Enzymes (P.D. Boyer, ed.) vol. 4, p.23. Academic Press, New York.

Claiborne, A. and Fridovich, I. (1979a) Biochemistry 18, 2324.

Claiborne, A. and Fridovich, I. (1979b) Biochemistry 18, 2329.

Clarke, J. and Shannon, L.M. (1976) Biochim. Biophys. Acta 427, 428.

Clarke, L., Hitzeman, R. and Carbon, J. (1979) Methods Enzymol. 68, 436.

Clausen, J. (1980) In: Immunochemical Techniques for the Identification and Estimation of Macromolecules. Vol. I pt. III of the series Laboratory Techniques in

Biochemistry and Molecular Biology (T.S. Work and E. Work, eds.). Elsevier Biomedical Press, Amsterdam.

Cleland, W.W. (1963) Biochim. Biophys. Acta *67*, 188.

Cleland, W.W. (1970) In: The Enzymes (P.D. Boyer, ed.) vol. 2. p. 1. Academic Press, New York.

Click, R.E., Benck, L. and Alter, B.J. (1972) Cell. Immunol. *3*, 264.

Clyne, D.H., Norris, S.H., Modesto, R.R., Pesce, A.J. and Pollak, V.E. (1973) J. Histochem. Cytochem. *21*, 233.

Cohen, E. (1974) Ann. New York Acad. Sci. *234*, 1.

Cohn, E.J. and Edsall, J.T. (1943) Proteins, amino acids and peptides. Reinhold, New York.

Cohn, M. and Torriani, A.M. (1952) J. Immunol. *69*, 471.

Collins, C., Hu, M., Crowl, C., Kabakoff, D.S., Singh, P. (1979) Clin. Chem. *25*, 1093.

Comoglio, S. and Celada, F. (1976) J. Immunol. Methods *10*, 161.

Conradie, J.D., Vorster, B.J. and Kirk, R. (1981) J. Immunoassay *2*, 109.

Conradie, J.D., Govender, M. and Visser, L. (1983) J. Immunol. Methods *59*, 289.

Conroy, J.M. and Esen, A. (1984) Anal. Biochem. *137*, 182.

Conway de Macario, E., Macario, A.J.L. and Jovell, R.J. (1983) J. Immunol. Methods *59*, 39.

Cook, R.D. and Wellington, D.G. (1978) Data Handling for Syva EMIT (TM) assays. Syva Company, Palo Alto, Ca.

Cook, C.E., Twine, M.E., Meyers, M., Amerson, E., Kepler, J.A. and Taylor, G.F. (1976) Res. Commun. Chem. Pathol. Pharmacol. *13*, 497.

Coons, A.H. (1961) J. Immunol. *87*, 499.

Córdoba, F. González, C. and Rivera, P. (1966) Biochim. Biophys. Acta *127*, 151.

Corfield, A.P., Parker, T.L. and Schauer, R. (1979) Anal. Biochem. *100*, 221.

Cornish-Bowden, A. (1975) Biochem. J. *149*, 305.

Cornish-Bowden, A. (1979) Fundamentals of Enzyme Kinetics. Butterworths, London.

Costello, S.M., Felix, R.T. and Giese, R.W. (1979) Clin Chem. *25*, 1572.

Coulter, H.D. and Terracio, L. (1977) Anat. Rec. *187*, 477.

Cramer, M. and Braun, D.G. (1974) J. Exptl. Med. *139*, 1513.

Craven, G.R., Steers, E., Jr. and Anfinsen, C.B. (1965) J. Biol. Chem. *240*, 2468.

Cremer, N.E., Cossen, C.K., Hanson, C.V. and Shell, G.R. (1982) J. Clin. Microbiol. *13*, 226.

Croce, C.M., Linnenbach, A., Hall, W., Steplewski, Z. and Koprowski, H. (1980) Nature *288*, 488.

Crook, N.E. and Payne, C.C. (1980) J. Gen. Virol. *46*, 29.

Culling, C.F.A. (1974) Handbook of Histopathological and Histochemical Techniques. 3rd ed. Butterworths, London.

Curran, R.C. and Gregory, J. (1977) Experienta *30*, 1400.

Cursons, R.T.M. (1982) Am. J. Clin. Pathol. *77*, 459.

Curtis, J. and Bourne, F.J. (1971) Biochim. Biophys. Acta *236*, 319.

Czok, R. and Bücher, T. (1961) Adv. Prot. Chem. *15*, 315.

Dales, S., Gomatos, P.J. and Hsu, K.C. (1965) Virology *25*, 193.

D'Alisa, R. and Erlanger, B.F. (1976) J. Immunol. *116*, 1629.

Dalziel, K. (1957) Acta Chem. Scand. *11*, 1706.

Dandliker, W.B., Alonso, R., De Saussure, V.A., Kierszenbaun, F., Levison, S. and Schapiro, H.C. (1967) Biochemistry *6*, 1460.

Danielsson, B., Mattiasson, B. and Mosbach, K. (1979) Pure Appl. Chem. *51*, 1443.

Davies, M.E., Barrett, A.J. and Hembry, R.M. (1978) J. Immunol. Methods *21*, 305.

Davis, B.J. (1964) Ann. New York Ac. Sci. *121*, 404.

Davis, J.M., Pennington, J.E., Kubler, A.-M. and Conscience, J.-F. (1982) J. Immunol. Methods *50*, 161.

Day, E.D. (1972) Advanced Immunochemistry. 477 pp. Williams and Wilkins Co., Baltimore.

Debray, H., Decout, D., Strecker, G., Spik, G. and Montreuil, J. (1981) Eur. J. Biochem. *117*, 41.

Deelder, A.M. and De Water, R. (1981) J. Histochem. Cytochem. *29*, 1273.

Deinhardt, F. and Gust, I.D. (1982) Bull. WHO *60*, 661.

De Jong, P.J. (1983) J. Clin. Microbiol. *17*, 928.

Delacroix, D. and Vaerman, J.P. (1979) Mol. Immunol. *16*, 837.

De la Llosa, P., El Abed, A. and Roy, M. (1980) Can. J. Biochem. *58*, 745.

De Lean, A., Munson, P.J. and Rodbard, D. (1978) Am. J. Physiol. *235* (2) E97.

Delincée, H. (1977) In: Electrofocusing and Isotachophoresis (B.J. Radola and D. Graesslin, eds.) p. 181. Walter de Gruyter, Berlin.

Den Hollander, F.C., Van Weemen, B.K. and Woods, G.F. (1974) Steroids 23, 549.

DeMoss, R.D., Gunsalus, I.C. and Bard, R.C. (1953) J. Bacteriol. *66*, 10.

Denmark, J.R. and Chessum, B.S. (1978) Med. Lab. Sci. *35*, 227.

De Savigny, D. and Voller, A. (1980) J. Immunoassay *1*, 105.

De Savigny, D.H., Voller, A. and Woodruff, A.W. (1979) J. Clin. Pathol. 32, 284.

De Toledo, S.M., Haun, M., Bechara, E.J.H. and Durán, N. (1980) Anal. Biochem. *105*, 36.

Deutsch, H.F. and Morton, J.I. (1958) J. Biol. Chem. *231*, 1107.

Dévényi, T., Rogers, S.J. and Wolfe, R.G. (1966) Nature *210*, 489.

Dietzler, D.N., Weidman, N. and Tieber, V.L. (1980) Clin. Chim. Acta *101*, 163.

Dietzler, D.N., Leckie, M.P., Hoelting, C.R., Porter, S.E., Smith, C.H., and Tieber, V.L. (1983) Clin. Chim. Acta *127*, 239.

Dixon, M. and Webb, E.C. (1961) Adv. Prot. Chem. *16*, 197.

Dobbins Place, J. and Schroeder, H.R. (1982) J. Immunol. Methods *48*, 251.

Doellgast, G.J. and Plaut, A.G. (1976) Immunochemistry *13*, 135.

Dölken, G. and Klein, G. (1977) J. Natl. Cancer Inst. *50*, 1239.

Domin, B.A., Serabjit-Singh, C.J. and Philpot, R.M. (1984) Anal. Biochem. *136*, 390.

Dougherty, R.M., Marucci, A.A. and DiStefano, H.S. (1972) J. Gen. Virol. *15*, 149.

Dougherty, R.M., DiStefano, H.S. and Marucci, A.A. (1974) In: Viral Immunodiagnosis (E. Kurstak and R. Morisset, eds.) p. 89. Academic Press, New York.

Dresser, D.W. (1977) In: Immunochemistry: An Advanced Textbook. (L.E. Glynn and M.W. Steward, eds.) p. 602. John Wiley and Sons, Chichester, New York.

Dreyer, W.J. and Bennett, J.C. (1965) Proc. Natl. Acad. Sci. USA *54*, 864.

Druet, E., Mahieu, P., Foidart, J.M. and Druet, P. (1982) J. Immunol. Methods *48*, 149.

Dubois-Dalcq, M., McFarland, H. and McFarlin, D. (1977) J. Histochem. Cytochem. *25*, 1201.

Duggleby, R.G. and Morrison, J.F. (1978) Biochim. Biophys. Acta *526*, 398.

Duhamel, R.C., Schur, P.H., Brendel, K. and Meezan, E. (1979) J. Immunol. Methods *31*, 211.

Duhamel, R.C., Meezan, E. and Brendel, K. (1980) Mol. Immunol. *17*, 29.

Dyer, J.R. (1956) Methods Biochem. Anal. *3*, 111.

Dyson, G.M. and George, H.J. (1924) J. Chem. Soc. *125*, 1702.

Echols, H., Garen, A., Garen, S. and Torriani, A. (1961) J. Mol. Biol. *3*, 425.

Edelman, G.M., Cunningham, B.A., Gall, W.E., Gottlieb, P.D., Rutishauser, U. and Waxdal, M.J. (1969) Proc. Natl. Acad. Sci. USA *63*, 78.

Edgington, T.S. (1971) J. Immunol. *106*, 673.

Edmundson, A.B., Ely, K.R., Sly, D.A., Westholm, F.A., Powers, D.A. and Liener, I.E. (1971) Biochemistry *10*, 3554.

Ehrlich, P.H., Moyle, W.R., Moustafa, Z.A. and Canfield, R.E. (1982) J. Immunol. *128*, 2709.

Eisen, H.N. (1964) Methods Med. Res. *10*, 94.

Eisen, H.N. (1980) Immunology: An Introduction to Molecular and Cellular Principles of the Immune Responses. 2nd edition. Harper and Row Publ., Hogerstown, Md.

Eisen, H.N. and Siskind, G.W. (1964) Biochemistry *3*, 996.

Eisenthal, R. and Cornish-Bowden, A. (1974) Biochem. J. *139*, 715.

Ek, N. (1974) Acta Vet. Scand. *15*, 609.

Ekins, R.P. (1974) Br. Med. Bull. *30*, 3.

Ekins, R.P. (1976) Hormone Assays and their Clinical Application. 4th ed. p. 1–72. Churchill Livingstone, Edinburgh.

Ekins, R. (1979) In: Radioimmunology 1979. (C.A. Bizollon, ed.) p. 239. Elsevier/North-Holland Biomedical Press, Amsterdam.

Ekins, R. (1980) In: Immunoassays of the 80s (A. Voller, A. Bartlett and D. Bidwell, eds.) p. 5. Park University Press, Baltimore.

Ekins, R.P., Newman, G.B. and Riordan, J.C.H. (1968) In: Radioisotopes in Medicine: In Vitro Studies (R.L. Hayes, F.D. Goswitz and B.E.P. Murphy, eds.) p. 59. US Atomic Energy Commission (from Clearing House for Federal Scientific and Technical Information; CONF (1967) 1111) Nat. Bureau of Standards, Springfield, VA 22151.

Ellens, D.J. and Gielkens, A.L.J. (1980) J. Immunol. Methods *37*, 325.

Elveback, L.R. and Taylor, W.F. (1969) Ann. New York Ac. Sci. *161*, 538.

Elwing, H. and Nygren, H. (1979) J. Immunol. Methods *31*, 101.

Elwing, H., Lange, S. and Nygren, H. (1980) J. Immunol. Methods *39*, 247.

Engvall, E. (1976) Lancet (ii) 1410.

Engvall, E. (1978) Scand. J. Immunol. *8* (Suppl. 7), 25.

Engvall, E. (1980) Methods Enzymol. *70*, 419

Engvall, E. and Perlmann, P. (1971) Immunochemistry *8*, 871.

Engvall, E., Jonsson, K. and Perlmann, P. (1971) Biochim. Biophys. Acta *251*, 427.

Ephrussi, B. and Weiss, M.C. (1969) Sci. American *220* (4), 26.

Erickson, P.F., Minier, L.N. and Lasher, R.S. (1982) J. Immunol. Methods *51*, 241.

Erlandsen, S.L., Parsons, J.A., Burke, J.P., Redick, J.A., Van Orden, D.E. and Van Orden, L.S. (1975) J. Histochem. Cytochem. *23*, 666.

Erlandsen, S.L., Hegre, O.D., Parsons, J.A., McEvoy, R.C. and Elde, R.P. (1976) J. Histochem. Cytochem. *24*, 883.

Erlanger, B.F. (1980) Methods Enzymol. *70*, 85.

Erlanger, B.F., Borek, F., Beiser, S.M. and Lieberman, S. (1957) J. Biol. Chem. *228*, 713.

Erlanger, B.F., Borek, F., Beiser, S.M., and Lieberman, S. (1959) J. Biol. Chem. *234*, 1090.

Escribano, M.J., Haddada, H. and De Vaux Saint Cyr, Ch. (1982) J. Immunol. Methods *52*, 63.

Esen, A., Conroy, J.M. and Wang, S.-Z. (1983) Anal. Biochem. *132*, 462.

Espersen, F. and Schiøtz, P.O. (1981) Acta Pathol. Microbiol. Scand. Section C *89C*, 93.

Eveleigh, J.W. and Levy, D.E. (1977) J. Solid Phase Biochem. *2*, 44.

Exley, D. and Abuknesha, R. (1978) FEBS Lett. *91*, 162.

Exley, D., Johnson, M.W. and Dean, P.D.G. (1971) Steroids *18*, 605.

Ey, P.L., Prowse, S.J. and Jenkin, C.R. (1978) Immunochemistry *15*, 429.

Faith, A., Pontesilli, O., Unger, A., Panayi, G.S. and Johns, P. (1982) J. Immunol. Methods *55*, 169.

Falini, B., Tabilio, A., Zuccaccia, M. and Martelli, M.F. (1980) J. Immunol. *39*, 111.

Fanciullo, R.A., Huber, N., Izutsu, A., Pirio, M.R., Buckley, N., Singh, P., Gushaw, J.B., Miller, J.G. and Schneider, R.S. (1978) Clin. Chem. *24*, 1056.

Farr, A.G. and Nakane, P.K. (1981) J. Immunol. Methods *47*, 129.

Farrah, S.R., Shah, D.O. and Ingram, L.O. (1981) Proc. Natl. Acad. Sci. USA *78*, 1229.

Farrar, J.J., Koopman, W.J. and Fuller-Bonar, J. (1977) J. Immunol. *119*, 47.

Fazekas de St. Groth, S. and Scheidegger, D. (1980) J. Immunol. Methods *35*, 1.

Feder, N. (1971) J. Cell Biol. *51*, 339.

Feinstein, A. and Beale, D. (1977) In: Immunochemistry: An Advanced Textbook (L.E. Glynn and M.W. Steward, eds.) p. 263. John Wiley and Sons, Chichester, New York.

Feinstein, A. and Munn, E.A. (1969) Nature (N.Y.) *224*, 1307.

Feldmann, M. (1974) Contemp. Top. Mol. Immunol. *3*, 57.

Feldmann, M. and Basten, A. (1972) J. Exptl. Med. *136*, 722.

Feldmann, M. Greaves, M.F., Parker, D.C. and Rittenberg, M.B. (1974) Eur. J. Immunol. *4*, 591.

Felgner, P. (1978) Zbl. Bakt. Hyg., I. Abt. Orig. A *242*, 100.

Fernandez, A.A., Stevenson, G.W., Abraham, G.E. and Chiamori, N.Y. (1983) Clin. Chem. *29*, 284.

Fernley, H.N. (1971) In: The Enzymes (P.D. Boyer, ed.) vol. 4. p. 417. Academic Press, New York.

Ferrua, B., Maiolini, R. and Masseyeff, R. (1979) J. Immunol. Methods *25*, 49.

Ferrua, B., Vincent, C., Revillard, J.P., Pettazi, G., Maiolini, R., Viot, G. and Masseyeff, R. (1980) J. Immunol. Methods *36*, 149.

Ferrua, B., Milano, G., Ly, B., Guennec, J.Y. and Masseyeff, R. (1983) J. Immunol. Methods *60*, 257.

Fey, H. (1981) J. Immunol. Methods *47*, 109.

Fields, H.A., Davis, C.L., Dreesman, G.R., Bradley, D.W. and Maynard, J.E. (1981) J. Immunol. Methods *47*, 145.

Findlay, J.W.A., Butz, R.F. and Welch, R.M. (1977) Res. Commun. Chem. Pathol. Pharmacol. *17*, 595.

Finn, F.M., Titus, G., Montibeller, J.A. and Hofmann, K. (1980) J. Biol. Chem. *255*, 5742.

Finley, P.R., Williams, R.J. and Byers III, J.M. (1976) Clin. Chem. *22*, 911.

Fleming, A. (1922) Proc. Roy. Soc. *B93*, 306.

Ford, D.J., Radin, R. and Pesce, A.J. (1978) Immunochemistry *15*, 237.

Forghani, B., Dennis, J. and Schmidt, N.J. (1980) J. Clin. Microbiol. *12*, 704.

Forsgren, A. (1968) J. Immunol. *100*, 927.

Forsgren, A.. Sjöquist, J. (1966) J. Immunol. *97*, 822.

Fowler, A.V. and Zabin, I. (1977) Proc. Natl. Acad. Sci. USA *74*, 1507.

Fraenkel-Conrat, H., Snell, N.S. and Ducay, E.D. (1952) Arch. Biochem. Biophys. *39*, 80.

Frankel, M. and Gerhard, W. (1979) Mol. Immunol. *16*, 101.

Freedman, M.H., Grossberg, A.L. and Pressman, D. (1968) J. Biol. Chem. *243*, 6186.

Freiman, D.G., Goldman, H. and Kaplan, N. (1962) J. Histochem. Cytochem. *10*, 520.

Fridovich, I. (1963) J. Biol. Chem. *238*, 3921.

Friguet, B., Djavadi-Ohaniance, L., Pages, J., Bussard, A. and Goldberg, M. (1983) J. Immunol. Methods *60*, 351.

Gabriel, A., Jr. and Agnello, V. (1977) J. Clin. Invest. *59*, 990.

Galanaud, P. (1979) Immunol. Rev. *45*, 141.

Galfrè, G., Milstein, C. and Wright, B. (1979) Nature *277*, 131.

Gallati, H. and Brodbeck, H. (1982) J. Clin. Chem. Clin. Biochem. *20*, 221.

Gallyas, F., Görcs, T. and Merchenthaler, I. (1982) J. Histochem. Cytochem. *30*, 183.

Garcia-Pardo, A., Lamm, M.E., Plaut, A.G. and Frangione, B. (1979) Mol. Immunol. *16*, 477

Garcia-Pardo, A., Lamm, M.E., Plaut, A.G. and Frangione, B. (1981) J. Biol. Chem. *256*, 11734.

Garen, A. and Levinthal, C. (1960) Biochim. Biophys. Acta *38*, 470.

Gebauer, C.R. and Rechnitz, G.A. (1982) Anal. Biochem. *124*, 338.

Genta, V.M. and Bowdre, J.H. (1982) J. Clin. Microbiol. *16*, 168.

Geoghegan, W.D., Struve, M.F. and Jordon, R.E. (1983) J. Immunol. Methods *60*, 61.

Gerber, H.A., Schaffer, T. and Hess, M.W. (1975) Immunochemistry *12*, 847.

Gershon, R.K. and Kondo, K. (1971) Immunology *18*, 723.

Gershon, R.K., Eardley, D.D., Durum, S., Green, D.R., Shen, F.-W., Yamauchi, K., Cantor, H. and Murphy, D.B. (1981) J. Exptl. Med. *153*, 1533.

Gershoni, J.M. and Palade, G.E. (1982) Anal. Biochem. *124*, 396.

Gershoni, J.M. and Palade, G.E. (1983) Anal. Biochem. *131*, 1.

Gershoni, J.M., Palade, G.E., Hawrot, E., Klimowicz, D.W. and Lentz, T.L. (1982) J. Cell Biol. *95*, 422a(21046).

Geschwind, I.I. and Li, C.H. (1957) Biochim. Biophys. Acta *25*, 171.

Giallongo, A., Kochoumian, L. and King, T.P. (1982) J. Immunol. Methods *52*, 379.

Gibbons, I., Skold, C., Rowley, G.L. and Ullman, E.F. (1980) Anal. Biochem. *102*, 167.

Gibson, W. (1981) Anal. Biochem. *118*, 1.

Gilbert, D. (1978) Nature *272*, 577.

Gill, T.J., Kunz, H.W. and Papermaster, D.S. (1967) J. Biol. Chem. *242*, 3308.

Ginsburg, V., ed. (1972) In: Methods Enzymol., vol 28, section III. Academic Press, New York.

Givol, D., Strausbauch, P.H., Hurwitz, E., Wilchek, M., Haimovich, J., and Eisen, H.N. (1971) Biochemistry *10*, 3461.

Glad, C. and Grubb, A.O. (1978) Anal. Biochem. *85*, 180.

Glad, C. and Grubb, A.O. (1981) Anal. Biochem. *116*, 335.

Glaser, L. and Brown, D.H. (1955) J. Biol. Chem. *216*, 67.

Glatthaar, B.E., Barbarash, G.R., Noyes, B.E., Banaszak, L.J. and Bradshaw, R.A. (1974) Anal. Biochem. *57*, 432.

Glauert, A.M. and Glauert, R.H. (1958) J. Biophys. Biochem. Cytol. *4*, 191.

Glazer, A.N., DeLange, R. and Sigman, D.S. (1975) Selected Methods and Analytical Procedures. North-Holland, Amsterdam.

Goding, J.W. (1976) J. Immunol. Methods *13*, 215.

Goding, J.W. (1978) J. Immunol. Methods *20*, 241.

Goding, J.W. (1980) J. Immunol. Methods *39*, 285.

Gold, A.P. and Balding, P. (1975) Receptor-specific proteins, plant and animal lectins. 440 pp. American Elsevier, New York.

Gold, P. and Freedman, S.O. (1965) J. Exptl. Med. *122*, 467.

Goldstein, L. (1972) Biochemistry *11*, 4072.

Goldstein, I.J. and Hayes, C.E. (1978) Adv. Carbohydr. Chem. Biochem. *35*, 127.

Goldstein, D.J., Rogers, C.E. and Harris, H. (1980) Proc. Natl. Acad. Sci. USA *77*, 2857.

Golub, E.S. (1981) The Cellular Basis of the Immune Response. 330 pp. Sinauer Ass., Inc. Sunderland, Mass.

Goodman, M.G. and Weigle, W.O. (1977) J. Exptl. Med. *145*, 437.

Gonwa, T.A., Peterlin, P.M. and Stobo, J.D. (1983) Adv. Immunol. *34*, 71.

Gordon, A.H. (1975) Electrophoresis of Proteins in Polyacrylamide and Starch Gels. 216 pp. Vol. 1. pt. 1. In: Laboratory Techniques in Biochemistry and Molecular Biology (T.S. Work and E. Work, eds.) Elsevier/North-Holland, Amsterdam.

Gordon, L.K. (1981) J. Immunol. Methods 44, 241.

Gordon, M.A., Edwards, M.R. and Tompkins, V.N. (1962) PNS 109, 96.

Gosling, J.P. (1980) In: Immunoenzymatic assay techniques (R. Malvano, ed.) p. 259. Martinus Nijhoff, The Hague.

Goudswaard, J., van der Donk, J.A., Noordzij, A., Van Dam, R.H. and Vaerman, J.-P. (1978) Scand. J. Immunol. 8, 21.

Graham, R.C., Jr., Karnovsky, M.J., Shafer, A.W., Glass, E.A. and Karnovsky, M.L. (1967 J. Cell Biol. 32, 269.

Grassetti, D.R. and Murray, J.F., Jr. (1967) Arch. Biochem. Biophys. 119, 41.

Green, A.A. (1931) J. Biol. Chem. 93, 495.

Green, N.M. (1963) Biochem. J. 89, 609.

Green, N.M. (1965) Biochem. J. 94, 23C.

Green, N.M. (1971) Biochem. J. 125, 781.

Green, N.M. (1975) Adv. Prot. Chem. 29, 85.

Green, N.M. and Toms, E.J. (1970) Biochem. J. 118, 67.

Gregory, E.M., Yost, F.J., Jr., Rohrbach, M.S. and Harrison, J.H. (1971) J. Biol. Chem. 246, 5491.

Gregory, E.M., Rohrbach, M.S. and Harrison, J.H. (1971) Biochim. Biophys. Acta 243, 489.

Gripenberg, M., Linder, E., Kurki, P. and Engvall, E. (1978) Scand. J. Immunol. 7, 151.

Gripenberg, M.F., Wafin, F., Isomali, H. and Linder, E. (1979) J. Immunol. Methods 31, 109.

Griswold, W.R. and Nelson, D.P. (1984) J. Immunoassay 5, 71.

Groome, N.P. (1980) J. Clin. Chem. Clin. Biochem. 18, 345.

Gros, C., Petit, O. and Dray, F. (1976) Prot. Biol. Fluids Proc. Coll. 24, 763.

Gross, S.J., Grant, J.D., Wong, S.R., Schuster, R., Lomax, P. and Campbell. D.H. (1974) Immunochemistry 11, 453.

Grossi, C.E. and von Mayersbach, H. (1964) Acta Histochemistry 19, 382.

Grube, D. (1980) Histochemistry 66, 149.

Grube, D. and Weber, E. (1980) Histochemistry 65, 223.

Gruhn, W.B. and McDuffie, F.C. (1979) J. Immunol. Methods 29, 227.

Grzanna, R., Molliver, M.E. and Coyle, J.T. (1978) Proc. Natl. Acad. Sci. USA 75, 2502.

Guesdon, J.-L. and Avrameas, S. (1977) Immunochemistry 14, 443.

Guesdon, J.-L. and Avrameas, S. (1980) J. Immunol. Methods 39, 1.

Guesdon, J.-L., Ternynck, T. and Avrameas, S. (1979) J. Histochem. Cytochem. 27, 1131.

Guesdon, J.-L., Jouanne, C. and Avrameas, S. (1983) J. Immunol. Methods 58, 133.

Guilbault, G.G. (1976) Handbook of Enzymatic Methods of Analysis. Marcel Dekker, New York.

Gurd, F.R.N. (1967) Methods Enzymol. 11, 532.

518   PRACTICE & THEORY OF ENZYME IMMUNOASSAYS

Gurvich, A.E., Kuzozela, O.B. and Tumaneva, A.E. (1961) Biokhimiya 26, 934.
Guthrie, R.D. (1961) Adv. Carbohydr. Chem. 16, 105.
György, P., Rose, C.S. and Tomarelli, R. (1942) J. Biol. Chem. 144, 169.

Haase, A.T., Stowring, I., Harris, J.D., Traynor, B., Ventura, P., Peluso, R., Brahic, M. (1982) Virology 119, 339.
Habeeb, A.F.S.A. (1966) Anal. Biochem. 14, 328.
Habeeb, A.F.S.A. and Hiramoto, R. (1968) Arch. Biochem. Biophys. 126, 16.
Haden, B.H., McNeil, K.G., Huber, N.A., Khan, W.A., Singh, P. and Schneider, R.S. (1976) Clin. Chem. 22, 1200.
Haeckel, R., Collombel, C., Geary, T.D., Mitchell, F.L., Nadeau, R.G., and Okuda, K. (1980) Clin. Chim. Acta 103, 249.
Haggerty, C., Jablonski, E., Stav, L. and DeLuca, M. (1978) Anal. Biochem. 88, 162.
Halbert, S.P., Bastomsky, C.H. and Anken, M. (1983) Clin. Chim. Acta 127, 69.
Hales, C.N. and Randle, P.J. (1963) Biochem. J. 88, 137.
Hales, C.N. and Woodhead, J.S. (1980) Methods Enzymol. 70, 334.
Hamaguchi, Y., Kato, K., Fukui, H., Shirikawa, I., Ishikawa, E., Kobayashi, K. and Katunuma, N. (1976) J. Biochem. 80, 895.
Hamaguchi, Y., Yoshitake, S., Ishikawa, E., Endo, Y. and Ohtaki, S. (1979) J. Biochem. 85, 1289.
Hames, H.D. (1981) In: Gel Electrophoresis of Proteins: A Practical Approach. (B.D. Hames and D. Rickwood, eds.) p. 219. IRL Press Ltd, London and Washington.
Hames, B.D. and Rickwood, D. (eds.) (1981) Gel Electrophoresis of Proteins: A Practical Approach. 290 pp. IRL Press Ltd, London and Washington DC.
Hanlon, J. (1978) New Scientist, May 11, 352.
Harboe, M. and Fölling, I. (1974) Scand. J. Immunol. 3, 471.
Harboe, N.M.G. and Ingild, A. (1983) Scand. J. Immunol. 17 (suppl. 10), 345.
Harbury, H.A. and Loach, P.A. (1959) Proc. Natl. Acad. Sci. USA 45, 1344.
Hardy, P.M., Nichols, A.C. and Rydon, H.N. (1976) J. Chem. Soc. Perkin Trns. 1 9, 958.
Harper, J.R. and Orengo, A. (1981) Anal. Biochem. 113, 51.
Harris, C.C., Yolken, R.H., Krokan, H. and Hsu, I.C. (1979) Proc. Natl. Acad. Sci. USA 76, 5336.
Haschke, R.H. and Friedhoff, J.M. (1978) Biochem. Biophys. Res. Comm. 80, 1039.
Hawkes, R., Niday, E. and Gordon, J. (1982) Anal. Biochem. 119, 142.
Hayat, M. (1970) In: Principles and Techniques of Electron Microscopy. Van Nostrand Reinhold Co., New York.
Hebert, G.A., Pittman, B. and Cherry, W.B. (1967) J. Immunol. 98, 1204.
Heck, F.C., Williams, J.D. and Pruett, J. (1980) J. Clin. Microbiol. 11, 398.
Heggeness, M.H. and Ash, J.F. (1977) J. Cell Biol. 73, 783.
Heitzmann, H. and Richards, F.M. (1974) Proc. Natl. Acad. Sci. USA 71, 3537.
Hellsing, K. and Richter, W. (1974) J. Immunol. Methods 5, 147.
Hendry, R.M. and Herrmann, J.E. (1980) J. Immunol. Methods 35, 285.
Heney, G. and Orr, G.A. (1981) Anal. Biochem. 114, 92.

Heppel, L.A., Harkness, D.R. and Hilmoe, R.J. (1962) J. Biol. Chem. *237*, 841.

Herbert, W.J. (1966) Nature *210*, 747.

Herbert, W.J. (1973) In: Handbook of Experimental Immunology (D.M. Weir, ed.) 2nd ed. appendix 2 and 3. Blackwell Scientific Publications, Oxford.

Herrmann, J.E., Hendry, R.M. and Collins, M.F. (1979) J. Clin. Microbiol. *10*, 210.

Hersh, L.S. and Yaverbaum, S. (1975) Clin. Chim. Acta *63*, 69.

Herzog, V. and Fahimi, H.D. (1973) Anal. Biochem. *54*, 554.

Heusser, C.H., Stocker, J.W. and Gisler, R.H. (1981) Methods Enzymol. *73*, 406.

Hevey, R., Bonacker, L.H. and Sparacio, R. (1976) In: Immunoenzymatic Techniques (G. Feldman, P. Druet, J. Bignon and S. Avrameas, eds.) p. 191. Elsevier/North-Holland, Amsterdam.

Hildebrandt, A.G. and Roots, I. (1975) Arch. Biochem. Biophys. *171*, 385.

Hoffmann, M.K. (1980) Immunol. Rev. *49*, 79.

Hofmann, K., Wood, S.W., Brinton, C.C., Montibeller, J.A. and Finn, F.M. (1980) Proc. Natl. Acad. Sci. USA *77*, 4666.

Hogg, R.J. and Davidson, G.P. (1982) Austr. Paediatr. J. *18*, 184.

Holbeck, S.L. and Nepom, G.T. (1983) J. Immunol. Methods *60*, 47.

Holbrook, J.J. and Wolfe, R.G. (1972) Biochemistry *11*, 2499.

Horejsi, J. and Smetana, R. (1956) Acta Med. Scand. *155*, 65.

Hornby, W.E., Lilly, M.D. and Crook, E.M. (1968) Biochem. J. *107*, 673.

Hsu, S.-M. and Raine, L. (1981) J. Histochem. Cytochem. *29*, 1349.

Hsu, S., Raine, L. and Fanger, M. (1981) J. Histochem. Cytochem. *29*, 577.

Huang, S.N. (1975) Lab. Invest. *33*, 88.

Hughes-Jones, N.C., Gardner, B. and Telford, R. (1964) Immunology *7*, 72.

Hunter, W.M. (1980) UK Patent Spec. 1 566 098 (30.4.80). See also: Hunter, W.M. and Budd, P.S. (1981) J. Immunol. Methods *45*, 255.

Hunter, W.M., McKenzie, I. and Bacon, R.R.A. (1980) In: Immunoassays for the 80s (A. Voller, A. Bartlett and D. Bidwell, eds.). p. 155. Park University Press, Baltimore.

Imagawa, M., Yoshitake, S., Ishikawa, E., Niitsu, Y., Urushizaki, I., Kanazawa, R., Tachibana, S., Nakazawa, N. and Ogawa, H. (1982a) Clin. Chim. Acta *121*, 277.

Imagawa, M., Yoshitake, S., Hamaguchi, Y., Ishikawa, E., Niitsu Y., Urushizaki, I., Kanazawa, R., Tachibana, S., Nakazawa, N. and Ogawa H. (1982b) J. Appl. Biochem. *4*, 41.

Imoto, T., Johnson, L.N., North, A.C.T., Phillips, D.C. and Rupley, J.A. (1972) In: The Enzymes (P.D. Boyer, ed.). vol. 7. p. 666. Academic Press, New York.

Inbar, D., Hochman, J. and Giool, D. (1972) Proc. Natl. Acad. Sci. USA *69*, 2659.

Inganäs, M., Johansson, S.G. and Bennick, O. (1980) Scand. J. Immunol. *12*, 23.

Inman, J.K. (1974) Methods Enzymol. *34*, 30.

Inouye, S., Matsuno, S. and Yamaguchi, H. (1984) J. Clin. Microbiol. *19*, 259.

Iscove, N.N. and Melchers, F. (1978) J. Exptl. Med. *147*, 923.

Iscove, N.I. and Schreier, M.H. (1979) In: Immunological Methods (I. Lefkovits and B. Pernis, eds.). vol. 1. p. 279. Academic Press, New York.

Ishaque, A., Milhausen, M. and Levy, H.R. (1974) Biochem. Biophys. Res. Commun. 59, 894.

Ishikawa, E. and Kato, K. (1978) Scand. J. Immunol. (Suppl.) 8, 43.

Ishikawa, E., Yamada, Y., Hamaguchi, Y., Yoshitake, S., Shiomi, K., Ota, T., Yamamoto, Y. and Tanaka, K. (1978) In: Enzyme-labeled Immunoassay of Hormones and Drugs (S.B. Pal, ed.). p. 43. Walter de Gruyter, Berlin.

Ishikawa, E., Hamaguchi, Y. and Imagawa, M. (1980) J. Immunoassay 1, 385.

Ishikawa, E., Imagawa, M., Hashida, S., Yoshitake, S., Hamaguchi, Y., and Ueno, T. (1983) J. Immunoassay 4, 209.

Isobe, Y., Chen, S.-T., Nakane, P.K. and Brown, W.R. (1977) Acta Histochem. Cytochem. 10, 161.

Ito, J.I., Wunderlich, A.C., Lyons, J., Davis, C.E., Gurney, D.G. and Braude, A.I. (1980) J. Inf. Dis. 142, 532.

Izutsu, A., Pirio, M.R., Buckley, N., Singh, P., Gushaw, J.B., Miller, J.G. and Schneider, R.S. (1978) Clin. Chem. 24, 1055.

Izutsu, A., Leung, D., Araps, C., Singh, P., Jaklitsch, A. and Kabakoff, D.S. (1979) Clin. Chem. 24, 1055.

Jackson, S., Sogn, J.A. and Kindt, T.J. (1982) J. Immunol. Methods 48, 299.

Jackson, S., Chused, T.M., Wilkinson, J.M., Leiserson, W.M. and Kindt, T.J. (1983) J. Exptl. Med. 157, 34.

Jahn, R., Schiebler, W. and Greengaard, P. (1984) Proc. Natl. Acad. Sci. USA 81, 1684.

Jansen, E.F., Tomimatsu, Y. and Olson, A.C. (1971) Arch. Biochem. Biophys. 144, 394.

Jasiewicz, M.L., Schoenberg, D.R. and Mueller, G.C. (1976) Exp. Cell Res. 100, 213.

Jaton, J.-C., Brandt, D.C. and Vassali, P. (1979) In: Immunological Methods (I. Lefkovits and B. Pernis, eds.). vol. 1 p. 43. Academic Press, New York.

Jensenius, J.C., Andersen, I., Hau, J., Crone, M. and Koch, C. (1981) J. Immunol. Methods 46, 63.

Jerne, N.K. (1974) Ann. Immunol. (Paris) 125C, 373.

Jessen, K.R. (1983) In: Immunocytochemistry: Practical Applications in Pathology and Biology (J.M. Polak and S. Van Noorden, eds.). p. 169. Wright PSG, Bristol.

Jessen, K.R., Saffrey, M.J., Van Noorden, S., Bloom, S.R., Polak, J.M., and Burnstock, G. (1980) Neuroscience 5, 1717.

Jirgensons, B. (1952) Arch. Biochem. Biophys. 39, 261.

Johnson, L.N. and Phillips, D.C. (1965) Nature 206, 761.

Jollès, P. and Paraf, A. (1973) Chemical and Biological Basis of Adjuvants. Springer Verlag, Berlin.

Jollès, J., Jauregui-Adell, J., Bernier, I. and Jollès, P. (1963) Biochim. Biophys. Acta 78, 668.

Jonak, Z.L. and Kennett, R.H. (1982) cited by Reading (1982).

Joseph, S.A. and Sternberger, L.A. (1979) J. Histochem. Cytochem. 27, 1430.

Josephson, L. (1981) cited by Parsons (1981).

Jovin, T.M. (1973) Ann. New York Acad. Sci. 209, 477.

Joyce, B.G., Read, F.F. and Fahmy, D.R. (1977) Steroids *29*, 761.

Ju, S.-T., Benacerraf, B. and Dorf, M.E. (1980) J. Exptl. Med. *152*, 170.

Jue, R., Lambert, J.M., Pierce, L.R. and Traut, R.R. (1978) Biochemistry *17*, 5399.

Jung, K. and Köhler, A. (1980) Clin. Chim. Acta *101*, 1.

Jung, K. and Pergande, M. (1980) Clin. Chim. Acta *102*, 215.

Kabakoff, D.S. (1980) In: Enzyme-immunoassay (E.T. Maggio, ed.). p. 71. CRC Press Inc, Boca Raton, Fa.

Kabakoff, D.S. and Greenwood, H.M. (1982) Recent Adv. Clin. Biochem. *2*, 1.

Kabakoff, D.S., Leung, D. and Singh, P. (1978) Clin. Chem. *24*, 1055.

Kakita, K., O'Connell, K. and Permutt, M.A. (1982) Diabetes *31*, 648.

Kappler, J.W. and Marrack, P.C. (1976) Nature *262*, 797.

Karush, F. (1962) Adv. Immunol. *2*, 1.

Kato, K., Hamaguchi, Y., Fukui, H. and Ishikawa, E. (1975) J. Biochem. *78*, 423.

Kato, H., Haruyama, Y., Hamaguchi, Y. and Ishikawa, E. (1978) J. Biochem. *84*, 93.

Kato, K., Umedo, Y., Suzuki, F. and Kosaka, A. (1980) Clin. Chim. Acta *102*, 261.

Kay, E. Shannon, L.M. and Lew, J.Y. (1967) J. Biol. Chem. *242*, 2470.

Kearney, J.F., Radbruch, A., Liesegang, B. and Rajewsky, K. (1979) J. Immunol. *123*, 1548.

Keilin, D. and Hartree, E.F. (1948) Biochem. J. *42*, 221.

Keller, D.F. (1971) G-6-PDH Deficiency. 67 pp. CRC Press, Cleveland, Ohio.

Kendal, A. (1980) Summarized in: McIntosh et al., J. Infect. Dis. *142*, 793.

Kendall, C., Ionescu-Matiu, I. and Dreesman, G.R. (1983) J. Immunol. Methods *56*, 329.

Kennedy, J.H., Kricka, L.J. and Wilding, P. (1976a) Clin. Chim. Acta *70*, 1.

Kennedy, J.H., Kricka, L.J. and Wilding, P. (1976b) Prot. Biol. Fluids Proc. Coll. *24*, 787.

Kennedy, R.C., Melnick, J.L. and Dreesman, G.R. (1984) Science *223*, 930.

Kenny, G.E. and Dunsmoor, C.L. (1983) J. Clin. Microbiol. *17*, 655.

Kessler, S.W. (1976) J. Immunol. *117*, 1482.

Kessler, S.W. (1981) Methods Enzymol. *73*, 442.

Khan, S.A.K. and Jacob, T.M. (1977) Nucl. Acids Res. *4*, 3007.

Kilburn, D.G. and Levy, J.G. (1980) Cancer Immunol. Immunother. *8*, 71.

King, E.L. and Altman, C. (1956) J. Phys. Chem. *60*, 1375.

Kitagawa, T. and Aikawa, T. (1976) J. Biochem. *79*, 233.

Kitagawa, T., Fujitake, T., Taniyama, H. and Aikawa, T. (1978) J. Biochem. *83*, 1493.

Kitagawa, T. and Kanamazu, T. (1978) In: Enzyme-labeled Immunoassay of Hormones and Drugs (S.B. Pal, ed.). p. 59. Walter de Gruyter, Berlin.

Kittler, J.M., Meisler, N.T., Viceps-Madore, D., Cidlorwski, J.A., Thanassi, J.W. (1984) Anal. Biochem. *137*, 210.

Klein, J. (1979) Science *203*, 516.

Klein, J. (1982) Immunology. The Science of Self-nonself Discrimination. John Wiley and Sons, Chichester, New York.

Kleppe, K. (1966) Biochemistry 5, 139.
Klinman, N. and Press, J. (1975) Transplant. Rev. 24, 41.
Klotz, I.M. and Heiney, R.E. (1962) Arch. Biochem. Biophys. 96, 605.
Klotz, J.L. (1982) Methods Enzymol. 84, 194.
Knowles, J.R. (1972) Acc. Chem. Res. 5, 155.
Knudsen, K.A., Rao, P.E., Damsky, C.H. and Buck, C.A. (1981) Proc. Natl. Acad. Sci. USA 78, 6071.
Kobayashi, K., Vaerman, J.-P., Bazin, H., Lebacq-Verheyden, A.-M and Heremans, J.F. (1973) J. Immunol. 111, 1590.
Kobayashi, Y., Ogihara, T., Amitani, K., Watanabe, F., Kiguchi, I., Ninomiya, I. and Kumahara, Y. (1978) Steroids 32, 137.
Koenig, R. (1981) J. Gen. Virol. 55, 53.
Koenig, R. and Paul, H.L. (1982) J. Virol. Methods 5, 113.
Köhler, G. (1976) Eur. J. Immunol. 6, 340.
Köhler, G. (1978) In: EMBO Laboratory Course on B-lymphocyte Fusion (Basel Institute for Immunology, Basel) p.1.
Köhler, G. (1981) In: Immunological Methods (I. Lefkovits and B. Pernis, eds.). vol. 2. p. 285. Academic Press, New York.
Köhler, G. and Milstein, C. (1975) Nature 256, 495.
Köhler, G. and Milstein, C. (1976) Eur. J. Immunol. 6, 511.
Kohlrausch, F. (1897) Ann. Phys. (Leipzig) 62, 511.
Konijn, A.M., Levy, R., Link, G. and Hershko, C. (1982) J. Immunol. Methods 54, 297.
Koprowski, H., Herlyn, D., Lubeck, M., DeFreitas, E. and Sears, H.F. (1984) Proc. Natl. Acad. Sci. USA 81, 216.
Korn, A.H., Feairheller, S.H. and Filachione, E.M. (1972) J. Mol. Biol. 65, 525.
Koshland, M.E. (1975) Adv. Immunol. 20, 41.
Koshland, D.E., Némethy, G. and Filmer, D. (1966) Biochemistry 5, 365.
Kraehenbuhl, J.P., Galardy, R.E. and Jamieson, J.D. (1974) J. Exptl. Med. 139, 208.
Kricka, L.J., Carter, T.J.N., Burt, S.M., Kennedy, J.H., Holder, R.L., Halliday, M.I., Telford, M.E. and Wisdom, G.B. (1980) Clin. Chem. 26, 741.
Krigbaum, W.R. and Kügler, F.R. (1970) Biochemistry 9, 1216.
Kristiansen, T. (1976) Scand. J. Immunol. (Suppl.) 3, 19.
Kronvall, G. and Frommel, D. (1970) Immunochemistry 7, 124.
Kronvall, G., Grey, H.M. and Williams, R.C., Jr. (1970) J. Immunol. 105, 1116.
Kronvall, G., Seal, U.S., Svensson, S. and Williams, R.C. (1974) Acta Pathol. Microbiol. Scand. B 82, 12.
Kubo, R.T., Zimmerman, B. and Grey, H.M. (1973) In: The Antigens (M. Sela, ed.). vol. 1 p. 417. Academic Press, New York.
Kuhlmann, W.D. and Peschke, P. (1982) Histochemistry 75, 151.
Kuhlmann, W.D., Avrameas, S. and Ternynck, T. (1974) J. Immunol. Methods 5, 33.
Kun, E., Eanes, R.Z. and Volfin, P. (1967) Nature 214, 1328.
Kuramitsu, H.K. (1966) Biochem. Biophys. Res. Commun. 23, 329.
Kurstak, E., Tijssen, P., Kurstak, C. and Morisset, R. (1975) Ann. New York Acad.

Sci. *254*, 369.

Kurstak, E., Tijssen, P. and Kurstak, C. (1977) In: Comparative Diagnosis of Viral Diseases (E. Kurstak and C. Kurstak, eds). vol. 2, p. 402. Academic Press, New York.

Kurstak, E., de Thé, G., Van den Hurk, J., Charpentier, G., Kurstak, C., Tijssen, P. and Morisset, R. (1978) J. Med. Virol. *2*, 189.

Kurstak, E., Tijssen, P. and Kurstak, C. (1983) In: Control of Virus Diseases (E. Kurstak and R. Maruszyk, eds.). p. 477. Marcel Dekker, New York.

Kyle, R.A., Bieger, R.C. and Gleich, G.J. (1970) Med. Clin. North Amer. *54*, 917.

Labrousse, H., Guesdon, J.-L., Ragimbeau, J. and Avrameas, S. (1982) J. Immunol. Methods *48*, 133.

Laemmli, U.K. (1970) Nature *227*, 680.

Lamoyi, E. and Nisonoff, A. (1983) J. Immunol. Methods *56*, 235.

Landsteiner, K. (1945) The Specificity of Serological Reactions. Harvard University Press, Cambridge Massachusetts.

Landt, M., Boltz, S.C. and Butler, L.G. (1978) Biochemistry *17*, 915.

Langer, P.R., Waldrop, A.A. and Ward, D.C. (1981) Proc. Natl. Acad. Sci. USA *78*, 6633.

Langer-Safer, P.R., Levine, M. and Ward, D.C. (1982) Proc. Natl. Acad. Sci. USA *79*, 4381.

Langmuir, I. (1918) J. Am. Chem. Soc. *40*, 1361.

Langone, J.J. (1982) Adv. Immunol. *32*, 157.

Lauer, R.C. and Erlanger, B.F. (1971) Immunochemistry *11*, 533.

Lauer, R.C., Solomon, P.H., Nakanishi, K. and Erlanger, B.F. (1974) Experienta *30*, 558.

Lazdunski, U., Brouillard, J. and Ouellet, L. (1965) Can. J. Chem. *43*, 2222

Leary, J.J., Brigati, D.J. and Ward, D.C. (1983) Proc. Natl. Acad. Sci. USA *80*, 4045.

Ledbetter, J.A. and Herzenberg, L.A. (1979) Immunol. Rev. *47*, 63.

Leder, P. (1982) Scientific American *246* (May) 102.

Leduc, E.H. and Bernhard, W. (1967) J. Ultrastruct. Res. *19*, 196.

Leduc, E.H., Wicker, R., Avrameas, S. and Bernhard, W. (1969) J. Gen. Virol. *4*, 609.

Lee, C.-Y., Huang, Y.-S., Hu, P.-C., Gomel, V. and Menge, A.C. (1982) Anal. Biochem. *123*, 14.

Legocki, R.P. and Verma, D.P.S. (1981) Anal. Biochem. *111*, 385.

Lehrer, S.B. (1979) Immunology *36*, 103.

Lehtonen, O.-P. and Eerola, E. (1982) J. Immunol. Methods *54*, 233.

Lehtonen, O.-P. and Viljanen, M.K. (1980a) J. Immunol. Methods *36*, 63.

Lehtonen, O.-P. and Viljanen, M.K. (1980b) J. Immunol. Methods *34*, 61.

Lehtonen, O.-P. and Viljanen, M.K. (1982) Int. J. Bio-Med. Comp. *13*, 471.

Leinikki, P.O. and Passila, S. (1977) J. Infect. Dis. *136* (Suppl.), S294.

Leinikki, P.O., Shekarchi, I., Dorsett, P. and Sever, J.L. (1978) J. Clin. Microbiol. *8*, 419.

Lenhoff, H.M. and Kaplan, N.O. (1955) Methods Enzymol. *2*, 758.

Leonard, A. and Botis, S. (1975) Specialia *15*, 341.

Leslie, G.A. and Clem, L.W. (1972) J. Enzymol. Methods *130*, 1337.

Leung, D., Tsay, Y., Singh, P., Jaklitsch, A. and Kabakoff, D.S. (1979) Clin. Chem. *25*, 1094.

Levy, H.B. and Sober, H.A. (1960) Proc. Soc. Exptl. Med. Biol. *103*, 250.

Levy, A., Kawashima, K. and Spector, S. (1976) Life Sci. *19*, 1421.

Lifson, S. (1972) In: Protein–protein Interactions (R. Jaenicke, ed.). p. 3. Springer Verlag, New York.

Lin, H.J. and Kirsch, J.F. (1977) Anal. Biochem. *81*, 442.

Lind, I. (1974) Acta Pathol. Microbiol. Scand. Section B *82B*, 821.

Lindmark, R. (1982) J. Immunol. Methods *52*, 195.

Lindmark, R., Movitz, J. and Sjöquist, J. (1977) Eur. J. Biochem. *74*, 623.

Lindner, H.R., Peril, E., Fiedlander, A. and Zeitlin, A. (1972) Steroids *19*, 357.

Lis, H., Lotan, R. and Sharon, N. (1974) Ann. New York Ac. Sci. *234*, 232.

Litman, D.J., Hanlon, T.M. and Ullman, E.F. (1980) Anal. Biochem. *106*, 223.

Little, J.R. and Donahue, H. (1967) In: Methods in Immunology and Immunochemistry (C.A. Williams and M.A. Chase, eds.). vol. 2, p. 343. Academic Press, New York.

Littlefield, J.W. (1964) Science *145*, 709.

Livingston, D.M. (1974) Methods Enzymol. *34*, 723.

Locarnini, S.A., Coulepis, A.G., Stratton, A.M., Kaldor, J. and Gust, I.D. (1979) J. Clin. Microbiol. *9*, 459.

Löhr, G.W. and Waller, H.D. (1974) In: Methods of Enzymatic Analysis (H.U. Bergmeyer, ed.) p. 636. Academic Press, New York.

Loontiens, F.G., Wallenfels, K. and Weil, R. (1970) Eur. J. Biochem. *14*, 138.

Luft, J.H. (1961) J. Biophys. Biochem. Cytol. *9*, 409.

MacRitchie, F. (1972) J. Colloid Interface Sci. *38*, 484.

Madri, J.A. and Barwick, K.W. (1983) Laboratory Invest. *48*, 98.

Maehly, A.C. (1954) Methods Biochem. Anal. *1*, 358.

Mainland, D. (1971) Clin. Chem. *17*, 267.

Malvano, R., Boniolo, A., Dovis, M. and Zannino, M. (1982) J. Immunol. Methods *48*, 51.

Mancini, G., Carbonara, A.O. and Heremans, J.F. (1965) Immunochemistry *2*, 235.

Mandrell, R.E. and Zollinger, W.D. (1984) J. Immunol. Methods *67*, 1.

Mannik, M. and Downey, W. (1973) J. Immunol. Methods *3*, 233.

Manuelidis, L., Langer-Safer, P.R. and Ward, D.C. (1982) J. Cell Biol. *95*, 619.

Marchalonis, J.J. and Edelman, G.H. (1968) J. Mol. Biol. *32*, 453.

Marchesi, S.L., Steers, E., Jr. and Shifrin, S. (1969) Biochim. Biophys. Acta *181*, 20.

Marcu, K.B. (1982) Cell *29*, 719.

Margiolash, E., Smith, E.L., Kreil, G. and Tuppy, H. (1961) Nature *192*, 1125.

Marklund, S. (1973) Arch. Biochem. Biophys. *154*, 614.

Marklund, S., Ohlsson, P.-I., Opara, A. and Paul, K.-G. (1974) Biochim. Biophys. Acta *350*, 304.

Marks, V., O'Sullivan, M.J., Al-Bassam, M.N. and Bridges, J.W. (1978) In: Enzyme-linked Immunoassay of Hormones and Drugs (S.B. Pal, ed.) p. 419. Walter de Gruyter, Berlin.

Marshall, T. (1984) Anal. Biochem. *136*, 340.

Martin, L. N. (1982a) J. Immunol. Methods *50*, 319.

Martin, L. N. (1982b) J. Immunol. Methods *52*, 205.

Martin-Comin, J. and Robyn, C. (1976) J. Histochem. Cytochem. *24*, 1012.

Marucci, A.A. and Dougherty, R.M. (1975) J. Histochem. Cytochem. *23*, 618.

Marucci, A.A., Halliday, D. and Mueller, J.F. (1977) J. Parasitol. *63*, 170.

Mason, D.Y. and Sammons, R. (1978) J. Clin. Pathol. *31*, 454.

Mason, D.Y. and Sammons, R.E. (1979) J. Histochem. Cytochem. *27*, 832.

Mason, T.E., Phifer, R.F., Spicer, S.S., Swallow, R.A. and Dreskin, R.B. (1969) J. Histochem. Cytochem. *17*, 563.

Mason, D.Y., Bell, J.I., Christensson, B. and Biberfeld, P. (1980) Clin. Exptl. Immunol. *40*, 235.

Mason, D.Y., Abdulaziz, Z., Falini, B. and Stein, H. (1983) In: Immunocytochemistry: Practical Applications in Pathology and Biology (J.M. Polak and S. Van Noorden, eds.). p. 113. Wright PSG, Bristol.

Matthew, W.B. and Reichardt, L.F. (1982) J. Immunol. Methods *50*, 239.

Matthews, J.B. (1981) J. Clin. Pathol. *34*, 103.

Mattiasson, B. and Boirebaeck, C. (1980) In: Enzyme-immunoassay (E.G. Maggio, ed.) p. 213. CRC Boca Raton, FA.

Mattiasson, B. and Nilsson, H. (1977) FEBS Lett. *78*, 251.

Mattiasson, B., Boirebaek, C., Sanfridson, B. and Mosbach, K. (1977) Biochim. Biophys, Acta *483*, 221.

Mayor, H.D., Hampton, J.C. and Rosario, B. (1961) J. Biophys. Biochem. Cytol. *9*, 909.

Maze, M. and Gray, G.M. (1980) Biochemistry *19*, 2351.

Mazurkiewicz, J.E. and Nakane, P.K. (1972) J. Histochem. Cytochem. *20*, 967.

Mazza, G., Job, C. and Bouchet, M. (1973) Biochim. Biophys. Acta *322*, 218.

McCall, J.S. and Potter, B.J. (1973) Ultracentrifugation. Balliere Tindall, London.

McCracken, S. and Meighen, E.A. (1981) J. Biol. Chem. *256*, 3945.

McCarrity, G.J. and Coriell, L.L. (1971) In Vitro *6*, 257.

McGhee, J.R., Michalek, S.M. and Ghanta, V.K. (1975) Immunochemistry *12*, 817.

McKenzie, I.F.C. and Potter, T. (1979) Adv. Immunol. *27*, 179.

McLaren, A.D. and Packer, L. (1970) Adv. Enzymol. *33*, 245.

McLaren, M., Draper, C.C., Roberts, J.H., Minter-Goedbloed, E., Ligthart, G.S., Teesdale, C.H., Amin, M.A., Omer, A.H.S., Bartlett, A., and Voller, A. (1978) Ann. Trop. Med. Parasitol. *72*, 243.

McLean, I.W. and Nakane, P.K. (1974) J. Histochem. Cytochem. *22*, 1077.

McLellan, T. and Ramshaw, J.A.M. (1981) Biochem. Genet. *19*, 647.

McMichael, J.C., Greisiger, L.M. and Millman, I. (1981) J. Immunol. Methods *45*, 79.

Mehta, H.C. and MacDonald, D.J. (1982) Clin. Chim. Acta *121*, 245.

Mehta, P.D., Reichlin, M., Tomasi, T.B., Jr. (1972) J. Immunol. *109*, 1272.

Melamed, M.D. and Green, N.M. (1963) Biochem. J. *89*, 591.

Mepham, B.L., Frater, W. and Mitchell, B.C. (1979) Histochem. J. *11*, 345.

Mesulam, M.-M. (1978) J. Histochem. Cytochem. *26*, 106.

Mesulam, M.-M. and Rosene, D.L. (1979) J. Histochem. Cytochem. *27*, 763.

Metzger, H. (1970) Adv. Immunol. *12*, 57.

Meyerhoff, M.E. and Rechnitz, G.A. (1980) Methods Enzymol. *70*, 439.

Michaelis, L. and Menten, M.L. (1913) Biochem. Z. *49*, 333.

Millán, J.L. and Stigbrand, T. (1981) Clin. Chem. *27*, 2018.

Milhausen, M. and Levy, H.R. (1975) Biochemistry *5*, 453.

Miller, T.J. and Stone, H.O. (1978) J. Immunol. Methods *24*, 111.

Milon, A., Houdayer, M. and Metzger, J.J. (1978) Dev. Comp. Immunol. *2*, 699.

Milstein, C.P., Richardson, N.E., Deverson, E.V. and Feinstein, A. (1975) Biochem. J. *151*, 615.

Miner, K.M., Reading, C.L. and Nicolson, G.L. (1981) Invasion Metastasis *1*, 158.

Mitchison, N.A. (1981) Cell. Immunol. *62*, 258.

Modesto, R.R. and Pesce, A. J. (1971) Biochim. Biophys. Acta *229*, 384.

Modesto, R.R. and Pesce, A.J. (1973) Biochim. Biophys. Acta *295*, 283.

Mole, J.E., Bhown, A.S. and Bennett, J.C. (1977) Biochemistry *16*, 3507.

Molin, S.-O., Nygren, H. and Dolonius, L. (1978) J. Histochem. Cytochem. *26*, 412.

Molin, S.-O., Nygren, H., Dolonius, L. and Hansson, H.-A. (1978) J. Histochem. Cytochem. *26*, 1053.

Molinari, J.A., Ebersole, J.L. and Platt, D. (1974) Infect. Immun. *10*, 1207.

Monod, J., Changeux, J.-P. and Jacob, F. (1963) J. Mol. Biol. *6*, 306.

Monod, J., Wyman, J. and Changeux, J.-P. (1965) J. Mol. Biol. *12*, 88

Monsan, P., Puzo, G. and Mazarguil, H. (1975) Biochimie *57*, 1281.

Moriarty, G.C. and Halmi, N.S. (1972) J. Histochem. Cytochem. *20*, 590.

Morissey, B.W. (1977) Ann. New York Ac. Sci. *283*, 50.

Morissey, J.H. (1981) Anal. Biochem. *117*, 307.

Moroz, L.A., Joubert, J.R. and Hogg, J.C. (1974) J. Immunol. *112*, 1094.

Morris, R.E. and Saelinger, C.B. (1982) J. Immunol. Methods *49*, 237.

Morris, B.A., Robinson, J.O., Aherne, G.W. and Marks, V. (1974) J. Endocrinol. *64*, 6.

Morris, R.E., Thomas, P.T. and Hong, R. (1982) Human Immunol. *5*, 1.

Mosmann, T.R., Gallatin, M. and Langenecker, B.M. (1980) J. Immunol. *125*, 1152.

Mössner, E., Boll, M. and Pfleiderer, G. (1980) Hoppe Seyler's Z. Physiol. Chem. *361*, 543.

Mostov, K.E., Friedlander, M. and Blobel, G. (1984) Nature *308*, 37.

Mould, G.P., Aherne, G.W., Morris, B.A., Teale, J.D. and Marks, V. (1977) Eur. J. Metab. Pharmacol. *2*, 171.

Muilerman, H.G., Ter Hart, H.G.J. and Van Dijk, W. (1982) Anal. Biochem. *120*, 46.

Mulé, S.J., Bastons, M.L. and Jukofsky, D. (1974) Clin. Chem. *20*, 243.

Munson, P.J. and Rodbard, D. (1980) Anal. Biochem. *107*, 220.

Murphy, B.E.P. (1980) J. Immunoassay *1*, 413.

Nairn, R.C. (1976) Fluorescent Protein Tracing. 4th ed. Churchill Livingstone, London.

Nairn, R.C., Richmond, H.G. and Fothergill, J.E. (1960) Br. J. Med. *2*, 1341.

Naito, S. and Ueda, T. (1981) J. Biol. Chem. *256*, 10657.

Nakamura, S. and Fujiki, S. (1968) J. Biochem. *63*, 51.

Nakamura, S. and Hayashi, S. (1974) FEBS Lett *41*, 327.

Nakamura, S., Hayashi, S. and Hasumi, H. (1976) In: Flavins and Flavoproteins (T.P. Singer, ed.). p. 691. Elsevier/North-Holland, Amsterdam.

Nakane, P.K. (1968) J. Histochem. Cytochem. *16*, 557.

Nakane, P.K. and Kawaoi, A. (1974) J. Histochem. Cytochem. *22*, 1084.

Nakane, P.K. and Pierce, G.B., Jr. (1966) J. Histochem. Cytochem. *14*, 929.

Nakane, P.K. and Pierce, G.B. (1967) J. Cell Biol. *33*, 307.

Naot, Y., Barnett, E.V. and Remington, J.S. (1981) J. Clin. Microbiol. *14*, 73.

Naus, A.J., Kuppens, P.S. and Borst, A. (1977) Clin. Chem. *23*, 1624.

Neufeld, H.S., Conklin, C.J. and Towner, R.D. (1965) Anal. Biochem. *12*, 303.

Neumann, H. and Lustig, A. (1980) Eur. J. Biochem. *109*, 475.

Neumann, H., Kezdy, F., Hsu, J. and Rosenberg, I.H. (1975) Biochim. Biophys. Acta *391*, 292.

Neurath, A.R. and Strick, N. (1981) J. Virol. Methods *3*, 155.

Newman, P.F.J., Atkins, G.L. and Nimmo, I.A. (1974) Biochem. J. *143*, 779.

Ngo, T.T. and Lenhoff, H.M. (1980) Anal. Biochem. *105*, 389.

Ngo, T.T. and Lenhoff, H.M. (1981) Biochem. Biophys. Res. Commun. *99*, 496.

Ngo, T.T., Carrico, R.J., Boguslaski, R.C. and Burd, J.F. (1981) J. Immunol. Methods *42*, 93.

Nilsson, P., Bergquist, N.R. and Grundy, M.S. (1981) J. Immunol. Methods *41*, 81.

Nisonoff, A., Hopper, J.E. and Spring, S.R. (1975) The Antibody Molecule. Academic Press, New York.

Nomura, M., Imai, M., Usuda, S., Nakamura, T., Miyakawa, Y. and Mayumi, M. (1983) J. Immunol. Methods *56*, 13.

North, J.R. and Askonas, B.A. (1976) Eur. J. Immunol. *6*, 8.

Norwood, T.H., Zeigler, C.J. and Martin, G.M. (1976) Somatic Cell. Gen. *2*, 263.

Notani, G.W., Parsons, J.A. and Erlandsen, S.L. (1979) J. Histochem. Cytochem. *27*, 1438.

Nowinsky, R.C., Lostrom, M.E., Tam, M.R., Stone, M.R. and Burnett, W.N. (1979) Virology *93*, 111.

Numazawa, M., Haryu, A., Kurosaka, K. and Nambara, T. (1977) FEBS Lett. *79*, 396.

Nygren, H. (1982) J. Histochem. Cytochem. *30*, 407.

Nygren, H. and Hansson, H.A. (1981) J. Histochem. Cytochem. *29*, 266.

Nygren, H. and Stenberg, M. (1982) Scand. J. Clin. Lab. Invest. *42*, 355.

Ochoa, S. (1955) Methods Enzymol. *1*, 685.

Odell, W.O., Abraham, G., Raud, H.R., Swerdloff, R.S. and Fisher, D.A. (1969) Acta Endocrinol. *140 (Suppl.)*, 54.

Oellerich, M. (1980) J. Clin. Chem. Clin. Biochem. *18*, 197.

Oellerich, M., Külpmann, W.R., Haeckel, R. and Heyer, R. (1977) J. Clin. Chem. Clin. Biochem. *15*, 353.

Oellerich, M., Sybrecht, G.W. and Haeckel, R. (1979) J. Clin. Chem. Clin. Biochem. *17*, 299.

Oellerich, M., Haeckel, R., Haindl, H. (1982) J. Clin. Chem. Clin. Biochem. *20*, 765.

O'Farrell, P.H. (1975) J. Biol. Chem. *250*, 4007.

Ogihara, T., Miyai, K., Nishi, K., Ishibashi, K. and Kumahara, Y. (1977) J. Clin. Endocrin. Metab. *44*, 91.

Oi, V.T., Jones, P.P., Goding, J.W., Herzenberg, L.A. and Herzenberg, L.A. (1978) Curr. Top. Microbiol. Immunol. *81*, 115.

Okabayashi, T., Mihara, S., Repke, D.B. and Moffat, J.G. (1977) Cancer Res. *37*, 619.

O'Keefe, E. and Bennett, V. (1980) J. Biol. Chem. *255*, 561.

Olive, C. and Levy, H.R. (1971) J. Biol. Chem. *246*, 2043.

Oliver, D.G., Sanders, A.H., Hogg, R.D. and Hellman, J.W. (1981) J. Immunol. Methods *42*, 195.

Olmsted, J.B. (1981) J. Biol. Chem. *256*, 11955.

Opitz, H.-G., Opitz, U., Lemke, H., Hewlett, G., Schreml, W. and Flad, H.-D. (1977) J. Exptl. Med. *145*, 1029.

Ordronneau, P. and Petrusz, P. (1980) Am. J. Anat. *158*, 491.

Oreskes, I. and Singer, J.M. (1961) J. Immunol. *86*, 338.

Ornstein, L. (1964) Ann. New York Ac. Sci. *121*, 321.

Osserman, E.F. and Lawlor, D.P. (1966) J. Exptl. Med. *124*, 921.

Osterloh, J. and Butrimovitz, G.P. (1982) Clin. Chem. *28*, 327.

O'Sullivan, M.J., Gnemmi, E., Morris, D., Chieregatti, G., Simmons, M., Simmonds, A.D., Bridges, J.W. and Marks, V. (1978) FEBS Lett. *95*, 311.

O'Sullivan, M.J., Gnemmi, E., Chieregatti, G., Morris, D., Simmonds, A.D., Simmons, M., Bridges, J.W. and Marks, V. (1979) J. Immunol. Methods *30*, 127.

O'Sullivan, M.J., Gnemmi, E., Morris, D., Chieregatti, G., Simmonds, A.D., Simmons, M., Bridges, J.W. and Marks, V. (1979) Anal. Biochem. *100*, 100.

Otvos, J.P. and Armitage, I.M. (1980) Biochemistry *19*, 4021.

Otvos, J., Armitage, I.M., Chlebowski, J.F. and Coleman, J.E. (1979) J. Biol. Chem. *254*, 4707.

Owen, R.D. (1945) Science *102*, 400.

Pain, D. and Surolia, A. (1981) J. Immunol. Methods *40*, 219.

Palfree, R.G.E. and Elliott, B.E. (1982) J. Immunol. Methods *52*, 395.

Palmer, D.F. and Cavallero, J.J. (1980) In: Manual of Clinical Immunology (N.R. Rose and H. Friedman, eds.). 2nd ed., p. 1078. American Society Microbiology, Washington DC.

Palosua, T. and Milgrom, F. (1981) J. Immunol. Methods *47*, 171.

Papasian, C.J., Bartholomev, W.R. and Amsterdam, D. (1984) J. Clin. Microbiol. *19*, 347.

Pape, B.E., Whiting, R., Parker, K.M. and Mitra, R. (1978) Clin. Chem. *24*, 2020.

Pardue, H.L., Simon, R.K. and Halmstadt, H. V. (1964) Anal. Chem. *36*, 735.

Parham, P., Androlewicz, M.J., Brodsky, F.M., Holmes, N.J. and Ways, J.P. (1982) J. Immunol. Methods *53*, 133.

Park, H. (1978) J. Immunol. Methods *20*, 349.

Park, H. (1981) Lancet (ii) 1309.

Parker, C.W. (1976) Radioimmunoassay of Biologically Active Compounds. Prentice-Hall, Englewood Cliffs, NJ.

Parks, D.R., Bryan, V.M., Oi, V.T. and Herzenberg, L.A. (1979) Proc. Natl. Acad. Sci. USA *76*, 1962.

Parry, S.H. and Porter, P. (1978) Immunology *34*, 471.

Parsons, G.H., Jr. (1981) Methods Enzymol. *73*, 224.

Parsons, J.A., Erlandsen, S.L., Hegre, O.D., McEvoy, R.C. and Elde, R.P. (1976) J. Histochem. Cytochem. *24*, 872.

Passoneau, J.V. and Lowry, O.H. (1974) In: Methods of Enzymatic Analysis (H.U. Bergmeyer, ed.). p. 135. Academic Press, New York.

Patrick, C.C. and Virella, G. (1978) Immunochemistry *15*, 137.

Paul, K.-G. and Stigbrand, T. (1970) Acta Chem. Scand. *24*, 3607.

Pauwels, R., Bazin, H., Platteau, B. and Van der Straeten, M. (1977) J. Immunol. Methods *18*, 133.

Pearse, A.G.E. (1980) Histochemistry, Theoretical and Applied. 4th ed. 439 pp. Churchill Livingstone, Edinburgh.

Perper, R.J., Okimoto, J.T., Cochrum, K.C., Ramsey, N. and Najarian, J.S. (1967) Proc. Soc. Exptl. Biol. Med. *125*, 575.

Peskar, B.A., Peskar, B.M. and Levine, L. (1972) Eur. J. Biochem. *26*, 191.

Peterson, E.A. (1970) In: Laboratory Techniques in Biochemistry and Molecular Biology (T.S. Work and E. Work, eds.) vol. 2, pt. 2. 223 pp. Elsevier/North-Holland, Amsterdam.

Peterson, J., Harmon, K.M. and Niemann, C. (1948) J. Biol. Chem. *176*, 1.

Petrusz, P., DiMeo, P., Ordronneau, P., Weaver, C. and Keefer, D.A. (1975) Histochemistry *46*, 9.

Pfleiderer, G., Jeckel, D. and Wieland, T. (1956) Biochem. Z. *328*, 187.

Phelps, C., Forlani, L. and Antonini, E. (1971) Biochem. J. *124*, 605.

Phillips, D.C. (1966) Scientific American *215* (Nov.), 78.

Phillips, D.J., Reimer, C.B., Wells, T.W. and Black, C.M. (1980) J. Immunol. Methods *34*, 315.

Pickel, V.M., Joh, T.H. and Reis, D.J. (1976) J. Histochem. Cytochem. *24*, 792.

Pickel, V.M., Joh, T.H., Reis, D.J., Leeman, S.E. and Miller, R.J. (1979) Brain Res. *160*, 387.

Pinckard, R.N. (1978) In: Handbook of Experimental Immunology (D.M. Weir, ed.). 3rd ed. p. 17.12. Blackwell Scientific Publications, Oxford.

Platt, J.H., Shore, A.B., Smithyman, A.M. and Kampfner, G.L. (1981) J. Immunoassay *2*, 59.

Plattner, H., Wachter, E. and Gröbner, P. (1977) Histochemistry *53*, 223.

Pohl, D.A., Gibbons, J.J., Jr., Tsai, C.C. and Roodman, S.T. (1980) J. Immunol. Methods *36*, 13.

Pohl, D.A., Tsai, C.C. and Roodman, S.T. (1981) J. Immunol. Methods *40*, 313.

Poljak, R.J., Amzel, L.M., Avey, H.P., Chen, B.L., Phizackerley, R.P. and Saul, F. (1973) Proc. Natl. Acad. Sci. USA *70*, 3305.

Polak, J.M. and Van Noorden, S., eds. (1983) Immunochemistry: Practical Applications in Pathology and Biology. 396 pp. Wright PSG, Bristol.

Polsen, A., Potgieter, G.M., Largier, J.F., Mears, G.E.F. and Joubert, F.J. (1964) Biochim. Biophys. Acta *82*, 463.

Ponder, B.A.J. (1983) In: Immunocytochemistry: Practical Applications in Pathology and Biology (J.M. Polak and S. Van Noorden, eds.). p. 129. Wright PSG, Bristol.

Ponder, B.A. and Wilkinson, M.M. (1981) J. Histochem. Cytochem. *29*, 981.

Porstmann, B., Porstmann, T., Gaede, D., Nugel, E. and Egger, E. (1981) Clin. Chim. Acta *109*, 175.

Porstmann, B., Avrameas, S., Ternynck, T. Porstmann, T. Micheel, B. and Guesdon, J.-L. (1984) J. Immunol. Methods *66*, 179.

Porter, R.R. (1959) Biochem. J. *73*, 119.

Presswood, W.G. (1981) In: Membrane Filtration, Applications and Problems (B.J. Dulka, ed.) Marcel Dekker, New York.

Pronovost, A.D., Baumgarten, A. and Hsiung, G.D. (1981) J. Clin. Microbiol. *13*, 97.

Puget, K., Michelson, A.M. and Avrameas, S. (1977) Anal. Biochem. *79*, 447.

Pütter, J. (1974) In: Methods of Enzymatic Analysis (H.U. Bergmeyer, ed.) p. 685. Academic Press, New York.

Quiocho, F.A. and Richards, F.M. (1966) Biochemistry *5*, 4062.

Radaszkiewicz, T., Dragosics, B., Abdelfattahgad, M. and Denk, H. (1979) J. Immunol. Methods *29*, 27.

Radola, B.J. (1974) Biochim. Biophys. Acta *386*, 181.

Raff, M. C.(1970) Nature *226*, 1257.

Rahman, S.B., Semar, J.B. and Perlman, D. (1967) Appl. Microbiol. *15*, 970.

Rajkowski, K.M., Cittanova, N., Desfosses, B. and Jayle, M.F. (1977) Steroids *29*, 701.

Rathlev, T. and Franks, G.F. (1982) Am. J. Clin. Pathol. *77*, 705.

Raval, D.N. and Wolfe, R.G. (1963) Biochemistry *2*, 220.

Reading, C.L. (1982) In: Hybridomas and Cellular Immortality (J.P. Allison and H.T. Baldwin, eds.) Plenum Press, New York.

Reece, G. and Knott, D. (1973) In: Proceedings of On-line Symposium 1972. Brunel University, Uxbridge.

Reedman, B.M. and Klein, G. (1973) Int. J. Cancer *11*, 499.

Reggiardo, Z., Vasquez, E. and Schnaper, L. (1980) J. Immunol. Methods *34*, 55.

Reid, T.W. and Wilson, I.B. (1971) In: The Enzymes (P.D. Boyer, ed.). vol. 4. p. 373. Academic Press, New York.

Reif, A.E. (1969) Immunochemistry *6*, 723.

Reimer, C.B., Phillips, D.J., Black, C.M. and Wells, T.W. (1978) In: Immunofluorescence and Related Staining Techniques (W. Knapp, H. Holubar and G. Wick, eds.). p. 189. Elsevier/North-Holland, Amsterdam.

Reinhart, M.P. and Malamud, D. (1982) Anal. Biochem. *123*, 229.

Reiser, J. and Wardale, J. (1981) Eur. J. Biochem. *114*, 569.

Reisfeld, R.A., Lewis, U.J. and Williams, D.E. (1962) Nature *195*, 281.

Reithel, F.J. (1971) In: The Enzymes (P.D. Boyer, ed.). vol. 4. p. 1. Academic Press, New York.

Reithel, F.J., Robbins, J.E. and Gorin, G. (1964) Arch. Biochem. Biophys. *108*, 409.

Reynolds, H.Y. and Johnson, J.S. (1970) J. Immunol. *105*, 698.

Rhigetti, P.G. (1983) Isoelectric Focusing: Theory and Applications. In: Laboratory Techniques in Biochemistry and Molecular Biology (T.S. Work, and R.H. Burdon, eds.) 386 pp. Elsevier/North-Holland, Amsterdam.

Ricardo, M.J. and Cebra, J.J. (1977) Methods Enzymol. *46*, 492.

Richards, F.M. and Wyckoff, H.W. (1971) In: The Enzymes (P.D. Boyer, ed.) vol. 4. p. 647. Academic Press, New York.

Richards, F.F., Konigsberg, W.H., Rozenstein, W.H. and Varga, J.M. (1975) Science *187*, 130.

Richardson, M.D., Turner, A., Warnock, D.W. and Llewellyn, P.A. (1983) J. Immunol. Methods *56*, 201.

Rigby, P.W.J., Dieckmann, M., Rhodes, C. and Berg, P. (1977) J. Mol. Biol. *113*, 237.

Ringertz, N.R. and Savage, R.E. (1976) Cell Hybrids. Academic Press, New York.

Riordan, J.F. and Vallee, B.L. (1963) Biochemistry *2*, 1460.

Ritchie, D.G., Nickerson, J.M. and Fuller, G.M. (1981) Anal. Biochem. *110*, 281.

Robinson, J. and Cooper, J.M. (1970) Anal. Biochem. *33*, 390.

Robinson, P.J., Dunnill, P. and Lilly, M.D. (1971) Biochim. Biophys. Acta *242*, 659.

Rodbard, D. (1974) Clin. Chem. *20*, 1255.

Rodbard, D. (1978) In: Radioimmunoassay and Related Procedures in Medicine. Vol. II, p.21. International Academic Energy Agency, Vienna.

Rodbard, D. and Feldman, Y. (1978) Immunochemistry *15*, 71.

Rodbard, D. and McClean, S.W. (1977) Clin. Chem. *23*, 112.

Rodbard, D., Rayford, P.L., Cooper, J.A. and Ross, G.T. (1968) J. Clin. Endocrinol. *28*, 1412.

Rodbard, D., Ruder, H.J., Vaitukaitis, J.L. and Jacobs, H.S. (1971) J. Endocrin. Metab. *33*, 343.

Rodbard, D., Feldman, Y., Jaffe, M.L. and Miles, L.E.M. (1978) Immunochemistry *15*, 77.

Rodgers, R., Crowl, C.P., Eimstad, W.M., Hu, M.W., Kam, J.K., Ronald, R.C., Rowley, G.L. and Ullman, E.F. (1978) Clin. Chem. *24*, 95.

Rodning, C.B., Erlandsen, S.L., Coulter, H.D. and Wilson, I.D. (1978) J. Histochem. Cytochem. *26*, 223.

Rogers, H.J. and Garrett, A.J. (1963) Biochem. J. *88*, 6p.

Roitt, I. (1980) Essential Immunology. 4th ed. Blackwell Scientific Publications, Oxford.

Rojas-Espinosa, O., Dannenberg, A.M., Sternberger, L.A. and Tsuda, T. (1974) Am. J. Pathol. *74*, 1.

Rordorf, C., Gambke, C. and Gordon, J. (1983) J. Immunol. Methods *59*, 105.

Rose, M.E., Orlans, E. and Buttress, N. (1974) Eur. J. Immunol. *4*, 521.

Rosenthal, A.S. (1978) Immunol. Rev. *40*, 136.

Rook, G.A.W. and Cameron, C.H. (1981) J. Immunol. Methods *40*, 109.

Roth, J. (1982) In: Techniques in Immunochemistry (G.R. Bullock and P. Petrusz, eds). vol. 1, p. 107. Academic Press, London.

Rothman, F. and Byrne, R. (1963) J. Mol. Biol. 6, 330.

Rotman, B. (1961) Proc. Natl. Acad. Sci. USA 47, 1981.

Rotman, M.B. and Celada, F. (1968) Proc. Natl. Acad. Sci. USA 60, 660.

Rousseaux, J., Picque, M.T., Bazin, H. and Biserte, G. (1981) Mol. Immunol. 18, 639.

Rowe, D.S. and Fahey, J.L. (1965) J. Exptl. Med. 121, 171.

Rowe, D.S., Anderson, S.G. and Grub, B. (1970a) Bull. W.H.O. 43, 535.

Rowe, D.S., Anderson, S.G. and Tackett, L. (1970b) Bull. W.H.O. 43, 607.

Rowe, D.S., Tackett, L., Bennich, H., Ishikawa, K., Johansson, S.G.O., and Anderson, S.G. (1970c) Bull. W.H.O. 43, 609.

Rowley, G.L., Rubenstein, K.E., Huisjen, J. and Ullman, E.F. (1975) J. Biol. Chem. 250, 3759.

Ryal, R.G., Story, C.J. and Turner, D.R. (1982) Anal. Biochem. 127, 308.

Ryan, J.W., Day, A.R., Schultz, D.R., Ryan, U.S., Chung, A., Marborough, D.I. and Dorer, F.E. (1976) Tissue Cell 8, 111.

Rybycki, E.P. and Von Wechmar, M.B. (1981) Virology 109, 391.

Rubenstein, K.E., Schneider, R.S. and Ullman, E.F. (1972) Biochem. Biophys. Res. Commun. 47, 846.

Ruitenberg, E.J. and Brosi, B.J.M. (1978) Scand. J. Immunol. 8(Suppl. 7), 63.

Ruitenberg, E.J., Brosi, B.J.M. and Steerenberg, P.A. (1976) J. Clin. Microbiol. 3, 541.

Ruitenberg, E.J., Sekhuis, V.M. and Brosi, B.J.M. (1980) J. Clin. Microbiol. 11, 132.

Sabatini, D.D., Miller, F. and Barnett, R.J. (1964) J. Histochem. Cytochem. 12, 57.

Salik, S.E. and Cook, G.M.W. (1976) Biochim. Biophys. Acta 419, 119.

Salonen, E.-M. and Vaheri, A. (1981) J. Immunol. Methods 41, 95.

Sammons, D.W., Adams, L.D. and Nishizawa, E.E. (1981) Electrophoresis 2, 135.

Sandor, M. and Langone, J.J. (1981) Biochem. Biophys. Res. Commun. 100, 1326.

Sanger, F. (1945) Biochem. J. 39, 507.

Saunders, G.C. (1979) In: Immunoassays in the Clinical Laboratory (R.M. Nakamura, W.R. Dito and E.S. Tucker, eds.) p. 99. Alan R. Liss, New York.

Saunders, B.C., Holmes Siedle, A.G. and Stark, B.P. (1964) Peroxidase. 271 pp. Butterworths, London.

Saunders, G.C., Clinard, E.H., Bartlett, M.L. and Mort Sanders, W.M.J. (1977) J. Infect. Dis. 136, S258.

Sawyer, M., Osburn, B.I., Knight, H.D. and Kendrick, J.W. (1973) Am. J. Vet. Res. 34, 1281.

Scatchard, G. (1949) Ann. New York Ac. Sci. 51, 660.

Schalch, W. and Braun, D.G. (1979) In: Immunological Methods (I. Lefkovits and B. Pernis, eds.). vol. 1, p. 123. Academic Press, New York.

Scheidegger, J.J. (1955) Intern. Arch. Allergy Appl. Immunol. 7, 103.

Schick, A.F. and Singer, S.J. (1961) J. Biol. Chem. 236, 2477.

Schimpl, A. and Wecker, E. (1972) Nature New Biol. 237, 15.

Schneider, Z. (1980) Anal. Biochem. 108, 96.

Schneider, R.S., Lindquist, P., Wong, E.T., Rubenstein, K.E. and Ullman, E.F. (1973) Clin. Chem. *19*, 821.

Schneider, R.S., Bastiani, R.J., Leute, R.K. and Ullman, E.F. (1974) In: Immunoassays for Drugs Subject to Abuse (S.J. Mulé, I. Sunshine, M. Branle and R.E. Willette, eds.). p. 45. CRC Press, Boca Raton, FA.

Schottelius, D.D. (1978) In: Antiepileptic Drugs (C.E. Pippinger, J.K. Perry and H. Kutt, eds.) chapter 10. Raven Press, New York.

Schreffler, D.C. (1976) Transplant. Rev. *32*, 140.

Schreier, M.H. and Nordin, A.A. (1977) In: B and T Cells in Immune Recognition (F. Loor and G.E. Rolants, eds.) p. 127. John Wiley and Sons, Chichester, New York.

Schroeder, H.R., Carrico, R.J., Boguslaski, R.C. and Christner, J.E. (1975) Anal. Biochem. *72*, 283.

Schroeder, H.R., Vogelhut, P.O., Carrico, R.J., Boguslaski, R.C. and Bucker, R.T. (1976) Anal. Chem. *48*, 1933.

Schuit, H.R.E., Moree van der Linden, P.C., Hijmans, W. (1981) J. Immunol. Methods *47*, 321.

Schur, P. (1972) Prop. Clin. Immunol. *1*, 71.

Sedgwick, A.K., Ballow, M., Sparks, K. and Tilton, R.C. (1983) J. Clin. Microbiol. *18*, 104.

Seeman, P. (1967) J. Cell Biol. *32*, 55.

Segrest, J.P. and Jackson, R.L. (1972) Methods Enzymol. *28*, 54.

Sela, M. (1969) Science *166*, 1365.

Sela, M. (1973–1982) (ed.) The Antigens. vol. 1–6. Academic Press, New York.

Sela, M. and Fuchs, S. (1973) In: Handbook of Experimental Immunology (D.M. Weir, ed.) 2nd ed. p. 1.1. Blackwell Scientific Publications, Oxford.

Selsted, M.E. and Martinez, R.J. (1978) Infect. Immun. *24*, 460.

Selsted, M.E. and Martinez, R.J. (1980) Anal. Biochem. *109*, 67.

Sequin, R.J. and Kosicki, G.W. (1967) Can. J. Biochem. *45*, 659.

Sever, J.L. (1983) Curr. Top. Microbiol. Immunol. *104*, 57.

Sevier, E.D., David, G.S., Martinis, J., Desmond, W.J., Bartholomew, R.M. and Wang, R. (1981) Clin. Chem. *27*, 1797.

Shalev, A., Greenberg, A.H. and McAlpine, P.J. (1980) J. Immunol. Methods *38*, 125.

Shannon, L.M., Kay, E. and Lew, J.Y. (1966) J. Biol. Chem. *241*, 2166.

Shapiro, A.L., Viñuela, E. and Maizel, J.V. (1967) Biochem. Biophys. Res. Commun. *28*, 815.

Sharon, J., Morrison, S.L. and Kabat, E.A. (1979) Proc. Natl. Acad. Sci. USA *76*, 1420.

Shaw, W., Smith, J., Spierto, F.W. and Agnese, S.T. (1977) Clin. Chim. Acta *76*, 15.

Shechter, T., Schlesinger, J., Jacobs, S., Chang, K.-J. and Cuatrecasas, P. (1978) Proc. Natl. Acad. Sci. USA *75*, 2135.

Shek, P.N. and Howe, S.A. (1982) J. Immunol. Methods *53*, 255.

Shekarchi, I.C., Sever, J.L., Ward, L.A. and Madden, D.L. (1982) J. Clin. Microbiol. *16*, 1012.

Shekarchi, I.C., Sever, J.L., Lee, Y.J., Castellano, G. and Madden, D.L. (1984) J. Clin. Microbiol. *19*, 89.

Shin, S.-I. and Van Diggelen, O.P. (1977) In: Mycoplasma Infection of Cell Cultures (G.J. McGarrity, D.G. Murphy and W.W. Nichols, eds.) p. 191. Plenum Press, New York.

Shore, J.D. and Chakrabarti, S.K. (1976) Biochemistry *15*, 875.

Shugar, D. (1952) Biochim. Biophys. Acta *8*, 302.

Shulman, M.C., Wilde, D. and Köhler, G. (1978) Nature *276*, 269.

Siess, E., Wieland, O. and Miller, F. (1971) Immunology *20*, 658.

Signorella, A.P. and Hymer, W.C. (1984) Anal. Biochem. *136*, 372.

Simionescu, N. (1979) J. Histochem. Cytochem. *27*, 1120.

Simmonds, R.G., Smith, W. and Marsden, H. (1982) J. Immunol. Methods *54*, 23.

Simpson, R.T. and Vallee, B.L. (1970) Biochemistry *9*, 953.

Simpson, R.T., Vallee, B.L. and Tait, G.H. (1968) Biochemistry *7*, 4336.

Singer, I.I. (1974) In: Viral Immunodiagnosis (E. Kurstak and R. Morisset, eds.) p. 101. Academic Press, New York.

Singh, P., Leung, D.K. and Ullman, E.F. (1978) Int. Congr. Clin. Chem., Mexico City. 69 (abstract).

Sips, R. (1949) J. Chem. Phys. *16*, 490.

Sjödal, J. (1977) Eur. J. Biochem. *78*, 471.

Sjöquist, J., Meloun, B., Hjelm, H. (1972) Eur. J. Biochem. *29*, 572.

Skujins, V.J., Pukite, A. and McLaren, A.D. (1973) Mol. Cell. Biochem. *2*, 221.

Skurrie, I.J. and Gilbert, G.L. (1983) J. Clin. Microbiol. *17*, 738.

Smith, K.O. and Gehle, W.D. (1977) J. Infect. Dis. *136* (suppl.), S329.

Smith, K.O. and Gehle, W.D. (1980) Methods Enzymol. *70*, 388.

Smith, M.R., Devine, C.S., Cohn, S.M. and Lieberman, M.W. (1984) Anal. Biochem. *137*, 120.

Smithies, O. and Poulik, M.D. (1972) Proc. Natl. Acad. Sci. USA *69*, 2914.

Snedecor, G.W. and Cochran, W.G. (1967) Statistical Methods. 6th ed., 593 pp. Iowa State University Press, Ames, Iowa, USA.

Sofroniew, M.V. and Schrell, U. (1982) J. Histochem. Cytochem. *30*, 504.

Sophianopoulos, A.J. and Van Holde, K.E. (1964) J. Biol. Chem. *239*, 2516.

Soula, A., Laurent, N., Tixier, G. and Moreau, Y. (1982) Develop. Biol. Stand. *52*, 147.

Southern, E.M. (1975) J. Mol. Biol. *98*, 503.

Spaur, R.C. and Moriarty, G.C. (1977) J. Histochem. Cytochem. *25*, 163.

Speth, V., Wallach, D.F.H., Weidekamm, E. and Knüfermann, H. (1972) Biochim. Biophys. Acta *255*, 386.

Stanbridge, E.J. and Schneider, E.L. (1976) Tissue Cult. Assoc. Man. *2*, 371.

Stanworth, D.R. and Turner, M.W. (1973) In: Handbook of Experimental Immunology (D.M. Weir, ed.). 2nd ed. p. 10.1. Blackwell Scientific Publications, Oxford.

Stapley, E.O., Mata, J.M., Miller, I.M., Demmy, T.C., Woodruff, H.B. (1963) Antimicrob. Agents Chemotherap. *3*, 20.

Steensgaard, J., Steward, M.W. and Frich, J.R. (1980) Mol. Immunol. *17*, 689.

Steers, E., Jr., Cuatrecasas, P. and Pollard, H.B. (1971) J. Biol. Chem. *246*, 196.

Stefanini, M., De Martino, C. and Zamboni, L. (1967) Nature *216*, 173.

Stein, H., Bank, A., Tolksdorf, G., Lennert, K., Rodt, H. and Gordes, J. (1980) J. Histochem. Cytochem. *28*, 746.

Steinbuch, M. and Audran, R. (1969) Arch. Biochem. Biophys. *134*, 279.

Steiner, A.L., Kipnis, D.M., Utiger, R. and Parker, C. (1969) Proc. Natl. Acad. Sci. USA *64*, 367.

Steinitz, M., Izak, G., Cohen, S., Ehrenfeld, M. and Flechner, I., (1980) Nature *287*, 443.

Stellwag, E.J. and Dahlberg, D. (1980) Nucl. Acids Res. *8*, 299.

Sternberger, L.A. (1969) Mikroskopie *25*, 346.

Sternberger, L.A. (1979) Immunocytochemistry. 2nd ed. John Wiley and Sons, Inc. Chichester, New York.

Sternberger, L.A. and Joseph, S.A. (1979) J. Histochem. Cytochem. *27*, 1424.

Sternberger, L.A., Hardy, P.H., Jr., Cuculis, J.J. and Meyer, H.G. (1970) J. Histochem. Cytochem. *18*, 315.

Sternberger, N.H., Tabira, T., Kies, M.W. and Webster, H. de F. (1977) Transact. Ann. Soc. Neurochem. *8*, 157.

Steward, M.W. (1977) In: Immunochemistry: An Advanced Textbook (L.E. Glynn and M.W. Steward, eds.) p. 223. John Wiley and Sons, Chichester, New York.

Stone, M.J. and Metzger, H. (1969) J. Immunol. *102*, 222.

Straus, W. (1971) J. Histochem. Cytochem. *19*, 682.

Strauss, A.W., Alberts, A.W., Hennessy, S. and Vagelos, P.R. (1975) Proc. Natl. Acad. Sci. USA *72*, 4366.

Streefkerk, J.G. (1972) J. Histochem. Cytochem. *20*, 829.

Streefkerk, J.G., Manjula, B.N. and Glaudemans, C.P.J. (1979) J. Immunol. *122*, 537.

Symington, J., Green, M. and Brackmann, K. (1981) Proc. Natl. Acad. Sci. USA *78*, 177.

Sueoka, N. and Cheng, T.-Y. (1962) J. Mol. Biol. *4*, 161.

Sund, H. and Weber, K. (1963) Biochem. Z. *337*, 24.

Suter, M. (1982) J. Immunol. Methods *53*, 103.

Swoboda, B.E.P. and Massey, V. (1965) J. Biol. Chem. *240*, 2209.

Tandon, A., Zahner, H. and Lemmler, G. (1979) Tropenmed. Parasitol. *30*, 189.

Tanford, C. (1978) Science *200*, 1012.

Tanford, C. and Wagner, D. (1954) J. Am. Chem. Soc. *76*, 3331.

Tasheva, B. and Dessev, G. (1983) Anal. Biochem. *129*, 98.

Tateishi, K., Yamamoto, H., Ogihara, T. and Hayashi, C. (1977) Steroids *30*, 25.

Taurog, J.D. (1981) Ann. Neurol. *9* (suppl.), 107.

Telegdi, M., Wolfe, D.V. and Wolfe, R.G. (1973) J. Biol. Chem. *248*, 6484.

Ternynck, T. and Avrameas, S. (1977) Immunochemistry *14*, 767.

Terouanne, B., Nicolas, J.C., Descomps, B. and Crastes de Paulet, A. (1980) J. Immunol. Methods *35*, 267.

Theorell, H. (1942) Arch. Kemi Mineral. Geol. *16A*, 2.

Theorell, H. and Akesson, A. (1941) J. Am. Chem. Soc. *63*, 1818.

Thomas, P.S. (1980) Proc. Natl. Acad. Sci. USA *77*, 5210.

Thomas, W.R., Turner, K.J., Eadie, M.E. and Yadeo, M. (1972) Immunology *22*,

401.

Thorne, C.J.R. and Kaplan, N.O. (1963) J. Biol. Chem. *238*, 1861.

Tiggeman, R., Plattner, H., Rasched, I., Baeuerle, P. and Wachter, E. (1981) J. Histochem. Cytochem. *29*, 1387.

Tijssen, P. and Kurstak, E. (1974) In: Viral Immunodiagnosis (E. Kurstak and R. Morisset, eds.) p. 125. Academic Press, New York.

Tijssen, P. (1985) In: Detection of Bacterial Antigen for the Rapid Diagnosis of Infectious Diseases (R.B. Kohler, ed.), chapt. 8, CRC Press, Boca Raton, FL (in press).

Tijssen, P. and Kurstak, E. (1977) In: Comparative Diagnosis of Viral Diseases (E. Kurstak and C. Kurstak, eds.) vol. 2, p 489. Academic Press, New York.

Tijssen, P. and Kurstak, E. (1979a) Intervirology *11*, 261.

Tijssen, P. and Kurstak, E. (1979b) Anal. Biochem. *99*, 97.

Tijssen, P. and Kurstak, E. (1981) J. Virol. *37*, 17.

Tijssen, P. and Kurstak, E. (1983) Anal. Biochem. *128*, 26.

Tijssen, P. and Kurstak, E. (1984) Anal. Biochem. *136*, 451.

Tijssen, P., Su, D.-M. and Kurstak, E. (1982) Arch. Virol. *74*, 277.

Tom, H., Schneider, R.S., Ernst, R., Khan, W., Singh, P. and Kabakoff, D.S. (1979) Clin. Chem. *25*, 1094.

Tonegawa, S. (1983) Nature *302*, 575.

Tonks, H.B. cited by Palmer and Cavallero (1980).

Torriani, A. (1968) Methods Enzymol. *12B*, 212.

Towbin, H., Staehelin, T. and Gordon, J. (1979) Proc. Natl. Acad. Sci. USA *76*, 4350.

Tracey, D.E., Liu, S.H. and Cebra, J.J. (1976) Biochemistry *5*, 624.

Tramu, G., Pillez, A. and Leonardelli, J. (1978) J. Histochem. Cytochem. *26*, 322.

Traut, R.R., Bollen, A., Sun, T.-T., Hershey, J.W.B., Sundberg, J. and Pierce, L.R. (1973) Biochemistry *12*, 3266

Trevan, M.D. (1980) Immobilized Enzymes. 138 pp. John Wiley and Sons, Chichester, New York.

Trowbridge, I.S. (1978) J. Exptl. Med. *148*, 313.

Tubbs, R.R. and Shebani, K. (1981) J. Histochem. Cytochem. *29*, 684.

Ullman, E.F. and Maggio, E.T. (1980) In: Enzyme-immunoassay (E.T. Maggio, ed.) p. 105. CRC Press, Inc. Boca Raton, Fa.

Ullman, E.F., Blakemore, J., Leute, R.K., Eimstad, W. and Jaklitsch, A. (1975) Clin. Chem. *21*, 1011.

Ullman, E.F., Yoshida, R., Blakemore, J., Maggio, E.T. and Leute, R.K. (1979) Biochim. Biophys. Acta *567*, 66.

Ullmann, A., Goldberg, M.E., Perrin, D. and Monod, J. (1968) Biochemistry *7*, 261.

Unanue, E.R. (1981) Adv. Immunol. *31*, 1.

Unanue, E.R. and Askonas, B.A. (1968) J. Exptl. Med. *127*, 915.

Underdown, B.J., De Rose, J. and Plaut, A. (1977) J. Immunol. *118*, 1816.

Ungar-Waron, H. and Sela, M. (1966) Biochim. Biophys. Acta *124*, 147.

Uotila, M., Ruoslahti, E. and Engvall, E. (1981) J. Immunol. Methods *42*, 11.

Vacca, L.L., Rosario, S.L., Zimmerman, E.A., Tomashefsky, P., Ng, P.-Y. and Hsu, K.C. (1975) J. Histochem. Cytochem. *23*, 208.

Vallee, B.C., Hoch, F.L., Adestein, S.J. and Wacker, W.E.C. (1956) J. Am. Chem. Soc. *78*, 5879.

Van Belle, H. (1972) Biochim. Biophys. Acta *289*, 158.

Vandesande, F. (1979) J. Neuroscience Methods *1*, 3.

Vandesande, F. and Dierickx, K. (1975) Cell Tiss. Res. *164*, 153.

Van Furth, R. (1980) In: Mononuclear Phagocytes, functional aspects. (R. Van Furth, ed.) p. 1. Martinus Nijhoff, The Hague.

Van Heyningen, V., Brock, D.J.H. and Van Heyningen, S. (1983) J. Immunol. Methods *62*, 142.

Van Kamp, G.J. (1979) J. Immunol. Methods *27*, 301.

Van Lente, F. and Galen, R.S. (1980) In: Enzyme-immunoassay (E.G. Maggio, ed.) p. 135. CRC Press, Boca Raton, Fa.

Van Loon, A.M. and Van der Veen, J. (1980) J. Clin. Pathol. *33*, 635.

Van Noorden, S. and Polak, J.M. (1983) In: Immunocytochemistry: Practical Applications in Pathology and Biology (S. Van Noorden and J.M. Polak, eds.) p. 11. Wright PSG, Bristol.

Van Weemen, B.K. and Schuurs, A.H.W.M. (1971) FEBS Lett. *15*, 232.

Van Weemen, B.K. and Schuurs, A.H.W.M. (1972) FEBS Lett. *24*, 77.

Van Weemen, B.K. and Schuurs, A.H.W.M. (1975) Immunochemistry *12*, 667.

Van Weemen, B.K., Bosch, A.M.G., Dawson, E.C., van Hell, H. and Schuurs, A.H.W.M. (1978) Scand. J. Immunol. *8(suppl. 7)*, 73.

Varga, J.M., Lande, S. and Richards, F.F. (1974) J. Immunol. *112*, 1565.

Venitt, S. and Searle, C.E. (1976) INSERM Symposia Series 52, IARC Scientific Publications, no. 13. (INSERM Paris) p. 263.

Vidal, M.A. and Conde, F.P. (1980) J. Immunol. Methods *35*, 169.

Villarejo, M.A. and Zabin, I. (1974) J. Bacteriol. *120*, 466.

Viscidi, R., Laughon, B.E., Hanvanich, M., Bartlett, J.G. and Yolken, R.H. (1984) J. Immunol. Methods *67*, 129.

Volkman, D. and Fauci, A.S. (1981) Cell. Immunol. *60*, 415.

Voller, A., Bidwell, D.E. and Bartlett, A. (1979) A guide with abstracts of microplate applications (Dynatech Europe, Guernsey).

Voogd, C.E., Van der Stel, J.J. and Jacobs, J.J.J.A.A. (1980) J. Immunol. Methods *36*, 55.

Walberg, C.B. (1974) Clin. Chem. *20*, 305.

Wallace, E.F. and Wofsy, L. (1979) J. Immunol. Methods *25*, 283.

Wallenfels, K. and Weil, R. (1972) In: The Enzymes (P.D. Boyer, ed.) vol. 7, p. 617. Academic Press, New York.

Wallenfels, K. and Malhotra, O.P. (1960) In: The Enzymes (P.D. Boyer, H. Lardy and K. Myrbäck, eds.) vol. 4, p. 409. Academic Press, New York.

Wallenfels, K., Zarnitz, M.L., Laule, G., Bender, H. and Keser, M. (1959) Biochem. Z. *331*, 459.

Wallis, C., Melnick, J.L. and Gerba, C.P. (1979) Ann. Rev. Microbiol. *33*, 413.

Wang, A.-C. and Fudenberg, H.H. (1972) Nature New Biol. *240*, 24.

Walsh, B.J., Wrigley, C.W. and Baldo, B.A. (1984) J. Immunol. Methods 66, 99.

Walter, K. and Schütt, C. (1974) In: Methods of enzymatic analysis (H.U. Bergmeyer, ed.) p. 856. Academic Press, New York.

Watkins, W.B. (1977) J. Histochem. Cytochem. 25, 61.

Weber, G. (1975) Adv. Prot. Chem. 29, 1.

Weber, K. and Osborn, M. (1969) J. Biol. Chem. 244, 4406.

Weber, K., Sund, H. and Wallenfels K. (1964) Biochem. Z. 339, 498.

Webster, H. de F., Reier, P.J., Kies, M.W. and O'Connell, M. (1974) Brain Res. 79, 132.

Wedding, R.T., Hansch, C. and Fukuto, T.R. (1967) Arch. Biochem. Biophys. 121, 9.

Wei, R. and Riebe, S. (1977) Clin. Chem. 23, 1386.

Weigand, K., Alpert, E., Keutmann, H. and Issenbacher, K.J. (1980) Comp. Biochem. Physiol. 67B, 115.

Weigand, K., Birr, C. and Suter, M. (1981) Biochim. Biophys. Acta 670, 424.

Weiner, W. (1957) Br. J. Haematol. 3, 276.

Weinheimer, P.F., Mestecky, J. and Acton, R.T. (1971) J. Immunol. 107, 1211.

Weir, E.E., Pretlow II, T.G., Pitts, A. and Williams, E.E. (1974) J. Histochem. Cytochem. 22, 51.

Welinder, K.G. (1979) Eur. J. Biochem. 96, 483.

Welinder, K.G. and Smillie, L.B. (1972) Can. J. Biochem. 50, 63.

Welinder, K.G. and Mazza, G. (1977) Eur. J. Biochem. 73, 353.

Wellington, D. (1980) In: Enzyme-immunoassay (E.T. Maggio, ed.) p. 249. CRC Press, Inc., Boca Raton, Fa.

White, P.J. and Hoch, S.O. (1981) Biochem. Biophys. Res. Commun. 102, 365.

Wide, L. and Porath, J. (1966) Biochim. Biophys. Acta 130, 257.

Williams, C.A. and Chase, M.A. (1967) Methods in Immunology and Immunochemistry. vols. I and II. Academic Press, New York.

Williams, D.E. and Reisfeld, R.A. (1964) Ann. New York Acad. Sci. 121, 373.

Williams, M.R., Maxwell, D.A.G. and Spooner, R.L. (1975) Res. Vet. Sci. 18, 314.

Williamson, A.R., Salaman, M.R. and Kreth, H.R. (1973) Ann. New York Ac. Sci. 209, 210.

Willingham, M.C. (1983) J. Histochem. Cytochem. 31, 791.

Willingham, M.C., Yamada, S.S. and Pastan, I. (1978) Proc. Natl. Acad. Sci. USA 75, 4359.

Willstätter, R. and Stoll, A. (1917) Liebigs Ann. Chem. 416, 21.

Wilson, M.B. and Nakane, P.K. (1978) In: Immunofluorescence and Related Techniques (W. Knapp, H. Holubar and G. Wick, eds.). p. 215. Elsevier/North-Holland, Amsterdam.

Winchester, R. (1980) Summarized in J. Infect. Dis. 142, 793.

Wofsy, L., Baker, P.C., Thompson, K., Goodman, J., Kimura, J. and Henry, C. (1974) J. Exptl. Med. 140, 523.

Wojtkowiak, Z., Briggs, R.C. and Hnilica, L. S. (1983) Anal. Biochem. 129, 486.

Wolfe, R.G. and Neilands, J.B. (1956) J. Biol. Chem. 221, 61.

Woodhead, J.S., Addison, G.M. and Hales, C.N. (1974) Br. Med. Bull. 30, 44.

Woodhead, J.S., Kemp, H.A., Nix, A.B.J., Rowlands, R.J., Kemp, K.W., Wilson,